Medicine

General and Systematic Pathology

WITHDRAWN

For Elsevier:
Commissioning Editor: Timothy Horne
Development Editor: Barbara Simmons
Project Manager: Emma Riley
Designer: Stewart Larking
Illustrations Manager: Merlyn Harvey

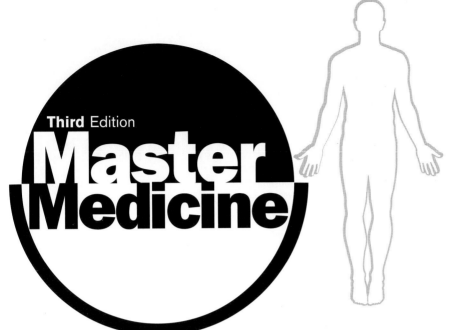

Third Edition

Master Medicine

General and Systematic Pathology

A core text with self-assessment

Paul Bass
BSc MD FRCPath
Consultant in Histopathology and Honorary Clinical Senior Lecturer, Southampton University Hospitals NHS Trust, Southampton, UK

Norman Carr
MB BS FRCPath FRCPA
Professor of Anatomical Pathology, Graduate School of Medicine, University of Wollongong, New South Wales, Australia

Susan Burroughs
BSc BM FRCPath
Consultant in Histopathology, Salisbury NHS Foundation Trust, Salisbury, UK

Claire Way
BSc MBChB MRCPath
Consultant in Histopathology, Queen Alexandra Hospital, Portsmouth, UK

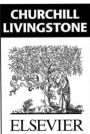

CHURCHILL LIVINGSTONE

ELSEVIER

Edinburgh London New York Oxford Philadelphia St Louis Sydney Toronto 2009

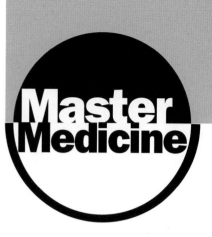

CHURCHILL
LIVINGSTONE
ELSEVIER

© 2009, Elsevier Limited. All rights reserved.

Pathology
© Pearson Professional Limited 1997
© 2004, Elsevier Limited. All rights reserved.

Systematic Pathology
© 2005, Elsevier Science Limited. All rights reserved.

Pathology
First edition 1997
Second edition 2004

Systematic Pathology
First edition 2005

ISBN 978-0-08-045129-9

British Library Cataloguing in Publication Data
A catalogue record for this book is available from the British Library

Library of Congress Cataloging in Publication Data
A catalog record for this book is available from the Library of Congress

Note
Neither the Publisher nor the Authors assumes any responsibility for any loss or injury and/or damage to persons or property arising out of or related to any use of the material contained in this book. It is the responsibility of the treating practitioner, relying on independent expertise and knowledge of the patient, to determine the best treatment and method of application for the patient.

The Publisher

ELSEVIER   your source for books,
            journals and multimedia
            in the health sciences
www.elsevierhealth.com

Working together to grow
libraries in developing countries
www.elsevier.com | www.bookaid.org | www.sabre.org
ELSEVIER BOOK AID International Sabre Foundation

The
publisher's
policy is to use
**paper manufactured
from sustainable forests**

Printed in China

Contents

Dedication

For Paulina, Aaron, David and Abraham, without whose forbearance this book would never have been written.
PB

For Mark
CW

And for Nicola, Chris and Anne, for their support and inspiration.
NC

Acknowledgements

We would like to thank the following for their helpful comments and for allowing us to adapt some of the pathology material used by Southampton medical students: Professor George Stevenson, Dr David Jones, Dr Bridget Wilkins, Dr Patrick Gallagher, Dr Steve George and Dr Shaoli Zhang.

Using this book

Learning pathology

How much do I need to know?

Pathology is the study of disease processes and is the link between the basic sciences and the practice of medicine. Thus, a good understanding of pathological principles is essential to all clinicians. However, because of the exponential increase in scientific knowledge and the increasing emphasis in medical courses on topics such as communication, clinical skills, ethics and professional development, students have no time to waste while trying to master the huge knowledge base that they have to learn and understand. Modern curriculum models, such as integrated or problem-based learning, can be particularly challenging in this respect, because pathology may not be taught as a recognisable 'course' and it can be difficult for students to identify core subject matter. Therefore, it is more necessary than ever for students to sort out what is important from what is less important. This book has been designed to help students with this task.

In preparing this book, we have concentrated on core material and we have eliminated a lot of detail which will be found in larger pathology textbooks. The rationale is that a large text, no matter how well written, is difficult to study from without prior knowledge of the subject. Students trying to use a large text can find it very difficult to identify the essential basic principles and core facts; they 'cannot see the wood for the trees'. On the other hand, short revision 'crammers' consisting largely of lists encourage simple retention of facts rather than understanding, and they are unlikely to be of use unless you are already familiar with the material. This book is designed to tread a middle ground. It contains all the information that we believe you need for a basic understanding of pathology, without confusing detail, but with enough explanation so that even complex concepts can be understood.

Using this book

Studying this text will provide you with the building blocks required for your ward-based and postgraduate studies. Larger textbooks can be used for reference or if you wish to study topics in more depth, but it should not be necessary to read them from cover to cover. The self-assessment questions will provide feedback on your progress and emphasise important points.

We hope this book will help you develop the skills of deep learning which will form the basis of a lifetime of learning. All those involved in medical care learn until they retire. There is no doubt that the majority of students find it easier to remember and understand basic science if they can see its relevance. The use of clinical examples and case histories in this book is designed to make the subject more interesting, memorable and understandable.

Self-assessment

We have included a mixture of assessment methods for you to use. The answers which we provide will give you some idea of where your gaps are and will also help you to organise your answers effectively. Some of the answers contain new material or new examples of basic principles and are designed to build on the main text. We do not give comprehensive answers for the OSCE, short answer or viva questions, but suggest an outline answer and a way of approaching it to show that you can organise, prioritise and apply your knowledge in different situations.

Multiple choice questions

The multiple choice question is a popular form of assessment because the questions can be marked quickly and efficiently in large numbers by mechanical means. Well-constructed multiple choice questions can test knowledge, understanding and reasoning skills.

There are many formats for multiple choice, including the one best answer, true-false and extended matching item formats used in this book. True-false questions still have a place although they are used less often now because it is difficult to write clinically relevant questions that are clearly always true or always false. Questions in which the most appropriate response is selected are usually better because they allow for the 'shades of grey' that characterise clinical practice. In one best answer questions, the single most appropriate response is selected from a list of five possibilities, whereas in extended matching items questions the list is longer and is typically used for several questions.

Some multiple choice questions use negative marking, where points are deducted for wrong answers. This system is designed to prevent guessing. Nevertheless, studies have shown that you are, on average, more likely to be right than wrong if you have a hunch about the right answer, even if you are not sure. An over-cautious approach can result in answering too few questions to pass, so it is probably best to 'play your hunches'. If there is no negative marking, you should attempt all questions as you have nothing to lose.

Case histories (modified essay questions)

The case history questions in this book are a form of 'modified essay' question in which short responses are entered freehand by the examinee. They are more time-consuming to mark, since the responses have to be assessed manually. However, they are a good way of testing understanding in a clinically relevant context. Responses may be single words, sentences or brief explanations. What is required can usually be judged from the number of marks given to each section.

Objective Structured Clinical Examination (OSCE)

The OSCE is designed to test application of knowledge in clinical scenarios. Some OSCE scenarios may be obviously pathology based, for example discussing a blood test result. However, since pathology is the link between basic science and clinical practice, the demonstration of pathological knowledge is a component of the great majority of OSCEs. Regarding dress, the same principles apply to OSCEs as to vivas (see below). A professional appearance is appropriate.

Short answer questions

Short answer questions of the format 'Write short notes on . . .' test recall of facts on a specific topic. The examiners usually devise a prototype answer and marks are simply awarded for every item or cluster of items required. Start your answer with some kind of definition and go on from there. It is a good idea to use simple diagrams wherever possible. You can then refer to them in your explanation. Answers in the form of bullet point lists are usually allowed.

No extra points will be given for information which is not strictly relevant, therefore read the question critically and answer the question that is set. Unless the instructions for the paper indicate that different questions have different weights of marks, spend roughly the same amount of time on each question. There is sometimes a temptation to spend longer on questions that you believe you can answer particularly well, but this is unlikely to compensate fully for a question that is answered badly or not at all because of lack of time. It may be a good idea to start with the questions about which you feel less confident; as the pressure increases towards the end of the exam you can concentrate on your areas of strength.

Essay

The essay is an extended piece of writing that gives you a chance to show how much you understand and your ability to relate one area of knowledge to another. It also tests your ability to organise and present information logically and clearly. Some essays allow you to develop an argument rather than simply set down facts. It is a communication exercise, so marks may be given not just for factual content but for use of English, presentation (including handwriting) and structure of the essay, and how the points and arguments are expounded.

It is vital that you read the question carefully so that you answer the question that is set. Examiners will not award marks for irrelevant material, so don't waste your time presenting it. Use side headings (underlined) and diagrams. These help to make things clear and demonstrate organised thought processes to the examiner. Do not spend too long on an essay on a favourite topic, or you will have insufficient time for other questions.

Essays are time-consuming and difficult to mark, and are used less often than previously. Nevertheless, a well-set essay can test a variety of skills, and essay papers are still encountered in many medical schools and higher professional examinations.

Viva

The viva voce or oral examination used to be a common component of many examinations in medicine, both undergraduate and postgraduate. For many reasons, it is now much less common than it used to be. However, it is still encountered and so we have included viva topics in this book.

Vivas tend to test factual recall and bear some similarity to short answer questions. However, the viva can be a particularly alarming experience because you are performing in real-time in front of the examiners. All candidates find vivas stressful. Attention to a few basic principles will help even if you are asked a question about an unfamiliar topic.

Sometimes you will feel as though your mind has gone blank when the examiner asks a question. Don't panic; take a deep breath and think for a second or two before jumping in with the first thing that comes into your head. Try to imagine how you would start the answer if you were writing it down. A simple definition is often a good start. If you do not understand the question then say so and ask for it to be repeated. The viva is a two-way communication process and examiners cannot expect you to give your best if they do not express themselves clearly.

If the question requires an answer listing the causes of a disease, assemble your causes in order of importance. Do not put the most rare one at the top of the list. Common things occur commonly; for example, traumatic crushing of the coronary artery comes very low on the list of causes of myocardial infarction – atheromatous narrowing of the coronary arteries is by far the most common cause. It may help to assemble topics in a logical way that demonstrates your understanding of basic principles and also acts as an aide memoire so you don't forget important areas. For example, you can divide causes of intestinal obstruction into factors within the lumen, within the wall and outside the wall. Likewise, an intestinal polyp can be inflammatory, hamartomatous or neoplastic; neoplasms can be benign or malignant, primary or metastatic.

If you mention a rare disease, the examiner may ask you more about it. This is fine if you know the subject, but not if you don't, so try to keep the conversation to areas about which you are confident, at least initially. The days of examiners revelling in making candidates uncomfortable and even scoring points off them should be long past. Most examiners try to be empathic and sympathetic. Nevertheless, they are usually trying to determine the limits of your knowledge and understanding, so you will probably be asked some questions you cannot answer. If you do not know the answer, it is perfectly acceptable to say that you do not so the examiner can move on to a different area.

Vivas are formal occasions and formal dress is customary. The examiners will almost certainly have taken the trouble to look smart, and it is only polite to do the same. You will feel more confident if you look the part. On the other hand, if you are concerned that you might look unprofessional, you have one more thing to worry about.

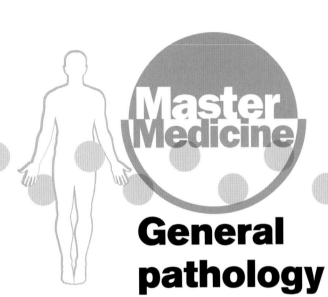

General
pathology

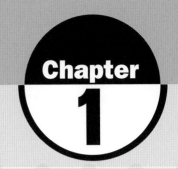

Pathology, health and disease

Chapter 1

Chapter overview

Pathology is the study of the structural and functional changes which occur in cells and tissues as a result of injuries, abnormal stimuli or genetic abnormalities, and the consequences for the organism. It provides the link between basic biological sciences and the practice of medicine. In broad terms, the study of pathology encapsulates the way we think about diseases and about their causes, prevention and classification. Together with epidemiology (the study of disease at the level of populations), an understanding of pathology allows rational and practical classification of diseases.

- Pathology is the study of disease processes.
- Epidemiology is the study of diseases at the level of populations and provides a broad context for understanding pathology.
- Both provide a useful framework for classifying and understanding mechanisms of disease.

1.1 Health, illness and disease

Learning objectives

You should:
- discuss the nature of health and disease
- discuss why and how disease is classified
- define and correctly use the terms aetiology, pathogenesis, congenital, genetic and acquired.

Health and disease

Producing an accurate and complete definition of disease is not straightforward. Disease is often said to be a state of physiological or psychological dysfunction, or an abnormal variation in the structure or function of a part of the body. There is a wide range of normality and the human body can readily adapt to changes in the environment (e.g. by an increase in haemoglobin at an altitude where oxygen levels are low). Disease can be defined as a state in which these limits of normality are over-reached. Definitions like

this one are 'naturalistic', and take the philosophical position that to have a disease is to fall outside the limits of normality, and that normality can be objectively defined. An alternative view is called 'normativism' and states that our ideas of what constitutes a disease are subjective and dependent on our personal and cultural values. For example, whether baldness is a disease depends on the cultural significance placed on hair loss. In some political contexts, political dissent has been considered a disease requiring psychiatric treatment. Whatever definition is used, the consequence of labelling someone as having a disease engages healthcare workers in a moral, ethical or professional obligation to intervene.

The World Health Organization defines health as a state of complete physical, mental and social wellbeing, and not merely the absence of disease or infirmity. Illness is the subjective state of not feeling well. Thus, it is possible to have a disease but not feel ill, because some diseases do not cause symptoms (a symptom is something noticed by the patient).

Classification of disease

Diagnosis uses concepts of disease classification to identify a disease in an individual patient (see Ch. 2). The aims of disease classification are to:

- determine the best treatment
- estimate the prognosis (expected future outcome)
- ascertain the cause, so the disease can be prevented in the future.

The most useful disease classifications are based on causes (aetiology) and underlying mechanisms (pathogenesis).

Aetiology

Diseases result from the interaction between individuals and their environment. The underlying cause is termed the aetiology. Some examples are:

- genetic: Down's syndrome (extra chromosome 21)
- infective: bacteria, viruses, fungi
- chemical (drugs and toxins): cirrhosis of the liver caused by alcohol damage; respiratory failure as a result of paraquat poisoning affecting lungs; skin rash due to penicillin
- radiation: post-irradiation cancer (e.g. squamous cell carcinoma developing in the skin of a breast irradiated for mammary carcinoma)

- mechanical: traumatic crush injury
- heat and cold: burns; frostbite
- metabolic: diabetes mellitus due to lack of insulin; gout due to deposition of uric acid crystals in joints
- nutritional: malnutrition; obesity; vitamin deficiency
- psychological: post-traumatic stress disorder due to witnessing a horrific event.

The causes of disease extend beyond pathological processes, however. Social and political factors may be of great importance, for example social stigmatisation of certain physical conditions, poverty, and government policy with respect to healthcare.

Idiopathic disease

In some instances, the underlying cause of a disease is obscure. Many euphemisms are used for this, including idiopathic, cryptogenic, essential and spontaneous. 'Cause unknown' is a simpler and more honest way of saying the same thing.

Pathogenesis (mechanisms of disease)

The pathogenesis of a disease is the mechanism by which the cause(s) interact with the target cells or tissues to produce pathological changes. There are a few fundamental processes that underlie most diseases:

- inflammation: response to injury in living vascularised tissue
- degeneration: deterioration of cell function resulting from metabolic disease or ageing
- neoplasia (oncogenesis): the process of transformation of cells from normal to the neoplastic, autonomous state in which the cells do not respond normally to factors controlling cell growth
- immune reactions: specific responses to foreign organisms or material.

Genetic, acquired and congenital disease

Broadly speaking, diseases can be classified into two categories: 'genetic' and 'acquired'. Genetic diseases are due to abnormalities in the genome. Most are inherited, i.e. passed from parent to offspring, but about 15–20% occur due to new mutations in the affected individual. Some, such as trisomy 21 (Down's syndrome), are evident at birth, whereas others, such as Huntington's disease and familial adenomatous polyposis, produce symptoms only in later life. Table 1 gives a classification of the main types of genetic disease. Acquired diseases are caused by environmental factors, such as a road traffic accident resulting in a bone fracture.

Although the classification of disease into genetic and acquired is conceptually useful, the distinction is blurred because genetic and environmental factors interact in the pathogenesis of most diseases. For example, although carcinoma of the lung is acquired due to environmental exposure to cigarette smoke, there are genetic factors that make some individuals more prone to developing the condition than others. Likewise, there are genetic components to the development of diabetes mellitus, but the individual's diet

determines the severity of the disease. Only a few diseases can be considered entirely genetic or acquired in nature.

The term congenital is used for a disease present at birth, even though it may not be recognised or recognisable at that time. Such diseases include not only genetic abnormalities but also diseases acquired due to environmental factors acting on the developing embryo and fetus. Examples of acquired congenital diseases are:

- cerebral palsy due to fetal hypoxia during delivery
- congenital rubella due to intrauterine infection with rubella virus (German measles)
- fetal alcohol syndrome due to intrauterine exposure to large amounts of ethanol.

1.2 Ways of thinking about diseases

Learning objectives

You should:

- use a framework for thinking about the characteristics of a disease
- distinguish morbidity from mortality
- define incidence and prevalence, and discuss the factors that affect them
- interpret relative risk, sensitivity and specificity.

It is useful to have a logical framework for thinking about diseases. One way of organising the information is to use the following headings:

- definition: clinical or pathological
- epidemiology: e.g. incidence, age/gender, geography, race
- aetiology
- underlying pathology: mechanisms of disease (pathogenesis) with consequent structural changes in tissues (macroscopic – visible to the naked eye; microscopic – seen only by using the microscope) and functional changes in tissues (pathophysiology)
- clinical features: symptoms and signs; special investigations
- differential diagnosis: other diseases which may be similar
- treatment: e.g. drugs, surgery, counselling
- complications: other diseases that can follow
- prognosis: natural history of disease, disease outcome.

Epidemiology

Epidemiology provides a wider context for the study, classification and diagnosis of diseases. Data recorded about incidence, prevalence, death rate, etc. relate to populations, rather than to individuals.

Knowledge of epidemiology is important for:

- providing clues to what may cause disease
- identifying risk factors and risk markers
- planning and executing disease prevention and health promotion
- providing adequate healthcare facilities

Table 1 Classification of the main types of genetic diseases

Type	Basis	Transmission pattern	Examples
Mendelian	Expression of mutation in a single gene	Autosomal dominant	Huntington's disease: due to an abnormality in a protein called huntingtin; affected individuals develop movement disorders and dementia in adulthood
			Marfan's syndrome: defective matrix protein fibrillin-1 causes abnormalities in the skeleton, cardiovascular system and eye
			Familial adenomatous polyposis: mutation of APC results in large numbers of neoplasms in the colon and elsewhere
		Autosomal recessive	Cystic fibrosis: abnormal transmembrane ion transport resulting from a defective transmembrane conductance regulator causes thick, sticky mucous secretions
			Sickle cell anaemia: a point mutation in the beta-haemoglobin chain causes deoxygenated haemoglobin molecules to undergo abnormal polymerisation
		X-linked	Haemophilia A: a defect in blood clotting factor VIII causes abnormal bleeding
			Duchenne's muscular dystrophy: abnormalities in the sarcolemma-associated protein dystrophin cause progressive weakness
Multifactorial	The combined action of two or more genes with additive effects	The severity of the disease is proportional to the number of deleterious genes	Hypertension Congenital heart disease Diabetes mellitus
Cytogenetic	An abnormal number of chromosomes, or major structural changes in chromosomes affecting many genes	Generally arise de novo	Trisomy 21 (an extra chromosome 21) causes Down's syndrome: characteristic facial appearances, single palmar crease, learning disabilities, increased risk of heart defects and other diseases
			Deletion of part of the long arm of chromosome 22 causes DiGeorge syndrome: congenital heart defects, T cell immunodeficiency, parathyroid hypoplasia, facial abnormalities, psychiatric problems
			Lack of an X chromosome (X0 phenotype) causes Turner's syndrome: infertility, short stature, neck webbing, etc.

One

- setting up population screening programmes
- evaluating healthcare interventions.

Diseases are often discussed in terms of their morbidity (degree of 'illness' involved) and mortality (risk of death as a result of the disease). Five-year and 10-year survival rates are often used as an expression of mortality. For example, in some types of lung cancer the poor prognosis is reflected in a 5-year survival rate of 0%.

Screening is the process whereby apparently healthy people are investigated in order to detect unrecognised disease. Although 'mass screening' is carried out (e.g. all babies are screened for phenylketonuria at birth), most screening programmes target certain 'at risk' groups. Thus, the screening programmes for female breast and cervical cancer target subgroups of the population who are most at risk, namely females of certain age groups. Screen-ing involves a relatively inexpensive diagnostic test, such as a cervical smear or mammogram, which picks up those with early, treatable forms or precursors of the disease. The test must be sensitive so it picks up as many cases as possible, but not over-sensitive so that 'false-positive' results occur. In a perfect test, the sensitivity (true positives) and specificity (true negatives) will each be 100%.

Incidence and prevalence

Incidence of a disease is the number of new cases occurring in a defined population over a defined time period. In contrast, prevalence is the number of cases found in a defined population at a particular time. Factors affecting incidence and prevalence include:

- time: how the disease varies over the course of time, e.g. historically or with the changing seasons

- place: how the disease varies geographically
- person: the personal characteristics of those who have the disease and how they differ from those who do not, e.g. in age, sex, occupation, race, social class, behaviour.

Changes in the incidence of disease with time may result from preventive measures, such as immunisation programmes, or may reflect changes in social conditions. For example, increased smoking has led to an increase in heart disease and lung cancer, better housing conditions in the early twentieth century led to a decrease in tuberculosis. The biggest drop in the number of cases of tuberculosis antedated BCG immunisation and antibiotics, and was mainly a result of better housing and social conditions.

Many diseases show significant geographical variations: in industrialised countries heart disease and cancer are common, whereas in developing countries malnutrition and infection are often the principal health problems. Different infectious agents are common in different geographical areas.

There are many well-documented associations between occupations and disease:

- coal miners – pneumoconiosis (coal-dust disease of the lungs)
- boilermakers and dockyard workers – asbestosis (asbestos-related scarring in the lungs); mesothelioma (asbestos-related malignant tumour of the pleura)
- rubber and dye workers – bladder cancer through the effect of chemicals
- those working in hardwood manufacturing – nasal cancer as a result of inhalation of wood dust.

Relative risk is a way of describing the degree of risk for developing a disease associated with a particular occupation, behaviour or other factor. It is the proportion of individuals exposed to the risk factor who develop the disease divided by the proportion that develops it in the rest of the population. Thus, if exposure to a certain chemical has a relative risk of 2 for developing a particular cancer, it means that exposed individuals are twice as likely to develop the cancer as unexposed individuals.

Self-assessment: questions

One best answer questions

1. Which of the following positions defines disease in terms of deviation from statistical normality?

   a. feminist
   b. homeopathic
   c. naturalistic
   d. normative
   e. sociopolitical

2. Which of the following is *not* a genetic disease?

   a. Down's syndrome
   b. congenital rubella
   c. familial adenomatous polyposis
   d. haemophilia A
   e. Huntington's disease

3. Which of the following is *not* considered when classifying a disease?

   a. aetiology
   b. pathogenesis
   c. response to treatment
   d. social context
   e. star sign

4. A researcher is studying a disease and finds that the relative risk of developing the disease for people who drink coffee is 0.5. Which of the following conclusions is most appropriate?

   a. coffee drinkers are four times as likely to develop the disease as those who do not drink coffee
   b. coffee drinkers are twice as likely to develop the disease as those who do not drink coffee
   c. those who do not drink coffee are twice as likely to develop the disease as coffee drinkers
   d. those who do not drink coffee are four times as likely to develop the disease as coffee drinkers
   e. coffee is the most likely cause of the disease

True-false questions

1. The following are correctly paired:

   a. idiopathic – cause unknown
   b. pathogenesis – direct cause of disease
   c. congenital – present at birth
   d. prognosis – likely disease outcome
   e. aetiology – mechanism of disease production

2. The following are examples of cytogenetic diseases:

   a. haemophilia (factor VIII deficiency)
   b. Down's syndrome
   c. sickle cell anaemia

   d. Münchhausen's syndrome
   e. Turner's syndrome

3. The following are correctly paired:

   a. incidence – number of cases in a population at a given time
   b. symptoms – features of an illness that the patient notices
   c. prevalence – number of new cases in a population over a given time
   d. morbidity – number of deaths in a population
   e. sensitivity of a screening test – number of patients with the disease who have a positive screening test

Case history

A 9-year-old boy with cystic fibrosis presents to his local hospital with a chest infection. He has chest pain and is coughing up foul smelling, green sputum.

1. What is cystic fibrosis?
2. What is the pathogenesis of the child's chest infection?

He is treated with antibiotics and makes a swift recovery.

3. What other therapy is likely to be of value in treating the chest infection?
4. What other problems might this patient develop?
5. What is the prognosis of the disease?

Short note questions

1. What factors may affect the incidence and prevalence of a disease?
2. What is meant by the term 'screening'? What factors influence the success of a screening programme?
3. What factors influence the prognosis of a disease?

Viva questions

1. What does 'congenital' mean? How does this differ from the term genetic?
2. How do aetiology and pathogenesis differ?
3. What type of disease may have a high incidence but a low prevalence (and vice versa)?

Self-assessment: answers

One best answer

1. c. Naturalism is the concept that disease is an objective deviation from normality. Although a useful concept in some circumstances, it does not take into account the cultural, social and even spiritual aspects of disease.

2. b. Congenital rubella is present at birth, but it is an infectious disease, not a genetic one. Despite the principle that virtually all diseases have genetic and environmental components to some extent, it is still useful to distinguish those in which one or the other is predominant.

3. e. This question is not as trite as it looks, because astrology is an important part of many non-Western medical traditions. However, it is not supported by scientific evidence and so the patient's star sign is not considered in pathology or epidemiology.

4. c. Coffee seems to have a protective effect for this disease; coffee drinkers develop it only half as often as other individuals.

True-false answers

1. a. **True.** Idiopathic, essential and primary are all terms used to mean cause unknown.
   b. **False.** Pathogenesis is the mechanism by which the causal agent(s) act upon the body systems to produce the disease.
   c. **True.** The term congenital means that the pathological process has affected the embryo or fetus. It is important to remember that the congenital disease/defect may not cause illness until months or years after birth (e.g. various forms of congenital heart disease).
   d. **True.** The prognosis of a disease is an estimate of its outcome.
   e. **False.** The aetiology of a disease is the causal agent.

2. a. **False.** Haemophilia is an inherited disorder of blood clotting but it is caused by a single gene mutation. The genetic defect is linked to the X chromosome and is carried by females and mainly expressed in disease form in males. The abnormality in the gene causes a defect in factor VIII production and thus the clotting cascade is interrupted and affected individuals have a bleeding tendency.
   b. **True.** Down's syndrome is a common chromosomal disorder. Most affected individuals (95%) have trisomy 21, i.e. an extra chromosome 21. Their total chromosome count is therefore 47. The remaining 5% have an extra copy of the long arm of chromosome 21 translocated to another chromosome. Two other common trisomies are trisomy 18 (Edward's syndrome) and trisomy 13 (Patau's syndrome).
   c. **False.** Sickle cell anaemia is caused by a point mutation in the haemoglobin gene that substitutes a valine for a glutamate in the beta-haemoglobin molecule. It is not associated with cytogenetic abnormalities.
   d. **False.** Patients with Münchhausen's syndrome have fictitious illnesses with frequent admissions to hospital, repeated investigations and sometimes surgery.
   e. **True.** Girls with Turner's syndrome typically have only one X chromosome, so the total number of chromosomes is 45. They are phenotypically female but are infertile and show some classic features such as a webbed neck and short stature.

3. a. **False.** Incidence is the number of new cases in a population over a given time.
   b. **True.** Symptoms are reported by the patient. Signs are the clinical manifestations of a disease which the clinician elicits.
   c. **False.** Prevalence is the number of cases in a population at any one time.
   d. **False.** The term morbidity relates to illness, not death (mortality).
   e. **True.** The sensitivity of a test is the number of individuals with the condition who test positive. In other words, it is the power of the test to correctly identify individuals who have the disease. In contrast, specificity is the ability of the test to correctly identify people who are well: it is the number of individuals free of the disease who have a negative result.

Case history answer

1. Cystic fibrosis is characterised by the production of abnormally sticky mucous secretions by exocrine glands. This causes blockage of the ducts in organs such as the pancreas, lung and reproductive tissues, leading to failure of function. Susceptibility to lung infections is a particular problem. The diagnosis can be made by the finding of raised concentrations of chloride and sodium in sweat. Cystic fibrosis is an autosomal recessive disease. The CF gene is located on the long arm of chromosome 7 and codes for a chloride ion-linked transmembrane regulator protein. Many different mutations of the CF gene have been described. The prevalence of carriage of the abnormal gene is very high (of the order of 1:25 Caucasians).

2. This case illustrates the relationship between pathogenesis and aetiology. The sputum is characteristic of bacterial infection; common

organisms isolated from patients with cystic fibrosis include *Staphylococcus aureus*, *Haemophilus influenzae* and *Pseudomonas aeruginosa*. The pathogenesis involves the following processes:

a. cystic fibrosis leads to retention of sticky secretions in the lung

b. these sticky secretions can then be colonised by bacteria, some of which will be pathogenic (disease causing)

c. multiplication of the pathogenic bacteria incites an inflammatory reaction

d. the large numbers of neutrophils that form part of the inflammatory reaction produce pus, hence the characteristics of the sputum.

3. In addition to antibiotic treatment, physiotherapy is indicated to help drain the secretions.

4. Patients with cystic fibrosis have numerous systemic problems. Recurrent lung infections could be associated with the development of bronchiectasis. Cor pulmonale can complicate the lung disease in cystic fibrosis. Failure of pancreatic function is common, and this patient is likely to require enzyme supplements. A few patients also require replacement insulin treatment. Liver failure may occur due to inspissated secretions obstructing the biliary tree. Most males exhibit congenital absence of the vas deferens bilaterally and are infertile.

5. Although the prognosis of cystic fibrosis is improving with better therapeutic regimens, and it may ultimately be cured by gene therapy, the disease still causes premature death; very few patients with cystic fibrosis survive beyond the age of 40.

Short note answers

Comment: For all the three questions, start with a definition of the term. Use bulleted lists as appropriate.

1. The main points to be covered in this answer are:

   a. definitions of incidence and prevalence

   b. general factors affecting them: time, place, person

   c. examples of each factor.

2. The main points to be covered in this answer are:

   a. definition of screening (this answers the first part of the question)

   b. the relationship between the natural history of a disease and the target population

   c. the acceptability of the screening method

   d. sensitivity and specificity in relation to false-negative and false-positive results

   e. cost.

Illustrate your answer with examples, e.g. the cervical and breast screening programmes.

3. The prognosis of a disease will vary for each patient and depends on:

   a. the nature of the disease

   b. how long the patient has had the disease

c. the general state of health of the patient: the presence of other diseases, and the nutritional status of the patient

d. the age of the patient

e. availability of diagnostic and treatment facilities

f. the response of the patient to the treatment available.

There are many examples of changing prognosis related to factors of an individual patient's status, e.g. *Candida* infection in a healthy individual is a minor illness, whereas in a person with human immunodeficiency virus (HIV) infection it may be fatal; influenza in a healthy 20-year-old is usually a self-limiting illness, whereas in an elderly bed-ridden patient it may be complicated by pneumonia and lead to death.

Viva answers

Comment: It is a good idea to start off with a definition of the subject or topic and then give examples in the same way as for a short answer question. However, the examiners may ask questions which may deflect you from a logical sequence, because they will be looking for depth and breadth of knowledge. You will have to keep prioritising and reorganising your knowledge as you go along.

1. Congenital disease is present at birth, but not necessarily inherited. Genetic disease is present in the genome of the individual from conception but will not necessarily manifest at birth. For example, fetal alcohol syndrome and haemophilia are both congenital, but only haemophilia is a genetic disorder.

2. Aetiology is the cause of a disease whereas pathogenesis is the underlying abnormal process that gives rise to the disorder. For example, in the disease tuberculosis:

   • The organism *Mycobacterium tuberculosis* is the aetiology.

   • The pathogenesis is delayed hypersensitivity response of T cells and macrophages to the organism, giving rise to the destructive granulomas that characterise tuberculosis (see Ch. 9).

3. Incidence is the number of cases occurring in a defined population over a stated period of time whereas prevalence is the number of cases in a defined population at a given time. The common cold has a high incidence, because many new cases occur during the course of, say, a year. However, it is a short-lived condition and so the prevalence at any particular time is relatively low compared with the incidence. On the other hand, the incidence of new cases of cystic fibrosis in any particular year is relatively low, but because patients usually live for many years the prevalence in the population will be higher.

The diagnostic process: from clinical reasoning to molecular biology

Chapter 2

Chapter overview

Patients present with symptoms, and a clinical examination elicits signs that suggest a diagnosis. Examination of specimens such as blood, urine, faeces and tissue samples in the various pathology laboratories helps confirm this diagnosis and monitor the treatment.

- Diagnosis involves clinical skills and laboratory tests.
- Specialist pathological techniques can aid in diagnosis.
- The autopsy has a place in auditing the quality of diagnosis in addition to determining cause of death.

2.1 Diagnosis

Learning objectives

You should:
- outline the principles of the diagnostic process
- identify the clinical laboratory disciplines.

Diagnosis is the act of recognising a disease in an individual patient and is based on clinical history, physical examination and investigation. The ability to integrate knowledge of the classification, epidemiology and mechanisms of disease processes, as discussed in Chapter 1, is essential. Making a diagnosis involves:

- taking a clinical history of symptoms: what the patient has noticed wrong (e.g. cough, breathlessness, pain)
- clinical examination for signs: what the doctor finds wrong on examination (e.g. lumps, rashes, abnormal lung sounds).

The clinician then works through a series of questions:

- Which organ system is most likely to be affected?
- Which category of disease do the signs and symptoms most likely suggest, e.g. inflammation, malignancy or poisoning?
- Do other factors such as race, age, sex, behavioural patterns or occupation of the patient provide clues to the diagnosis?

The diagnostic process involves testing a series of hypotheses based on the clinician's knowledge of the frequency of occurrence of the symptoms and signs in different disease states and on the probability of these occurring in the population from which the patient comes. A list of possible diagnoses is constructed, known as the differential diagnosis, beginning with the most likely disease and progressing to include diagnoses which are less likely but are important to exclude.

Special investigations are used to refine the list of differential diagnoses by providing evidence consistent with some diagnoses but excluding others. In a sense, they test the hypothesis that a particular disease process is present in a patient. Special investigations can include radiology, isotope scans, and tests of body fluids and tissue in the pathology laboratories. Reaching a diagnosis enables the clinician to start treatment and to give the patient some idea of the outcome of the disease (prognosis).

The clinical laboratory disciplines

As a clinical subject, pathology grew up in side rooms adjacent to hospital wards where simple diagnostic tests could be performed by nurses, medical students and doctors, and in the post-mortem room where the morphological changes associated with disease could be observed at autopsy. As the number and complexity of tests grew, hospitals required centralised laboratories, staffed by dedicated technical and medical personnel.

Nowadays, clinical pathology is divided into a number of disciplines, each with its own specialist practitioners:

- Clinical chemistry or chemical pathology: the investigation of metabolic disturbances by changes in the concentration of substances in body fluids.
- Haematology: the study of diseases of the blood and bone marrow.

- Histopathology, anatomical pathology or cellular pathology: the examination of structural changes in diseased tissues, macroscopically or microscopically.
- Immunology: the study of diseases of the immune system.
- Medical genetics: the study of the inheritance of disease.
- Microbiology: the detection and characterisation of bacteria, viruses, fungi and parasites.

2.2 Laboratory methods

Learning objectives

You should:
- describe the principles and purposes of techniques commonly used in pathology
- interpret the significance of technical terms used in pathology reports.

Histopathology

Histology

Basic histological techniques involve the processing of tissue specimens, so that they can be finely sliced and stained on a glass slide to be examined under the light microscope. Specimens can include biopsies (small pieces of tissue removed to make a diagnosis) and excision specimens (where a surgeon removes the diseased tissue as a therapeutic procedure). The tissue is first fixed in a preservative, usually formalin. It is then processed into paraffin wax, which supports the tissue while it is sliced into thin sections, typically 4–5 μm in thickness.

Most histopathology laboratories use the haematoxylin and eosin (H&E) stain routinely. The haematoxylin dye stains basic molecules blue, such as nucleic acids, while the eosin stains acidic molecules red, such as proteins. Pathologists commonly use terms such as basophilic and eosinophilic for materials that take up haematoxylin and eosin, respectively. Other stains may be used in addition to H&E for some specimens to demonstrate a particular substance or structure better than in an H&E section. Some of these special stains are highly specialised and used rarely; others are used commonly in pathology (Table 2).

Sometimes clinicians require a very urgent diagnosis during surgery. If so, small amounts of tissue can be frozen quickly and sectioned in an instrument called a cryostat, and looked at within a few minutes ('frozen sections'). Another use for frozen sections is to demonstrate fatty material in a specimen, because processing to paraffin wax dissolves any lipid out of the tissue.

It is also possible to look at tissues at a much higher magnification using the electron microscope. This technique, also known as ultrastructural examination, demonstrates cell structures at the level of organelles and smaller. It is relatively expensive and is generally used only in specific circumstances, such as the investigation of glomerular disease in renal biopsies. Viral particles in cells can be seen by electron microscopy.

Cytology

Sometimes it is easier or more efficient to take specimens of cells rather than whole pieces of tissue. Cells can be scraped from the surface (as in cervical smears), aspirated from various parts of the body through a fine needle, or separated from body fluids (such as urine, effusions or cerebrospinal fluid). The cells thus obtained can be placed

Table 2 Some stains used for specific diagnostic purposes

Stain	Principle	Examples of diagnostic use
Reticulin	Silver impregnation of reticulin fibres (predominantly type III collagen)	Demonstration of the architecture of tissues, e.g. lung and liver, by outlining the reticulin network around cells
Trichrome	Dye binds to collagen	Demonstration of fibrosis in inflammatory and neoplastic processes
Periodic acid–Schiff (PAS)	Reacts with sugars and macromolecules rich in sugar residues	Demonstration of substances such as glycogen, mucin and basement membranes
Perls'	Uses the Prussian blue reaction to demonstrate iron	Demonstration of iron deposits following inflammation or in haemochromatosis
Congo red	Dye is taken up by beta-pleated sheets	Demonstration of amyloid
Gram's	Uptake and retention of dyes depends on qualities of bacterial cell walls	Demonstrates bacteria and divides them into two groups: Gram-positive (stain dark blue) and Gram-negative (stain pink-red).
Ziehl–Neelsen (ZN)	Stains acid-fast bacilli	Demonstration of mycobacterial infection
Giemsa's	One of the Romanowsky family of stains that uses methylene blue and eosin	A routine stain for blood films and air-dried cytology specimens. Can also be used in tissue sections, for example to demonstrate certain parasites
Papanicolaou's	A mixture of dyes gives good cellular morphology	The routine stain for fixed cytology preparations, e.g. cervical smears

Two

directly on glass slides and stained to produce a cytological preparation, allowing abnormal cell morphology to be identified. Alternatively, the cells can be used for other techniques such as flow cytometry or detection of viral DNA.

Immunohistochemistry

Immunohistochemistry provides the pathologist with a powerful tool for demonstrating and identifying proteins, glycolipids and carbohydrates, which may be normal tissue constituents or produced as a result of a pathological process. Immunohistochemistry is based on the specificity of antibody-antigen binding. Monoclonal antibodies (antibodies having only one antigenic target) or polyclonal antibodies (a group of antibodies having a range of targets) can be made against a range of human antigens (Figure 1 and Ch. 7). Monoclonal antibodies are more specific. The antibodies can be applied to tissue sections or cytology preparations and will bind wherever their antigen is present. The antibody can be tagged either with an enzyme that catalyses a colour reaction or with a fluores-

cent dye. In this way the antibody and, by implication, the antigen can be visualised. A simple example is given in Figure 2.

Immunohistochemistry has enabled pathologists to learn much about the distribution of tissue antigens in both health and disease, and has increased the accuracy of diagnosis. Examples of diagnostic immunohistochemistry are given in Table 3.

Molecular biology techniques

New techniques for looking at chromosomes, genes, DNA, RNA and proteins are being developed continuously. Some are still research techniques, but others have entered diagnostic practice and are described in this section. Familiarity with the structure of DNA and the 'DNA-RNA-protein' pathway (Figure 3) will help in understanding the principles of molecular biology.

In situ hybridisation

Molecular techniques can be used to determine whether specific DNA or RNA sequences are present in a specimen.

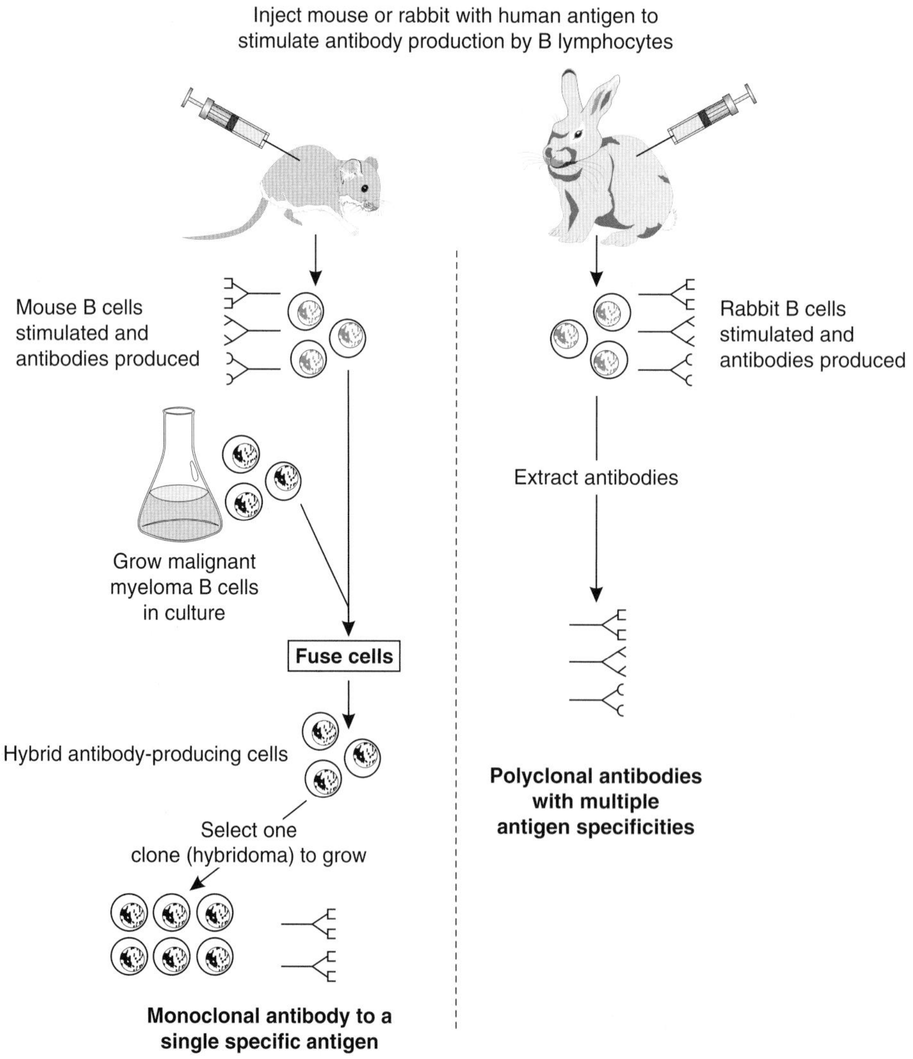

Figure 1 Monoclonal and polyclonal antibody production.

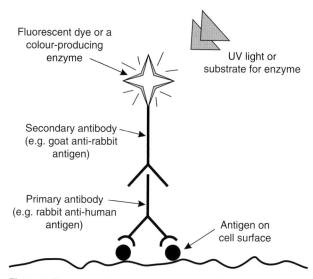

Figure 2 Illustration of basic immunohistochemical techniques to visualise antigens.

Table 3 Examples of diagnostic immunohistochemistry

Antibody	Diagnostic use
Chromogranin	This component of neurosecretory granules can be used to locate neuroendocrine cells in tissues. It is also found in neoplasms of neuroendocrine type, e.g. carcinoid tumours and pancreatic endocrine tumours
Cytokeratin	The expression of cytokeratin by a tumour may help differentiate between an epithelial and a non-epithelial neoplasm. Sometimes specific cytokeratins can suggest a primary site, e.g. CK20 is typically expressed by carcinomas of the large intestine
Desmin	This filamentous protein is found in muscle cells. Its expression in a neoplasm implies muscle differentiation
Immunoglobulin	Identification of immunoglobulin in neoplastic plasma cells can aid in the diagnosis of multiple myeloma; identification of immunoglobulin in the tissues can help determine the immune nature of a disease, e.g. immunoglobulin in the renal glomerulus in glomerulonephritis (see Chs 7 and 8)
S100	This protein is present in some cells (e.g. melanocytes, nerve cells and antigen-presenting cells), but not in others. It can be used to help determine the line of differentiation of neoplasms

A length of nucleic acid (the probe) with a complementary sequence to the DNA or RNA under study is constructed (see Box 1). The cDNA or cRNA probe is labelled with a radioisotope or a non-radioactive enzyme system and applied to a tissue section. Under the correct conditions the labelled probe will hybridise with its complementary

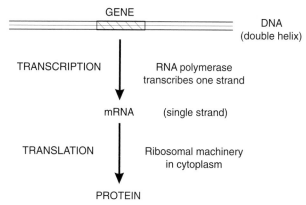

Figure 3 DNA-RNA-protein pathway.

Box 1 Principles of hybridisation

- DNA is double stranded
- Bonds between complementary bases hold strands together (cytosine–guanine; adenine–thymine)
- Heat/alkalinise DNA – separation of strands ('denaturation') occurs
- Cool separated strands – complementary double strands re-form
- Labelled complementary single-strand DNA can identify a DNA sequence (e.g. a gene) in intact cells or disrupted cell preparations

---

nucleic acid sequence in the tissue. The specimen is then washed, and if the probe has attached itself to the specimen it can be detected by its label. In this way, the locations, numbers or types of cells containing the DNA/RNA can be seen down the microscope. In the relatively new procedure of fluorescent in situ hybridisation (FISH), the probe is attached to a fluorescent marker.

Southern, northern and western blot analysis

These techniques are named as directional puns after Edward Southern who invented the first of these methods for examining DNA. In these techniques, DNA fragments (Southern blotting), mRNA fragments (northern) or polypeptides (western) are placed on an electrophoretic gel. The nucleic acid fragments or peptides then migrate through the gel according to their molecular size and separate into bands which are subsequently blotted onto nylon membranes and either hybridised with specific nucleic acid probes (Southern/northern) or visualised by labelled antibodies against the peptides (western).

Polymerase chain reaction (PCR)

This relatively simple technique is now widely used in molecular biology. It allows analysis of DNA or RNA from virtually any tissue specimen. Central to PCR is a chain reaction which amplifies the length of DNA under examination many million-fold. This increases the amount of the sequence to be identified to a level that can be detected

Two

easily in the laboratory. The three vital ingredients of the reaction are (Figure 4):

- The RNA/DNA to be examined (RNA needs to be converted into DNA by reverse transcription).
- Two oligonucleotides, usually 15–30 bases long, with sequences matching DNA sequences flanking the DNA fragment of interest. They give the amplification its specificity.
- A heat-stable DNA polymerase (typically *Taq* polymerase from the thermophilic organism *Thermus aquaticus*), which can withstand heating and synthesises DNA at high temperatures.

The mixture is heated, dissociating the double-stranded DNA and allowing the single strands to bind to the oligonucleotides. These oligonucleotides then act as primers for the polymerase and a new double-stranded DNA molecule is formed. Twice as much double-stranded DNA is then present and the cycle can be repeated. Each cycle doubles the amount of DNA in the area of interest, so at the end of several cycles (typically between 15 and 30) the area of interest will have been reproduced thousands or millions of times and there will be large amounts of DNA for analysis. The sensitivity of the technique is such that the DNA from a single cell can be amplified. The reaction has numerous applications:

- detection of genetic diseases, e.g. cystic fibrosis
- cross-matching tissues for transplantation (human leucocyte antigen (HLA) subtyping)
- detection of bacteria and viruses
- detection of abnormal genes linked with cancer.

Flow cytometry

Flow cytometers analyse cells as they flow one by one past one or more sensors. The cells are suspended in liquid (the sheath fluid), and as they flow through the machine they are illuminated with light, typically from a laser. From the degree and direction of scatter, information about the physical properties of each cell, such as size and shape, can be deduced. Further information can be obtained by labelling the cells with fluorescent antibodies; the laser causes any labelled cells to fluoresce, so cells with a specific antigen can be identified. Modern machines can analyse several thousand cells every second.

Flow cytometry is a powerful tool; haematologists use it to analyse blood cells, and histopathologists use it to analyse cells from cytological and histological specimens. In the latter case, the cells have to be disaggregated so they form a suspension in the sheath fluid.

DNA microarray analysis

A DNA microarray (DNA chip) is a collection of thousands of microscopic spots of DNA attached to a solid surface such as glass or a silicon chip. The process resembles Southern blotting in that when the DNA to be tested is exposed to the DNA chip, complementary strands will hybridise. The DNA attached to the substrate is called the probe, and the free DNA being tested is called the target. The probe may be a length of cDNA or an oligonucleotide synthesised from nucleic acid bases. Ways in which hybridisation can be detected include fluorescence, chemiluminescence and changes in conductivity in the silicone chip substrate. The result is that thousands of different genes from one sample can be analysed.

Although still essentially an experimental technique, DNA microarrays are expected to have applications in clinical diagnosis. For example:

- microbiological specimens could be screened for the presence of thousands of bacteria simultaneously, without the need for culture
- specific genetic mutations in cancers could be identified, helping accurate classification of the neoplasm and possibly allowing targeted gene therapy
- a potential application in forensic medicine is detection of single nucleotide polymorphisms that could link a sample to an individual person.

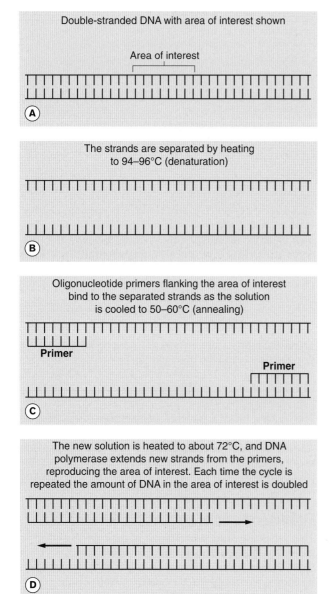

Figure 4 Polymerase chain reaction.

Microbiology

Microscopy and bacterial culture

Specimens for microbiological analysis are routinely examined under the microscope. Sometimes, there are enough organisms present for a provisional identification to be made. The Gram stain, Ziehl–Neelsen and Giemsa stains are often used (Table 2).

Culture is performed by inoculating a growth medium such as an agar plate with the specimen and then incubating it under conditions suitable for the growth of pathogenic bacteria. Any bacteria that grow can be isolated and identified by a combination of features, such as their morphology and biochemical profile. The sensitivity of the organism to various antibiotics can also be tested.

Detection of microbial antigens and nucleic acid

The presence of microbial antigens can be detected by using antibodies. For example, enzyme immunoassay uses antibodies fastened to a solid phase, such as the inside of a test tube, to trap antigens in a fluid. If the antigens are captured they can be detected by adding a labelled antibody of the same specificity. If the antigen is present, the labelled antibody will bind to it forming a 'sandwich'.

Microbiologists use molecular techniques to detect specific DNA or RNA from bacteria and viruses. PCR can be used to amplify microbial DNA so that even a single organism in the specimen can be detected. Although this sensitivity is one of the strengths of PCR, it is also a potential pitfall because contamination of the sample or the presence of clinically insignificant amounts of DNA could produce a false-positive reaction.

Serology

Serology is the detection of specific antibodies in a patient's blood. If antibodies to an organism are detected it provides indirect evidence of infection. However, the results of these tests require careful interpretation since a positive result could indicate past exposure to the organism rather than current infection.

A commonly used serological method is enzyme immunoassay. The principle is the same as described in the previous section except that the antigen is attached to the solid phase and is used to trap antibody in the fluid being tested.

Cytogenetics

The mainstay of morphological cytogenetics is the karyotype, which consists of the chromosomes numbered and arranged in sequence from largest to smallest. Classically, karyotyping is performed on chromosomes in metaphase obtained by treating cultured cells with colchicine, which disrupts the formation of the mitotic spindle. The chromosomes are stained with Giemsa's, resulting in a sequence of light and dark bands unique to each chromosome. The latest techniques use chromosomes in prometaphase because the banding pattern is visible more clearly. Changes in the number or structure of chromosomes can be used to diagnose cytogenetic diseases (see Ch. 1).

In comparative genomic hybridisation, changes in the number of copies of a segment of a chromosome can be detected. It is used in cancer cytogenetics and for the assessment of early embryos during in vitro fertilisation procedures. In principle, chromosomes from the patient are broken into small segments and labelled with a fluorochrome. Normal chromosomes act as a control; they are broken into similar segments and labelled with a different fluorochrome. A mixture of these chromosome fragments are hybridised to normal chromosome spreads on a microscope slide. If there is more or less of one segment in the patient's sample, the ratio of the intensities of the two fluorochromes along the chromosomes in the spreads will change. This finding represents regions of gain or loss of DNA sequences, such as duplications, amplifications or deletions.

2.3 The autopsy

Learning objectives

You should:
- discuss the purposes of the autopsy
- distinguish a hospital autopsy from a coroner's autopsy.

The word autopsy is derived from the Greek word for eye witness, and can be translated as 'seeing for oneself'. It is the examination of the body after death (post-mortem examination) and can involve histological, microbiological and other techniques in addition to the dissection and naked-eye examination of the organs.

Box 2 Deaths that come under the jurisdiction of the coroner in England and Wales

A death should be referred to the coroner if:

- the cause of death is unknown

- the deceased was not seen by the certifying doctor either after death or in the 14 days before death

- the deceased was not seen by a doctor during their last illness

- the death was violent, unnatural or suspicious

- the death may be due to an accident (whenever it occurred), suicide or an abortion

- the death may be due to self-neglect or neglect by others

- the death may be related to a medical procedure or treatment

- the death occurred during an operation or before recovery from the effects of an anaesthetic

- the death occurred during or shortly after detention in prison or police custody

- the deceased was detained under the Mental Health Act

- the death may be due to an industrial disease or related to the deceased's employment.

An important reason for autopsy examination is to determine the cause of death in cases where this is unknown. However, the autopsy can also have an important role in cases where it is believed the cause of death is clear – it is a form of audit that can identify conditions which were not apparent in life. Even nowadays, despite the sophisticated diagnostic techniques at the disposal of clinicians, autopsies regularly reveal significant unexpected findings. Conditions that would have changed patients' treatment had they been diagnosed during life often become apparent only at autopsy. In addition, the autopsy provides a unique opportunity for clinicopathological correlation, and thus has an important role in the education of medical students and doctors. Discussions between clinicians and pathologists about autopsy findings can lead to new insights into the causes and outcomes of disease, particularly diseases that have been described only recently.

Most countries have statutory procedures for investigating deaths that are suspicious or unnatural. In England and Wales, it is the responsibility of the coroner to investigate such deaths and to order an autopsy if one is required (see Box 2). If the case does not fall under the jurisdiction of the coroner, an autopsy can only be performed by obtaining fully informed consent from the next of kin; such cases are often called 'hospital autopsies' to distinguish them from coroners' autopsies. In the UK there are stringent regulations concerning the retention of tissues and organs at post mortem for further investigations, teaching or research. Other nations have similar regulations in place.

Self-assessment: questions

One best answer questions

1. In which of the following techniques is specific antigen-antibody binding a key step?
   a. Gram's stain
   b. immunohistochemistry
   c. karyotyping
   d. polymerase chain reaction (PCR)
   e. Southern blotting

2. Which of the following is most suitable for analysing thousands of different genes simultaneously?
   a. DNA microarray
   b. electron microscopy
   c. enzyme immunoassay
   d. flow cytometry
   e. polymerase chain reaction (PCR)

3. A doctor is examining a patient with high blood pressure. She suspects he may have a phaeochromocytoma (a tumour of the adrenal medulla that secretes adrenaline and noradrenaline) so she wishes to measure the levels of catecholamines in his urine. To which laboratory should she submit the urine specimen?
   a. chemical pathology
   b. cytogenetics
   c. haematology
   d. histopathology
   e. immunology

True-false questions

1. The following are correctly paired:
   a. haematoxylin uptake – eosinophilia
   b. DNA polymerase – polymerase chain reaction (PCR)
   c. tuberculosis – PAS stain
   d. serology – enzyme immunoassay
   e. high blood pressure – clinical sign

2. The following statements are correct:
   a. immunohistochemistry demonstrates the presence of antigens in tissues
   b. western blotting techniques are used to analyse DNA
   c. squamous cell carcinoma may produce cytokeratin intermediate filaments
   d. frozen sections are a rapid diagnostic technique which can be used intraoperatively
   e. in situ hybridisation techniques cannot be used to examine RNA in tissues

3. The following cases should be referred to the coroner under English law:
   a. a 90-year-old man falls down the stairs. He makes a good recovery, but a month later dies of subdural haemorrhage
   b. a 45-year-old man has a cardiac arrest during a coronary bypass operation and resuscitation is unsuccessful
   c. a 90-year-old woman is found dead in bed at her home address. Her doctor is unsure why she died
   d. a 22-year-old man is found dead in a hotel room. A note next to the body says he has taken tablets with the intention of killing himself
   e. a 50-year-old worker in a nuclear power station dies of leukaemia

Extended matching items questions (EMIs)

EMI 1

Theme: Laboratory procedures

A. Congo red stain
B. cytology
C. electron microscopy
D. karyotyping
E. immunohistochemistry
F. PAS stain
G. Perls stain
H. polymerase chain reaction
I. reticulin stain

Which of the above procedures is a pathologist most likely to use in the following scenarios?

1. A specimen of pleural fluid from a 75-year-old woman with a pleural effusion is sent to the laboratory. The request form states: 'Lung mass, ?malignant effusion.'
2. A pathologist examining a liver biopsy wants to delineate the architecture of the tissue to see if cirrhosis is present.
3. A pathologist wants to examine the internal structure of the mitochondria.
4. A rectal biopsy is received with a request form stating: 'Please test for amyloid.'
5. A pathologist examines a tumour and suspects it may be of smooth muscle type. She would like to determine whether it contains proteins typical of smooth muscle cells such as actin and desmin.
6. An infant with multiple congenital abnormalities dies a few hours after birth. The cause of death is unknown and an autopsy is performed. The pathologist suspects trisomy 13 (Patau's syndrome).

Case history question

Case history 1

A 63-year-old man has smoked 30 cigarettes a day for over 50 years and develops severe, band-like chest pain and breathlessness whenever he exerts himself climbing stairs or walking up a hill. The pain is associated with sweating and nausea. He goes to his general practitioner, who notices that the man has cold hands, a weak irregular pulse and abnormal heart sounds. A blood test reveals hypercholesterolaemia.

1. List the symptoms and signs in this case.
2. Why might the patient have these problems?
3. What factors in the history are likely to predispose to the development of this disease?

Objective structured clinical examination question (OSCE)

OSCE 1

You are the house officer caring for a 65-year-old man who worked as a roofer between the ages of 20 and 32. During this time, he was often exposed to asbestos. He was diagnosed as having malignant mesothelioma of the pleura 9 months ago and, despite treatment, died yesterday. His wife has just learnt that the case has been referred to the coroner and that an autopsy has been requested. She does not want an autopsy performed, and has asked to speak to you.

Short note questions

Write short notes on the following:

1. When could electron microscopic examination of tissues be of use diagnostically?
2. Describe the principles of the PCR reaction, and how it is used in diagnostic practice.

Viva question

1. What is the role of the autopsy in modern medicine?

Self-assessment: answers

One best answer

1. b. Immunohistochemistry detects antigens in tissue sections through specific antibody binding. Karyotyping and Gram staining rely on dyes to demonstrate chromosomes and bacteria, respectively. PCR and Southern blotting use DNA reactions.

2. a. The purpose of DNA microarrays is to analyse thousands of genes simultaneously. PCR amplifies only a single segment of DNA.

3. a. The chemical pathology laboratory measures the concentration of substances in blood, urine and other body fluids.

True-false answers

1. a. **False.** Substances that stain with haematoxylin are basophilic. A substance that stains with eosin is eosinophilic (or acidophilic).
   b. **True.** A heat-stable DNA polymerase is a key component of the PCR reaction.
   c. **False.** Tuberculosis is caused by *Mycobacterium tuberculosis*, which is an acid-fast bacillus which stains positively with the ZN stain. PAS stain does not demonstrate this particular organism.
   d. **True.** There are many variations on the theme of the enzyme immunoassay. Antibodies can be used to detect antigens and antigens can be used to detect antibodies, depending on how the test is configured. One application is serology, i.e. the detection of antibodies in the blood.
   e. **True.** High blood pressure (hypertension) is a clinical sign. Most patients will not know whether or not their blood pressure is normal unless it is measured, because high blood pressure is typically asymptomatic (without symptoms).

2. a. **True.** Immunohistochemical techniques exploit specific antigen-antibody binding to identify antigens in tissue sections.
   b. **False.** Western blot analysis is used for identification of peptides/proteins.
   c. **True.** Many cancers produce excessive quantities of certain cell products, which can be identified using histochemical or immunohistochemical techniques. For example, a malignant melanoma, a tumour of the pigment-containing cells of the epidermis (melanocytes) may produce excessive melanin which can be seen in diagnostic sections using a special silver stain (Masson–Fontana) or by immunostaining for S-100, a calcium-binding protein found in melanocytes. Similarly, squamous cancers produce cytokeratins, which are proteins found in most epithelial cells. Thus, cytokeratins are good markers of epithelial differentiation in tumours (see Ch. 12).
   d. **True.** The rapid frozen section is used by surgeons who require urgent confirmation of a diagnosis during surgery. They may alter their surgical procedure on this basis, e.g. knowing whether a tumour is benign or malignant may drastically alter the type of operation performed. Surgeons may also ask the pathologists to perform frozen sections on tissue resection margins during cancer operations, to ensure complete removal of the tumour.
   e. **False.** In situ hybridisation is a very useful technique which enables visualisation of specific DNA or RNA sequences in tissue sections. For example, it can be used to identify viral or bacterial RNA/DNA, such as the Epstein–Barr virus in malignant lymphoid tumours and human papilloma virus sequences in cervical cancer and pre-cancer.

3. a. **True.** The fall is an accident that represents a possible cause of the intracranial bleeding.
   b. **True.** Death during an operation is a coroner's case.
   c. **True.** If the cause of death is unknown, the doctor cannot complete a death certificate and the case needs to be referred to the coroner.
   d. **True.** This appears to be suicide.
   e. **True.** This could be an industrial disease.

EMI answers

EMI 1

Theme: Laboratory procedures

1. B. Typically, the specimen will be centrifuged to concentrate the cells in the fluid. Then the cells will be mounted on a glass slide, stained, and examined under the microscope to determine whether any of the cells show features of malignancy.

2. I. A reticulin stain is ideal for this purpose. A trichrome stain might also be of use in this case by demonstrating any fibrosis.

3. C. The electron microscope is required to examine the ultrastructure of cells.

4. A. Congo red is a good stain for amyloid. When the section is examined through crossed polarising filters, amyloid stained with Congo red exhibits apple-green birefringence. This finding increases the specificity of the reaction.

5. E. Immunohistochemistry is often used diagnostically in this way.

6. D. To detect a cytogenetic abnormality such as an extra chromosome 13, cells taken from the body can be cultured and karyotyped.

Case history answers

Case history 1

1. The patient's symptoms are chest pain, breathlessness, sweating and nausea on exertion. The signs of his illness elicited by his general practitioner are cold hands, abnormal pulse and heart sounds.

2. This is a very common clinical scenario in the Western world. The most likely pathogenesis is narrowing of the coronary arteries by atherosclerosis (furring of the arteries caused by a lipid-rich deposit in the vessel wall, see Ch. 6). This pathological process restricts the blood supply to the heart, thus compromising its function, particularly when the heart is stressed by the increased demands of exercise. The pain occurs when the oxygen demands of the heart are not matched by the supply of blood.

3. As in many diseases, both genetic and acquired processes have a role in the development of atherosclerosis. Inherited abnormalities of lipid metabolism can lead to early atherosclerosis, and the increased blood cholesterol is likely to be significant in this case. Many of the risk factors for atherosclerosis are acquired and can be controlled by alterations in lifestyle. Cigarette smoking is strongly associated with atherosclerosis, as in this case. Other factors predisposing to this condition are the patient's age (the incidence of coronary atherosclerosis increases with advancing age) and his sex (the incidence in men is higher than in women of the same age).

OSCE answers

OSCE 1

Comment: You should start by expressing sympathy and then explore the reasons for the patient's wife's request to see you. You should find out how much she already understands. You may need to explain that the mesothelioma was due to asbestos exposure during his employment and is therefore an industrial disease. There is often a long time delay between the exposure and the onset of the tumour, as in this case. The relatives cannot refuse the autopsy, since the case comes under the jurisdiction of the coroner and is thus a legal requirement.
You should explain that:

- the procedure will be performed by trained professionals who will be respectful

- the autopsy is designed to investigate fully the circumstances of the death

- it may help to answer any outstanding questions about the progress of the disease and its treatment.

Be prepared to answer questions about retention and disposal of tissue samples; if you don't know the details, agree to find out. She may wish to talk with a bereavement coordinator, chaplain or other member of the team, and you should be willing to facilitate this. Empathy and sensitivity will obviously be required throughout.

Short note answers

1. In microbiology, electron microscopy has applications in identifying viruses in specimens. It may also be of use in identifying some unusual bacteria and protozoa. In histopathology, it is used routinely in renal biopsies taken for investigation of glomerulonephritis. It can also be used to classify some tumours by identifying ultrastructural components in the cells (for example neurosecretory granules in neuroendocrine neoplasms), but immunohistochemistry has superseded the use of the electron microscope in this field for all but a few specific tumours.

2. *Comment*: A good answer would start by defining the PCR reaction as a technique which amplifies DNA. RNA can be amplified after conversion to complementary DNA by reverse transcriptase. Describe how repeated DNA strand separation, primer annealing and chain extension by heat-stable DNA polymerase are produced by cycles of heating and cooling. As a result, small amounts of DNA or RNA in the sample which otherwise might be too small to detect can be analysed. Examples of its use are to identify bacteria, viruses and other pathogens; abnormal genes in cancers; and inherited disease genes, such as those involved in muscular dystrophy or cystic fibrosis.

Viva answer

1. Even if a cause of death has been given on a death certificate, an autopsy can:

- detect conditions that were unsuspected during life (still a common occurrence despite the increasing use of modern diagnostic techniques), and thus act as a form of audit

- correlate clinical findings with pathological processes

- identify organs involved in 'new' diseases (e.g. HIV)

- be a valuable teaching resource

- provide data for research.

There are circumstances in which an autopsy may be required by law, for example to ascertain the cause of death where it is unknown, or in the investigation of unnatural deaths.

Cell growth and adaptation

Chapter 3

Chapter overview

In order to function appropriately, cells and tissues need to maintain a steady state (homeostasis). Within defined limits, cells are capable of adapting to a variety of stimuli which may upset normality. Cellular adaptation is the state between a normal unstressed cell and the overstressed injured cell. By definition, an adaptive process is one which is potentially reversible. This chapter covers:

- normal cell growth and the cell cycle
- reversible adaptive responses.

3.1 Normal cell growth

Learning objectives

You should:
- describe the characteristics of a stem cell
- use the terms labile, stable and permanent as they apply to cell populations
- describe the cell cycle and the fundamentals of its control.

Regeneration

Cells that are lost through death or injury need to be replaced. Furthermore, normal growth of tissues depends on a balance between the number of cells actively dividing and the number of cells dying. Therefore, tissues contain a population of cells capable of repeated mitotic division, called stem cells. Sometimes, differentiated cells can return to the cell cycle and divide to produce daughter cells. However, unless they take on the characteristics of stem cells, they cannot do so indefinitely. The reason is that the terminal ends of chromosomes called telomeres become slightly shorter with each cell division. Eventually, when the telomeres become too short, further mitotic division is not possible. In a sense, the telomeres act like a clock counting down the number of mitoses a cell is allowed. However, stem cells possess the enzyme telomerase, which reconstitutes the telomeres at each mitosis, allowing an infinite number of cell divisions. Most neoplastic cells (see Ch. 11) also possess telomerase, which explains why they too can divide indefinitely.

When a stem cell divides, it produces two daughter cells. One of these retains the characteristics of a stem cell so that it can divide again, but the other can differentiate and become a specialised cell of the tissue, such as an epithelial or connective tissue cell.

Traditionally, tissues have been divided into three types according to the nature of cell turnover they exhibit, namely: labile, stable and permanent. Labile tissues have a high cell turnover and show continuous mitotic activity, stable tissues contain cells with a longer lifespan and mitoses are rare or absent, and permanent tissues are incapable of any cell division. These concepts are useful when thinking about the way in which tissues respond to injury, and are defined in Box 3. (The term injury is used in a broad sense by pathologists to include any pathological alteration in the environment or integrity of a cell.)

In labile and stable tissues, stem cells can quickly replace dead cells within their population by cell division and replace them with cells of exactly the same type. This process is called regeneration (Figure 5). For example, removal of part of the liver triggers hepatocytes close to the area removed to enter the cell cycle, divide and replace the lost tissue. Successful regeneration of cell populations depends on an intact connective tissue matrix around the cells. If this matrix is destroyed, repair by fibrosis and scar formation is likely.

Repair

Permanent cells by definition cannot divide and replace lost cells by the same cell type. Instead, repair by fibrosis occurs (Figure 5). In this process, dead tissue is removed and scar tissue (collagen-rich fibrous tissue) fills the defect. The scar provides continuity and strength to the tissue but there is loss of the original specialised cell function. Repair, rather than regeneration, is also likely when labile or stable tissues show extensive injury that disrupts the normal architecture of the tissue or damages the connective tissue matrix. The mechanism of fibrosis is described in Chapter 10.

The cell cycle

The four main stages of the cell cycle (Figure 6) are:

- M phase: mitosis when the cell divides (about 1 hour)
- G1 phase: gap 1, the preparation for S phase

Box 3 Labile, stable and permanent tissues

- **Labile tissues**. These tissues contain stem cells that proliferate more or less continuously because the daughter cells have a short lifespan and need to be constantly replaced. Labile tissues have a high regenerative capacity. Examples are bone marrow, epidermis of the skin and the gut epithelium.

- **Stable tissues**. Although stable tissues also contain stem cells, the turnover is slow because the differentiated cells are long-lived. Therefore, a histological section of the tissue may not contain any mitoses. However, if the tissue is damaged and many cells are lost, the tissue can become highly active mitotically and regenerate itself. This can occur because the remaining stem cells are stimulated to divide, e.g. bone. Alternatively, in some tissues the differentiated cells can be stimulated to re-enter the cell cycle; an example is liver, in which it appears that liver cells can divide while retaining the characteristics of differentiated liver cells.

- **Permanent tissues**. These tissues only contain cells capable of division in fetal life. Therefore, cells lost after birth cannot be replaced. Examples of permanent cells are neurones and cardiac/skeletal muscle cells (although cardiac and skeletal muscle may be capable of limited proliferation under some circumstances).

- S phase: DNA synthesis
- G2 phase: gap 2, during which assembly of the apparatus for the distribution of chromosomes occurs.

In addition, a G0 phase of the cell cycle is recognised. This phase is non-proliferative and is known as growth arrest. Cells in G0 may re-enter the cell cycle at G1, thereby regaining the proliferative state. Locally active small-molecular-weight proteins called growth factors are important in stimulating this re-entry.

Stem cells are capable of going round the cell cycle indefinitely. In contrast, cells which undergo terminal differentiation cannot re-enter the cell cycle (Figure 6). In a permanent cell population, all the cells are terminally differentiated.

Control of the cell cycle

Growth factors

Growth factors are proteins of low molecular weight that have a similar mechanism of action to hormones. In general, the growth factor is produced by a cell, for example a macrophage, and acts either on the cell itself (autocrine action) or on a neighbouring cell (paracrine action) by linking to cell surface receptors. This interaction activates the receptor and triggers a series of cytoplasmic events usually involving phosphorylation-dephosphorylation of proteins. Ultimately, a signal reaches the nucleus where genes are switched on, new proteins produced and cell growth and division are initiated. Growth factors often have actions that go beyond effects on the cell cycle. They can also inhibit or promote apoptosis (programmed cell death, see Ch. 4), and can stimulate differentiation of cells.

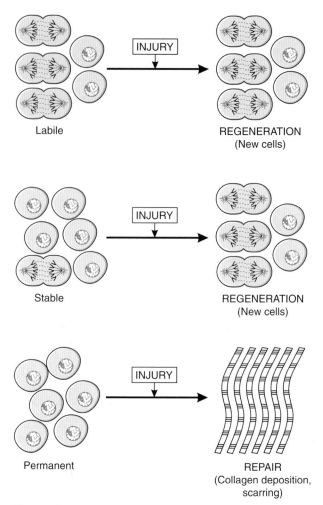

Figure 5 Regeneration and repair response to injury.

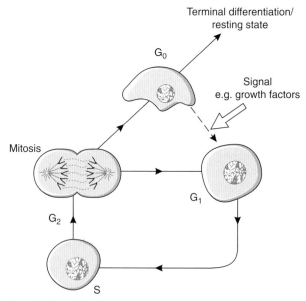

Figure 6 The cell cycle.

Cyclins

The cyclins are a family of proteins which coordinate the journey of cells through the different phases of the cell cycle. They form complexes with a protein kinase (phosphorylating) enzyme. The cellular concentration and activity of different cyclins varies through the cell cycle.

3.2 Cellular adaptation

Learning objectives

You should:
- define and use the terms atrophy, hypertrophy, hyperplasia and metaplasia
- give examples of these processes.

There are four main adaptive states (Figure 7):

- atrophy: shrinkage of an organ as a result of a decrease in cell size and/or number
- hypertrophy: enlargement of an organ as a result of increased cell size
- hyperplasia: enlargement of an organ through an increase in cell number
- metaplasia: change in tissue type as a result of replacement of one differentiated cell type by another.

These adaptations remain under the control of the complex web of genetic and environmental factors that control normal growth and development. In general, they are potentially reversible. Thus they differ from neoplasia, which is an irreversible process in which normal responses to control of growth and differentiation are lost.

Atrophy

Atrophy is a reduction in the mass of cells leading to a reduction in size of the tissue or organ. Two mechanisms can be involved: a reduction in the number of cells through apoptosis, and a reduction in the size of the cells.

Atrophy occurs in physiological circumstances, i.e. during normal growth and development, generally due to loss of endocrine stimulation. For example, the fall in circulating oestrogen after the menopause causes shrinkage of the endometrium, breast tissue, mucosal lining of the vagina, etc.

There are many ways in which atrophy occurs pathologically, i.e. as a result of a disease process:

- denervation, e.g. wasting of muscle caused by a lack of nerve stimulation, for example in poliomyelitis
- reduced blood supply, e.g. shrinkage of brain caused by atherosclerosis of carotid arteries
- inadequate nutrition, e.g. wasting of muscles and major organs in starvation
- decreased workload (disuse), e.g. wasting of muscles and bone (osteoporosis) after immobilisation of a limb in a plaster cast
- pressure, e.g. due to an adjacent tumour or cyst
- loss of endocrine stimulation, e.g. infarction of the pituitary gland results in atrophy of the tissues dependent on pituitary hormones, including the thyroid gland and adrenal gland.

Cell structural components are reduced in atrophy. There are:

- fewer mitochondria
- reduction in the amount of endoplasmic reticulum
- fewer cytoplasmic filaments.

The metabolic rate is reduced in atrophy. There is:

- less amino acid uptake
- less oxygen consumption
- less protein synthesis.

In atrophy, there is an increase in the number of autophagic vacuoles (intracellular dustbins) which contain fragments of intracellular debris such as organelles awaiting destruction. Lysosomes fuse with these vacuoles and discharge their digestive enzymes, which digest the material in the vacuole. Proteins destined for degradation are conjugated with the protein ubiquitin, which marks the protein for destruction in a specialised proteolytic organelle, called a proteasome.

Lipofuscin granules are yellow/brown in colour and represent non-digestible fragments of lipids and phospholipids combined with protein within autophagic vacuoles. They are commonly seen in ageing cells, particularly in the liver and myocardium.

Hypertrophy and hyperplasia

An organ or tissue can enlarge due to an increase in the number of constituent cells or to an increase in the size of

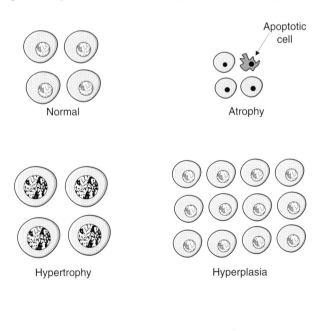

Figure 7 The four main types of cell adaptation.

the cells. The term hypertrophy is used to describe an increase in mass due to an increase in cell size, whereas hyperplasia is an increase in mass due to an increase in cell number. In practice, hypertrophy and hyperplasia commonly occur together. However, hyperplasia requires that the cells be capable of division. Therefore, it can only occur in labile and stable cell populations. Permanent cell populations can only enlarge by hypertrophy. Both hypertrophy and hyperplasia are reversible processes. If the cause is removed, the tissue can return towards normal.

Bodybuilders and athletes provide a good example of hypertrophy: muscle hypertrophy in response to increased workload. Individual cells increase in size as a result of an increase in their structural components, leading to an overall increase in the mass of the organ.

In general, hypertrophy and hyperplasia are due to increased mechanical demand or to stimulation by hormones and/or growth factors. In the case of muscle cells, both types of signal promote hypertrophy, i.e. mechanical stress on the tissue, such as increased stretch, and the release of growth factors due to increased blood flow. As a result, the expression of genes is altered, causing protein synthesis to increase and protein degradation to decrease. Some of the changes shown by hypertrophic muscle cells include increased synthesis of membrane components and myofilaments, increased ATP synthesis and increased enzyme activity. In the skeletal muscles, athletic training will have these effects. In the heart, increased workload due to increased cardiac output or increased resistance to outflow causes hypertrophy. However, there is a limit beyond which the muscle cannot enlarge any further; the limiting factors for maximum muscle size are poorly understood but seem to involve the nutrient and blood supply available for oxidative phosphorylation.

The term compensatory hypertrophy or compensatory hyperplasia is used when tissue is lost through disease or surgical resection and the remaining tissue enlarges. An example is seen in the heart if part of the muscle is lost through myocardial infarction. The undamaged muscle cells become hypertrophic to compensate, at least partially, for the loss of muscle in the infarcted area. The term compensatory hyperplasia is analogous; it refers to hyperplasia in the remaining tissue after some of the tissue is lost. It is seen when the liver regenerates after partial hepatectomy.

Hypertrophy and hyperplasia can be physiological (normal) or pathological (abnormal).

Physiological

- Skeletal muscle hypertrophy in the bodybuilder or athlete.
- Hypertrophy and hyperplasia of myometrial smooth muscle causing enlargement of the pregnant uterus.
- Hypertrophy and hyperplasia of the breasts during lactation.
- Compensatory hypertrophy and hyperplasia of the remaining kidney after the other kidney is removed.

Pathological

- Cardiac muscle hypertrophy as a result of working against an increased peripheral resistance in hypertension (high blood pressure).
- Bladder smooth muscle hypertrophy and hyperplasia caused by increased resistance to outflow (e.g. due to an enlarged prostate gland).
- Hyperplasia of the adrenal gland due to excess secretion of adrenocorticotrophic hormone (ACTH) by a pituitary neoplasm.
- Hyperplasia of the gastric epithelium in response to chemical irritation.
- Hyperplasia of the prostate gland due to an abnormal response to androgens.

Although both hyperplastic and neoplastic tissues show an increase in cell numbers, it is important to distinguish these conditions from each other (see Ch. 10). Unlike neoplastic cells, hyperplastic cells respond normally to the regulatory factors that control cell growth, and hyperplasia is a potentially reversible process. Nevertheless, some types of pathological hyperplasia predispose to the development of neoplasia.

Endoplasmic reticulum

Hypertrophy of smooth endoplasmic reticulum, i.e. hypertrophy at the subcellular level, can also occur. Drugs such as phenobarbital cause an increase in the activity of the mixed function oxidase system of liver cells, which results in increased metabolism of other agents. In some instances, this is therapeutically beneficial, in others it can lead to poisoning of the liver cells by toxic metabolites.

Metaplasia

Metaplasia is the term used when one differentiated tissue is replaced by another. It is a potentially reversible change, in that if the cause of the metaplasia is removed the tissue may revert to normal. It is generally seen in epithelia, usually as a response to chronic physical or chemical irritation.

Metaplasia is a response to a change in the environment of the tissue, and is typically an adaptive response that produces a tissue more able to withstand an adverse environment. A common type of metaplasia is the replacement of glandular or transitional epithelium by stratified squamous epithelium, which is often better able to withstand mechanical or chemical irritation. For example:

- bronchial (pseudo-stratified ciliated columnar) epithelium changes to squamous epithelium in smokers
- transitional bladder epithelium changes to squamous epithelium in people with bladder stones and infection.

Sometimes stratified squamous epithelium changes into glandular epithelium. This occurs in the lower oesophagus in patients with gastro-oesophageal reflux. The reflux of the acidic gastric contents into the oesophagus injures the oesophageal squamous epithelium, which changes into a mucus-secreting glandular epithelium; the mucus protects the oesophageal lining from the acidic gastric juice.

Metaplasia occurs at the level of the stem cell, which produces daughter cells that differentiate into the new type of epithelium. The differentiation of tissues depends on a complex network of interactions between the cell and cytokines, growth factors, hormones, the surrounding matrix, and adjacent cells. Like hyperplastic cells, metaplastic cells respond normally to these various stimuli. However, some types of metaplasia predispose to the development of neoplasia. Thus, squamous cell carcinoma can arise in metaplastic squamous epithelium in the airways, and adenocarcinoma can arise in metaplastic glandular epithelium in the lower oesophagus.

Three

Self-assessment: questions

One best answer questions

1. Which of the following components of the cell cycle constitute interphase?
   a. G0, G1, G2
   b. G0, S, G2
   c. G0, G1, M
   d. G1, S, M
   e. G1, S, G2

2. Which of the following is *not* a typical characteristic of stem cells?
   a. can divide indefinitely
   b. found in labile and stable tissues
   c. permanently in G0 phase
   d. respond to factors regulating cell growth
   e. show telomerase activity

3. A researcher is using liver cells in tissue culture to investigate intracellular digestion. By blocking the action of substance X, she finds that proteins destined for destruction are not digested but simply accumulate in the cell. However, other cell functions continue as normal. What is the most likely identity of substance X?
   a. ATP
   b. cyclin
   c. lipofuscin
   d. potassium
   e. ubiquitin

4. Which of the following is most likely to produce atrophy?
   a. excess intake of food
   b. increased blood flow through the tissue
   c. increased functional demand
   d. loss of innervation through nerve damage
   e. reduced pressure on the tissue

True-false questions

1. The following are correctly paired:
   a. hepatocytes – permanent cells
   b. adult neuronal loss – neuronal regeneration
   c. cell cycle – stem cells
   d. renal epithelial cells – stable cells
   e. hyperplasia – permanent cells

2. The following statements are correct:
   a. atrophy involves oncosis of cells
   b. smokers' bronchial epithelium is usually atrophic
   c. growth factors may inhibit cell growth or division
   d. metaplasia inevitably leads to neoplasia
   e. the lactating breast shows epithelial hyperplasia

3. A 58-year-old woman has abnormal vaginal bleeding due to endometrial hyperplasia. Which of the following statements is/are true?
   a. the hyperplasia will persist indefinitely after the cause is removed
   b. a likely cause is increased oestrogen production by an ovarian tumour
   c. an ultrasound examination is likely to show the endometrium is thinner than normal
   d. there is an increased risk of endometrial neoplasia
   e. histological examination of the endometrium will show an increase in the number of cells

Extended matching items questions (EMIs)

EMI 1

Theme: Responses to cell injury

A. atrophy
B. hyperplasia
C. hypertrophy
D. metaplasia
E. neoplasia
F. repair

For each of the following scenarios, which of the above pathological processes is principally responsible?

1. An ophthalmologist examines the eye of a patient with vitamin A deficiency and finds the conjunctiva to be lined by keratinising squamous epithelium.

2. A patient with stenosis of the aortic valve dies. At autopsy, the heart is found to weigh 50% more than normal.

3. As a result of infarction of the pituitary gland, a patient has an abnormally low level of ACTH. An ultrasound examination of the adrenal glands shows they are both smaller than normal.

4. A man aged 70 years has urinary outflow obstruction, and part of the prostate gland is surgically resected and submitted for histopathological examination. The pathologist finds that the prostate cells are of normal size but increased in number.

Case history questions

Case history 1

A 4-year-old boy is treated for leukaemia (uncontrolled, neoplastic proliferation of bone marrow white cells) with cytotoxic drugs which block the cell cycle and destroy the leukaemic cells. Unfortunately, these drugs also affect the normally rapidly dividing cells of the body.

1. Which of the three cell types in the body (labile, stable or permanent) are most likely to be affected by the treatment?

2. What symptoms and signs may the cytotoxic drugs cause in this patient?

3. Why are these drugs that block the cell cycle usually given in episodic doses (pulses) with a drug-free interval between treatments?

Case history 2

A 79-year-old woman falls over at home, injuring her left hip. She is taken to hospital, and on clinical examination and X-rays she is found to have fractured the neck of her left femur. Her bones appear less dense than normal on the X-ray and the radiologist suspects osteoporosis. She is otherwise reasonably fit and well for her age. Therefore she is operated on and the fracture fixed with internal screws and a plate. After the operation, she makes good recovery but is rather slow to mobilise. She requires extensive physiotherapy but eventually she can go home, walking with the aid of a stick.

1. What are the main risk factors for osteoporosis?

2. Why is it important for the patient to become mobile as quickly as possible postoperatively?

Self-assessment: answers

One best answer

1. e. Interphase is the period between mitoses in the cell cycle. It is the variability in the length of time of G1 which is mainly responsible for the difference in cell cycle time. The time taken for mitosis (0.5–1 hour) is fairly constant in most stem cells.

2. c. Stem cells go round the cell cycle repeatedly; a cell permanently in G0 (arrest) phase does not divide. All the other statements are true.

3. e. Ubiquitin binds to proteins destined for proteolysis in proteasomes. Failure of this function would specifically prevent the cell from recognising proteins destined for destruction. The other responses are incorrect. Inhibition of ATP would have a global effect on cell metabolism, not just proteolysis; the cyclins control passage through the cell cycle; lipofuscin is the non-digestible remains of lipids and phospholipids combined with protein; and potassium is an electrolyte.

4. d. Denervation is a cause of atrophy. Note that increased blood flow and increased functional demand are likely to produce hypertrophy and/or hyperplasia. A reduction in food intake will produce atrophy of fat and other body components.

True-false answers

1. a. **False.** Hepatocytes are a stable cell population. They can enter the cell cycle and divide in order to replace lost cell numbers.

   b. **False.** Neurones are permanent cells (terminally differentiated) which do not enter the cell cycle. Lost neurones cannot be replaced by new ones in the adult central nervous system.

   c. **True.** Stem cells go round the cell cycle indefinitely. At each division, one of the daughter cells can differentiate. The line of differentiation is controlled by interactions with cytokines, growth factors, hormones, the surrounding matrix and adjacent cells.

   d. **True.** The renal tubular epithelial cells are good examples of stable cells. This is clinically relevant in acute renal failure due to renal tubular damage, because regeneration of the renal tubular cells will allow renal function to return to normal.

   e. **False.** Permanent cells such as neurones and cardiac muscle cells do not divide. Hyperplasia can therefore only occur in labile or stable cell populations.

2. a. **False.** Atrophy may involve death by apoptosis (individual programmed cell death) but oncosis does not occur (see Ch. 4).

   b. **False.** Smoking leads to squamous metaplasia of the glandular bronchial epithelium. Metaplasia is the process where a differentiated epithelium is replaced by another differentiated cell type.

   c. **True.** Although many growth factors are mitogenic, i.e. they stimulate cells to divide, others inhibit cell growth. Some growth factors can either promote or inhibit growth, depending on the presence of other factors involved in regulating growth and differentiation. It is the balance between the various types of growth factor that contributes to the stability of a cell population.

   d. **False.** Metaplasia is a reversible adaptive response. Removal of the adverse stimulus will result in restitution of the normal tissue. In some cases, a persistent stimulus will lead to neoplastic change. In cigarette smokers, the metaplastic squamous bronchial epithelium becomes increasingly abnormal and eventually squamous cell carcinoma develops.

   e. **True.** In pregnancy, there is a massive hormonal stimulus to the breast epithelium, which leads to physiological hyperplasia and milk production. When hormone levels return to normal, lactation ceases and the epithelium returns to normal. Hyperplasia is a reversible process. After completion of lactation, the superfluous cells will be removed by apoptosis.

3. a. **False.** Hyperplasia is potentially reversible.

   b. **True.** Excess oestrogen stimulation is the usual cause of endometrial hyperplasia. Ovarian tumours are a possible source of abnormal oestrogen secretion, and they are particularly likely to be responsible in post-menopausal women.

   c. **False.** Hyperplasia causes an increase in mass of the tissue. An ultrasound of the uterus is likely to show a thickened endometrium, and this can be a useful diagnostic test.

   d. **True.** There is an increased risk of endometrial adenocarcinoma.

   e. **True.** This is the definition of hyperplasia.

EMI answers

EMI 1

Theme: Responses to cell injury

1. D. This is an example of metaplasia. The normal mucus-secreting epithelium of the conjunctiva has been replaced by another type of epithelium.

2. C. The mass of the heart has increased as a response to the increased workload required to force the blood through the narrowed aortic valve. Cardiac muscle is a permanent tissue for practical purposes, and so the increase in mass in solely due to enlargement of the cells, i.e. hypertrophy.

3. A. The loss of hormonal stimulation has caused atrophy of the adrenal glands.

4. B. The definition of hyperplasia is an increase in the mass of the tissue due to an increase in cell number.

Case history answers

Case history 1

1. The labile cells are most likely to be affected by the treatment. Cytotoxic agents are used in the treatment of some cancers. They act by blocking the cell cycle at various points, preventing cell division. It is not usually possible to target the drugs specifically at the cancer cells, and normal populations of labile cells, such as in the bone marrow, gut epithelium and skin, will also be killed.

2. This example of a child with acute leukaemia shows how knowledge of the cell cycle and understanding of cell turnover and proliferation is fundamental to clinical medicine. The effects of cytotoxic drugs are entirely predictable. Normal labile cells, as well as tumour cells, will be destroyed by the cytotoxic drugs. The child will lose his hair (labile hair root cells) and may have gastrointestinal upsets as a result of destruction of gut epithelium. Loss of bone marrow stem cells may lead to anaemia (insufficient red cells), bleeding tendency (insufficient platelets) and infection (insufficient white cells).

3. Cytotoxic drugs are often given in 'pulses' with drug-free intervals. The drug-free period between treatments allows some restoration of normal, labile cell numbers, particularly normal bone marrow stem cells. If cytotoxic drugs were given without a break the normal stem cells could be wiped out before the tumour cells were destroyed.

Case history 2

1. *Comment*: Osteoporosis is an extremely common and important condition in which there is reduction of total bone mass, i.e. bone atrophy, which causes weakening. It is most common in elderly women and predisposes to fractures. Osteoporosis may be localised to a single bone, e.g. after immobilisation in a plaster cast, or affect many bones in a generalised way. It is the latter form which is seen in the elderly. Post-menopausal women are especially at risk. In its advanced stages, osteoporosis may be seen on X-rays as pallor or thinning of the bones. The pathogenesis of the disease is not completely understood.

   The main risk factors and associated conditions are:

   - increasing age
   - lack of oestrogen (post-menopausal women)
   - immobilisation either after fracture or paralysis
   - corticosteroid therapy, where increased bone resorption probably occurs.

2. It is important for this woman to become mobile as quickly as possible postoperatively to prevent further worsening of the osteoporotic process through disuse atrophy, which might lead to further fractures. The patient needs to develop muscle tone in her legs to prevent disuse atrophy of the muscles from immobilisation and the development of venous stasis and deep vein thrombosis. In addition, there are important social reasons for her to regain mobility and return home to an independent life.

Cell injury

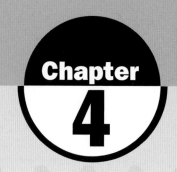

Chapter

4

Chapter overview

Cell injury may be reversible (sublethal) or irreversible (lethal). Reversible injury may require cellular adaptation but the cell survives. Irreversible injury leads to death of the cell. When cell death occurs in the living body, the term necrosis is used. At the cellular level, there are many processes that can lead to necrosis. In most cases, the process can be classified as one or other of two main mechanisms: apoptosis and oncosis. In contrast, autolysis is used to imply cell death that has not occurred in a living body.

4.1 Processes involved in cell injury

Learning objectives

You should:
- list the main causes of cell injury and give examples
- distinguish reversible from irreversible cell injury
- discuss the principal mechanisms of cell injury
- describe how the consequences of injury depend on cell-related factors and on cause-related factors.

Causes of cell injury

The causes of both reversible and irreversible cell injury are similar. Many of those listed below may result initially in reversible injury, from which the cell can recover if allowed time to repair itself. However, if the injury is of sufficient severity, the cell reaches a 'point of no return' and irreversible injury culminating in cell death will occur.

Possible causes of cell injury include:

- hypoxia (lack of oxygen), e.g. myocardial ischaemia (reduced blood flow to, and therefore oxygenation of, the heart) as a result of narrowing of the coronary arteries

- immunological mechanisms, e.g. thyroid damage caused by autoantibodies (antibodies produced by the body against its own tissues)
- infection by microorganisms, e.g. bacterial, viral, fungal infections (such as tuberculous infection of the lung or damage to respiratory mucosa by influenza virus)
- genetic abnormalities, e.g. Duchenne's muscular dystrophy or sickle cell disease
- physical agents, e.g. radiation (such as sunburn due to UV light damage to the skin), trauma, heat, cold
- chemicals, e.g. damage to liver cells by alcohol.

Mechanisms of cell injury

The structure and metabolic functions of the cell are interdependent. Therefore, although an injurious agent may target a particular aspect of cell structure or function, this will rapidly lead to wide-ranging secondary effects. Recognised mechanisms of cell injury include:

- cell membrane damage
  - *complement-mediated lysis via the membrane attack complex (MAC)*
  - *bacterial toxins*
  - *free radicals*
- mitochondrial damage leading to inadequate aerobic respiration
  - *hypoxia*
  - *cyanide poisoning*
- ribosomal damage leading to altered protein synthesis
  - *alcohol in liver cells*
  - *antibiotics in bacterial cells*
- nuclear damage
  - *viruses*
  - *radiation*
  - *free radicals.*

Free radicals and cell membrane damage

Free radicals are highly reactive atoms or molecules which have an unpaired electron in an outer orbit. They can be produced in cells by a variety of processes, including normal metabolic oxidation reactions and drug metabolism. Radiation and many organic poisons induce free radicals. Most clinically important free radicals are derived from oxygen, e.g. superoxide and hydroxyl ions. Free radicals can injure cells by generating chain reactions, producing further free radicals, which cause cell membrane damage by cross-linking of proteins and by critical alterations of lipids.

Ion transporter function and intracellular calcium

A large proportion of a cell's energy consumption is used by the ion transporter mechanisms ('membrane pumps'). Failure of adenosine triphosphate (ATP) synthesis, usually because of hypoxia, can result in failure of these mechanisms. Consequently, there is a rise in intracellular calcium and sodium ions and a reduction in intracellular potassium ions. If the endoplasmic reticulum is damaged, sequestered calcium is released, resulting in a further increase in intracellular calcium.

Raised intracellular calcium can have a number of effects. It may initiate the caspase cascade (see below) causing apoptosis. It can also activate proteases and phospholipases, causing further damage to cell cytoskeleton and membranes and thus contribute to necrosis.

Consequences of cell injury

The consequences of cell injury depend on both the characteristics of the injured cell and the injurious agent.

Cell features

Certain features of cells make them more vulnerable to serious sequelae of cell injury. Specialised cells that are enzyme rich or have special organelles within the cytoplasm may be more vulnerable. The presence of specialised proteins within a cell may make it prone to certain types of injurious agent.

Cell state

Cells that have an inadequate supply of oxygen, hormones or growth factors or lack of essential nutrients may be more prone to injury.

Regenerative ability

The potential of a cell population to enter the cell cycle and divide is important in the response of tissues to injury. Damaged areas in tissues made of cells which can divide may be restored to normal, while populations of permanent cells will be incapable of regeneration.

Injury features

In addition, the character of the injury will also affect the severity of the damage.

Type of injury

The injury may be ischaemic, toxic, traumatic, etc. Some cells will be more susceptible to particular injurious agents than others. For example, hypoxia has a greater effect on heart muscle cells than connective tissue cells.

Intensity

The greater the intensity, the greater the probability of damage. For example, a bone can withstand a bending force up to a certain level, but if the force exceeds the strength of the bone then the bone will break. Likewise, a cell may survive partial hypoxia but not complete lack of oxygen (anoxia).

Exposure time

The length of time of exposure to a toxin or reduced oxygen concentration will affect the chance of a cell surviving the insult. Even relatively resistant cells will be damaged if the duration of exposure is prolonged.

Reversible cell injury

Within limits, cells can accommodate derangements in their metabolism through compensatory mechanisms. However, they may show morphological changes. Under the light microscope, cellular swelling and fatty change are associated with reversible cell injury. Cellular swelling, also known as ballooning or hydropic degeneration, is due to osmotic swelling of cells as they accumulate an excess of small molecules and ions in their cytoplasm. Fatty change is seen when the injured cell cannot process lipids normally and results in the accumulation of fat globules in the cytoplasm (discussed further in Ch. 13).

The ultrastructural changes associated with reversible cell injury can be seen under the electron microscope and include:

* distortion of microvilli and blebbing of the plasma membrane
* cytoplasmic vacuolation
* swelling of mitochondria and endoplasmic reticulum
* clumping of nuclear chromatin.

Irreversible cell injury

Irreversible injury implies that the cell cannot survive and will die by one of the mechanisms discussed in the next section. If the damage is not too severe, death is likely to occur by apoptosis via the intrinsic pathway, but more severe damage causes death by oncosis.

When does reversible injury become irreversible? The exact 'point of no return' is difficult to identify, although massive caspase activation and loss of mitochondrial transmembrane potential are among those that have been proposed. Irreversible injury is associated with an influx of calcium and the release of calcium sequestered in endoplasmic reticulum, which activates enzymes that further degrade the constituents of the cell.

The morphological changes of irreversible cell injury take time to develop. It may be 8–12 hours before the appearance of abnormalities that are recognisable at the light microscopic or macroscopic level.

4.2 Cell death

Learning objectives

You should:
* use the terms autolysis, apoptosis, oncosis and necrosis
* describe the features distinguishing oncosis from apoptosis and give examples of these processes
* describe the characteristics of the five major types of necrosis.

Autolysis implies death of cells that does not occur in the living body. When cell death does occur in the living body, the term necrosis is used. Although there are many pathways to cell death at the cellular level, they tend to fall into one of two main types: apoptosis and oncosis. The term infarct is used for a zone of necrosis caused by lack of oxygen due to insufficient blood flow.

Autolysis

The term 'autolysis' has been used in different ways, but pathologists use it to describe the changes that occur in cells after death of an organism or after surgical removal. When an organism dies, the cells are degraded by the post-mortem release of digestive enzymes from lysosomes as the cell membranes break down. A similar process occurs when tissue is removed from the organism. Cells and tissues showing these changes are autolytic. Prompt preservation of tissues in a fixative such as formalin prevents autolysis after surgical removal.

Apoptosis

Apoptosis is also known as programmed cell death. It can occur in normal tissues, for example as a means of regulating the number of cells in a tissue or organ, and during embryological development. It is also seen in pathological processes. In pathological circumstances, apoptosis follows irreversible cell injury that is not sufficiently severe to damage cell membranes. If cell membrane damage does occur, death is likely to be by oncosis (see next section).

Examples of physiological apoptosis

- Embryogenesis: e.g. formation of digits from the limb buds.
- Menstrual cycle: endometrial cell loss during menstruation.
- Breastfeeding: reversal of changes in the lactating breast once breastfeeding is finished.
- Immune cell development: deletion of lymphocytes that may react with the body's own tissues.

Examples of pathological apoptosis

- Any of the injurious agents that can cause necrosis will cause apoptosis if the injury is insufficient to cause cell death by oncosis. For example, severe loss of oxygen in the heart muscle causes oncosis, but lesser degrees of hypoxia cause death by apoptosis.
- Viral illness: infected cells can die through apoptosis, e.g. in viral hepatitis, histological sections of the liver show apoptosis of hepatocytes.
- Acquired immune deficiency syndrome (AIDS): loss of lymphocytes occurs by apoptosis.

In addition, in neoplasms the balance between apoptosis and cell proliferation is disturbed, so that cell proliferation exceeds apoptosis. Thus, in a sense tumours suffer from a lack of apoptosis.

Apoptosis is triggered through one of two main pathways, both of which activate the caspases, a cascade of proteolytic enzymes responsible for the processes of apoptosis. The first is the intrinsic (mitochondrial) pathway, in which pro-apoptotic molecules are released from mitochondria into the cytoplasm. The second is the extrinsic (death receptor) pathway, in which transmembrane receptors bind to their ligand and thereby initiate cell signalling mechanisms. An example of the extrinsic pathway is seen in cells killed by cytotoxic T cells. The T cells express Fas ligand on their cell membranes; when this ligand binds to the Fas receptor on a cell it initiates apoptosis.

The cell signalling pathways and enzyme-induced events involved in apoptosis are complex, but the caspases are central to the execution phase of the process. As seen in other enzyme cascade reactions, such as the complement system (see Ch. 5), this process serves to amplify the initial apoptotic signal. Some caspases activate other enzymes, while others have a direct effect on the structure of the cell by breaking down components of the cytoskeleton. Endonucleases break down DNA into regular fragments at internucleosomal sites, and phospholipases change the configuration of cell membranes.

Morphologically, apoptotic cells shrink and the nucleus condenses. The organelles and nucleus break up, and then the cell breaks into fragments called apoptotic bodies. These express ligands on their surface membranes that are recognised by other cells, which bind to the apoptotic bodies and engulf them by phagocytosis. It is not just macrophages and neutrophils that can phagocytose apoptotic bodies – cells of many different types are able to do so (Figure 8).

In contrast with oncosis, the cell membrane pumps remain viable and continue to function until the terminal stages of the process. Apoptosis does not provoke an inflammatory response.

The control of apoptosis is crucial in the process of neoplasia. Some genes involved in cancer formation (e.g. the bcl-2 oncogene) switch off apoptosis, thus allowing the neoplastic cells to live indefinitely.

Oncosis

Oncosis is a term that has been introduced relatively recently to describe the passive cell death of necrosis. It derives its name from the characteristic cellular swelling that differentiates the process morphologically from apoptosis, in which cells tend to shrink. It is a useful term that distinguishes between the concept of passive death and programmed (i.e. apoptotic) death at the cellular level. Unfortunately, the word is rather similar to 'oncogenesis' and 'oncotic', both of which mean completely different things (see Glossary).

Oncosis is characterised by cellular swelling and the breakdown of the cell membrane. It is always pathological. In oncosis, death occurs of a large number of cells in one area, as opposed to the selective cell death of apoptosis (Figure 9). These changes occur because of digestion and denaturation of cellular proteins, largely by release of hydrolytic enzymes from damaged lysosomes. The appearance of necrotic tissue depends in part on the balance between digestion and denaturation.

The principal differences between apoptosis and oncosis are summarised in Table 4. In many pathological circumstances, both processes are involved. For example, in myocardial infarction the damage at the centre of the infarct is

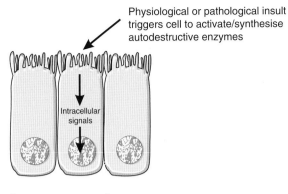

Physiological or pathological insult triggers cell to activate/synthesise autodestructive enzymes

Intracellular signals

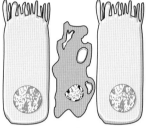

Triggered enzymes may cause changes in cell morphology

DNA cleavage
Cell shrinkage
Cell detachment

Surface signal

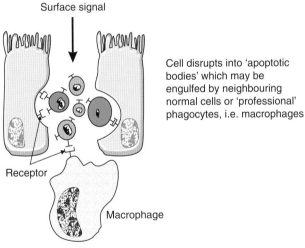

Cell disrupts into 'apoptotic bodies' which may be engulfed by neighbouring normal cells or 'professional' phagocytes, i.e. macrophages

Receptor

Macrophage

Figure 8 Apoptosis.

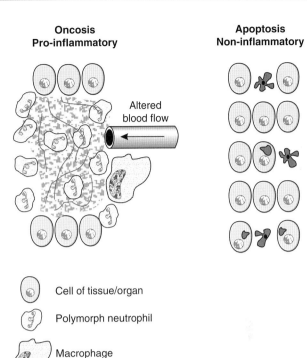

Oncosis
Pro-inflammatory

Altered blood flow

Apoptosis
Non-inflammatory

Cell of tissue/organ

Polymorph neutrophil

Macrophage

Apoptotic cell

Figure 9 Comparison of oncosis and apoptosis.

Table 4 Apoptosis versus oncosis

Apoptosis	Oncosis
Membrane integrity preserved	Membranes breached
No inflammation	Inflammatory response
Single cells	Contiguous cells
Active process; requires protein synthesis and consumes ATP	Passive process

mainly due to oncosis, but at the periphery (where the hypoxia is less severe) apoptosis is usually more important.

Necrosis

The term necrosis has been used in different ways. Originally, it simply meant the death of tissue in the living organism, but when apoptosis was first described, 'necrosis' was reserved for passive (non-apoptotic) cell death. However, macroscopic lesions produced by cell death, such as infarcts, are due to a combination of both passive and programmed cell death. Therefore, the term 'oncosis' was introduced recently for passive cell death, so that 'necrosis' can again be used for the structural changes associated with cell death in general, particularly at the level of tissues and organs. However, you will still encounter 'necrosis' being used specifically for oncosis in some places.

The consequences of necrosis include:

- cessation of function of a tissue or organ
- release of cellular components through damaged cell membranes; these can sometimes be detected in the blood and used as markers of the extent or timing of damage to a particular organ, e.g. cardiac enzymes and troponins after myocardial infarction
- initiation of the inflammatory response by areas of oncosis.

Types of necrosis

There are five main types of necrosis (Figure 10):

- coagulative
- caseous

Four

33

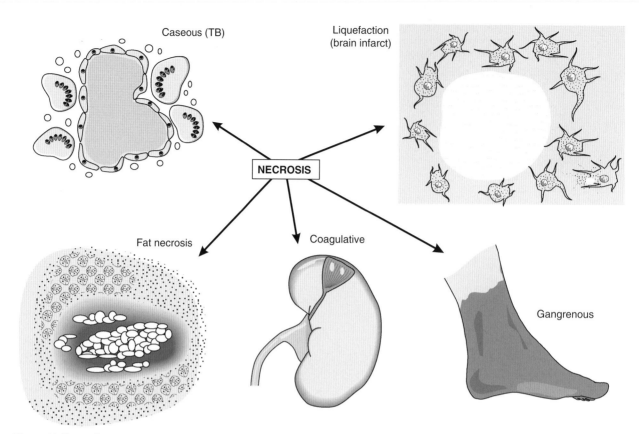

Figure 10 Types of necrosis.

- liquefaction
- fat
- gangrenous.

Coagulative necrosis

Denaturation of intracellular protein (analogous to boiling the white of an egg) leads to the pale firm nature of the tissues affected. The cells show the microscopic features of cell death but the general architecture of the tissue and cell ghosts remain discernible for a while. Coagulative necrosis is the commonest type of necrosis, typically seen in, for example, the kidney and heart.

Caseous necrosis

This cell death is characteristic of tuberculosis (TB) and is seen only rarely otherwise. The creamy white appearance of the dead tissue resembles cheese and is probably a result of the accumulation of the partly digested waxy lipid cell wall components of the tuberculous organisms. The tissue architecture is completely destroyed.

Liquefaction (colliquative) necrosis

This is characterised by tissue softening with destruction of architecture. The result is an accumulation of semi-fluid tissue. It is usually seen in the brain and spinal cord.

Fat necrosis

The necrosis of fat is distinctive because it is characterised by the presence of large numbers of foamy macrophages. They form when the dead adipocytes rupture and release fat, which is taken up by macrophages. The oily material in the macrophage cytoplasm gives the histological appearance of foam. The macrophages commonly form multinucleate giant cells (see Ch. 9). Sometimes, the liberated fat combines with calcium to produce soapy material in a process called saponification. Fat necrosis is encountered in the female breast as a result of trauma, or in the adipose tissue surrounding the pancreas in pancreatitis due to enzymes release from the diseased pancreas.

Gangrenous necrosis (gangrene)

This life-threatening condition occurs when coagulative necrosis of tissues is associated with superadded infection by putrefactive bacteria. Bacteria grow readily in necrotic tissue, so if tissues that have a resident bacterial population such as the intestine become necrotic, gangrene is likely to follow. Some bacteria are able to colonise living tissues and cause gangrene that way; an example is the contamination of a limb wound by *Clostridium* spp. derived from the soil. Gangrenous tissue is foul smelling and black. The bacteria produce toxins which destroy collagen and enable the infection to spread rapidly; it can reach the bloodstream and cause systemic infection and multi-organ failure. If fermentation occurs, gas gangrene ensues, characterised by the collection of gas within the gangrenous tissue.

Sometimes, the word gangrene is used to describe the necrotic death of part of a limb when there is little or no infection. In this case, the term 'dry gangrene' is used and the process resembles mummification.

Self-assessment: questions

One best answer questions

1. A patient presents with symptoms of a stroke. A computed tomography (CT) scan shows a cerebral infarction. Ten days after the onset of symptoms, the patient dies and an autopsy is performed. What is the pathologist most likely to observe in the brain?
   a. caseous necrosis
   b. fatty change
   c. fibrosis
   d. liquefactive necrosis
   e. normal appearances

2. A lymphocyte induces apoptosis in a cell infected with a virus. Which of the following is likely to occur *first* in this process?
   a. binding of Fas to Fas ligand
   b. cleavage of DNA by endonucleases
   c. initiation of the caspase cascade
   d. phagocytosis of apoptotic bodies
   e. widespread destruction of cell membranes

3. In which one of the following organs 1 week after an infarct is a pathologist most likely to observe complete loss of tissue architecture histologically?
   a. brain
   b. kidney
   c. liver
   d. lung
   e. spleen

True-false questions

1. The following statements are correct:
   a. caseous necrosis is characteristically caused by ischaemia
   b. carbon tetrachloride causes cell injury through free radicals
   c. ion pumps often fail in hypoxic cells
   d. the lung is a common site for gangrenous necrosis
   e. testicular torsion can cause venous infarction

2. Apoptotic cells:
   a. exclude vital dyes that enter cells across damaged plasma membranes
   b. provoke an acute inflammatory reaction
   c. may be phagocytosed by neighbouring cells
   d. contain enzymatically degraded nuclear fragments
   e. may occur in conjunction with oncosis

Case history questions

Case history 1

A 59-year-old man, a heavy smoker for much of his adult life, was brought into casualty at 4 am with a 3-hour history of crushing, band-like chest pain. He was seen immediately but died while being examined. His medical history included diet-controlled (type 2) diabetes mellitus, hypertension and intermittent claudication. He had had several attacks of chest pain in the 5 years before his death. A post-mortem examination was performed.

1. What is the likely cause of death?
2. At post mortem, the pathologist found no morphological evidence of acute myocardial infarction. Why was this?
3. What changes might have been present in the heart muscle and coronary arteries?
4. How do the medical and social history relate to this terminal event?

Essay question

1. Discuss the different types of necrosis that can be observed macroscopically. How does necrosis differ from autolysis?

Viva questions

1. Define infarction. How long does it take before morphological changes of infarction can be observed by a pathologist?
2. What are free radicals? How do they cause cell injury?

Self-assessment: answers

One best answer

1. d. The type of necrosis typically observed in the brain is liquefactive (colliquative). The changes would be well developed after 10 days. Fatty change is a sign of reversible injury, not infarction. Fibrosis does not generally occur in central nervous tissue (see Ch. 27).

2. a. The sequence of events is a, c, b, d. Widespread destruction of cell membranes is a feature of oncosis, not apoptosis.

3. a. The kidney, liver, lung and spleen generally undergo coagulative necrosis, unless there are unusual factors such as infection with tuberculosis causing caseation. Coagulative necrosis is characterised by relative preservation of tissue architecture, whereas liquefactive necrosis, which occurs typically in the brain, is characterised by complete loss of tissue architecture.

True-false answers

1. a. **False.** Caseous necrosis characteristically occurs as a response to *Mycobacterium* infection, e.g. TB.
   b. **True.** Carbon tetrachloride poisoning is one of the prototypic examples of free-radical-induced injury.
   c. **True.** This is an important factor contributing to hypoxic cell injury.
   d. **False.** Gangrenous necrosis usually occurs when a tissue/organ that has a resident population of bacteria dies. The organisms can then invade the tissues. The lung is normally sterile, so gangrene does not occur.
   e. **True.** Torsion (twisting) of the testis on its cord leads to obstruction to the venous drainage. The reduction in perfusion leads to infarction, which is markedly haemorrhagic due to the vascular congestion (see Ch. 6). Infarction of the testis can be prevented if the cord can be untwisted in time. Venous infarction can also be seen in the ovary and intestine.

2. a. **True.** One of the essential differences between an oncotic and apoptotic cell is that the latter remains 'alive' until late in the process. Therefore, dyes which enter dead cells across their damaged membranes are excluded by apoptotic cells.
   b. **False.** Apoptotic cells are disposed of by neighbouring cells or macrophages. No acute inflammation occurs; therefore there is no tissue damage.
   c. **True.** See answer (b).

d. **True.** Soon after apoptosis is triggered, nuclear material in the apoptotic cell is chopped up by endonucleases.

e. **True.** The processes of oncosis and apoptosis are not mutually exclusive and usually occur together in necrotic tissue. For example, in infarcts the apoptotic cells are typically found in areas where the hypoxia is less severe around the margins of the infarct. In these zones, the cells retain the ability to initiate apoptotic mechanisms when injury becomes irreversible. In contrast, the more severe hypoxia in the centre of the infarct causes significant cell membrane damage and thus oncosis.

Case history answer

Case history 1

1. The likely cause of death in this man is ischaemic heart disease caused by coronary artery atherosclerosis. The chest pain in this patient is quite characteristic of pain owing to an ischaemic myocardium (heart muscle deprived of blood supply and thus oxygen). Severe atherosclerosis of the coronary arteries would account for this.

2. The macroscopic (naked eye) and microscopic changes that characterise all forms of necrosis take time to develop. There is a significant lag, in this and in any case, between the onset of ischaemia and any changes in the myocardium that can be seen by the naked eye. This is not an unusual scenario at autopsy. A patient who has died instantly from myocardial ischaemia (clinically causing a lethal abnormal heart rhythm such as ventricular fibrillation) because of complete blockage of a coronary artery will have no visible evidence of acute infarction. If, however, the patient had lived for at least 8–12 hours after this event and then died, changes of myocardial necrosis would be seen (see Ch. 14).

3. The history of previous attacks of chest pain suggest past ischaemic events and the pathologist may find fibrosis (scarring) of the myocardium (cardiac muscle cells are permanent cells and regeneration cannot occur). The patient suffered from hypertension (high blood pressure); therefore hypertrophy of the myocardium is also likely. The normal heart weighs about 250–350 g, but in severe hypertension the weight can double as a consequence of hypertrophy of the left ventricular myocardium. Myocardium that has become pathologically hypertrophic in this way is more susceptible to ischaemia than a normal heart. The

coronary arteries will be atherosclerotic (see answers 2 and 4).

4. The pathological process that led to this man's death was atherosclerosis and he had several important risk factors for this, namely smoking, hypertension and type 2 diabetes mellitus. The fact that he had intermittent claudication (cramping pains in the calves, usually caused by exertion-induced muscle ischaemia and, therefore, lack of oxygen because of atherosclerotic limb arteries) emphasises the widespread nature of this process.

Essay answer

Comment: It is always worth starting with a brief definition of the matter in hand, i.e. necrosis is the death of cells within the living body. It would be appropriate to indicate that apoptosis and oncosis can contribute to necrotic lesions. However, the question does not ask for a description of cellular mechanisms, so details of oncosis and apoptosis at the cellular level would attract no marks. Likewise, a general discussion of irreversible cell injury would be a waste of time.

Then describe the five main types of necrosis, each under its own heading, describing the macroscopic (naked eye) appearances and giving examples of the causes:

- coagulative: denaturation of intracellular protein; commonest type of necrosis; wide range of causes, including ischaemia, physical causes and chemicals; typically there is preservation of cell outlines

- caseous: tissue architecture destroyed with a characteristic vital reaction around, typically including multinucleate giant cells; cell outlines are not apparent; prototype is infection with mycobacteria (although other conditions such as histoplasmosis can also cause caseation)

- liquefactive: accumulation of semi-fluid tissue typical of necrosis in the central nervous system; loss of cell outlines

- fat: adipocytes rupture releasing fats that are broken down; the oily material is ingested by macrophages to give a foreign body giant cell reaction or combine with calcium; can result from direct trauma, e.g. in the breast, or from pancreatic diseases, e.g. acute pancreatitis

- gangrenous: infection of necrotic tissue by putrefactive bacteria; characteristic smell and colour; toxins destroy collagen; fermentation produces gases; systemic infection can follow.

Diagrams to show you know what the different lesions look like would be appropriate.

Finally, autolysis is the death of cells and tissues after death or removal from the body. It differs from necrosis because there is no inflammation associated with it (inflammation requires a blood supply).

Viva answers

1. Infarction is the death of tissue within the living body due to ischaemia (lack of oxygen supply). It takes several hours before changes occur that can be recognised as irreversible cell injury either with the naked eye or the light microscope. In general, the tissue appears normal for about 8–12 hours.

2. Free radicals are highly reactive atoms or molecules which have an unpaired election. They can injure cells by generating a chain reaction of free radical production which causes cell membrane damage by cross-linking of proteins and alterations to membrane lipids.

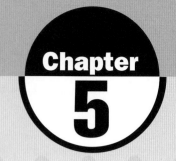

Cascades, haemostasis and shock

Chapter 5

Chapter overview

Cascade systems occur frequently in the body. They allow a rapid response to a stimulus because the inactive precursor molecules are already present. In addition, each step allows amplification of the response. The role of the caspase cascade in apoptosis has been discussed in Chapter 4; the complement and clotting cascades will be discussed in this chapter. Malfunction in any part of a cascade can lead to disease.

Shock is a complex series of changes which occur after severe and sudden diminution in the blood volume or cardiac output. The common feature of all causes of shock is insufficient circulating volume.

5.1 Principles of cascade systems

Learning objective

You should:
- describe the principles of cascade systems.

Enzyme cascades are involved in many processes in the body and are seen in immune, inflammatory and vascular events. They share the common underlying mechanism of cascade action in which the product of one reaction catalyses the subsequent reaction. For example, the blood plasma contains the components of four interlinked cascade systems that are involved in clotting and inflammation (see Table 5). Plasmin, a product of the fibrinolytic cascade, degrades the product of the clotting cascade and activates complement. Hageman factor, or factor XII, is a clotting factor which activates the complement, kinase and fibrinolytic systems (Figure 11). The caspase cascade has already been mentioned in Chapter 4.

At each step of the cascade, an inactive precursor is activated. Thus, the biologically inert components of the

cascade can be present in the body ready to be activated, in contrast with systems where the component molecules have to be synthesised by cells when they are required for action. Therefore, cascades allow a rapid response to a stimulus. Also, one activated enzyme can catalyse the activation of a large number of its substrate molecules, so amplification of the response occurs at each step. Furthermore, the activated components can have more than one action, allowing for a large number of possible final effects. In this way, a few molecules of an initiating substance can have huge consequences, as when activation of a small amount of caspase 8 by Fas ligand binding starts a series of reactions that kill the cell (see Ch. 4).

Another characteristic of cascades is that each step of the process can be promoted or inhibited by other factors, allowing for tight control of the cascade. Typically, the active constituents have a short half life and are rapidly broken down or inactivated, so the cascade can be rapidly 'switched off' if required.

In summary, the advantages of cascade systems are:

- amplification of the original stimulus
- rapid reaction
- a variety of different actions resulting from one initial stimulus
- modulation and control by a wide range of other factors.

5.2 The complement cascade

Learning objectives

You should:
- discuss the three pathways by which the complement cascade is triggered
- describe the role of complement in host defence.

Complement is a system of soluble molecules that forms an important part of the body's defence system against microbial infection. It is a cascade system and interacts with other components of the immune system (see Ch. 7).

Complement is activated via three pathways: the mannose-binding lectin (MBL, also known as mannan-

Table 5 The plasma cascade systems

	Activator(s)	Important end product(s)	Main functions
Kinin system	Exposed collagen activates factor XII	Bradykinin	Vasodilatation/hypotension, increased vascular permeability, stimulates pain receptors
Complement system	Antigen–antibody complexes (classical pathway); microbial endotoxin (alternative and MBL pathways)	C3a/C5a	Chemotaxis, increased vascular permeability, releases histamine from mast cells
		Membrane attack complex (C5–C9)	Cell lysis
		C3b	Opsonisation
Clotting system	Exposed collagen activates factor XII (intrinsic pathway); thromboplastin from damaged tissues activates factor VII (extrinsic pathway)	Thrombin	Production of fibrin clot, pro-inflammatory actions on leucocytes and other cells
Fibrinolytic system	Plasminogen activator from endothelium; activated factor XII	Plasmin	Lysis of fibrin clots by cleaving fibrin to form fibrin degradation products (FDPs), activation of complement cascade

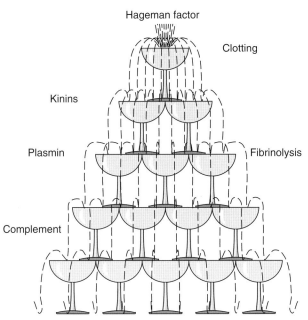

Hageman factor
Clotting
Kinins
Plasmin
Fibrinolysis
Complement

Figure 11 Cascades: illustrating the principles of activation and amplification.

Box 4 Complement cascade

Classical pathway
- Triggered by antigen–antibody complexes involving IgG or IgM

Alternative pathway
- Activated without IgG or IgM being present, e.g.:
  - bacterial endotoxin (surface lipopolysaccharide of Gram-negative bacteria)
  - snake venom
  - aggregated IgA

Complement assists in defence in three ways:

- **Triggering acute inflammation**: C3a, C5a, the anaphylatoxins, cause histamine-mediated vasodilatation and blood vessel leakage as well as acting as potent chemotaxins for neutrophils and monocytes
- **Helping phagocytosis** by coating foreign substances, e.g. bacterial cell walls, with protein (opsonisation)
- **Direct killing** of certain organisms: the membrane attack complex can kill some bacteria, e.g. *Neisseria* spp.

binding lectin), classical and alternative pathways. The MBL and alternative pathways are triggered by microbial substances and do not require the participation of B cells or T cells. Therefore, these pathways represent part of innate immunity (see Ch. 7). The classical pathway is triggered by antigen–antibody binding. Figure 12 shows the main steps of the classical and alternative pathways leading to the formation of the membrane attack complex. The MBL pathway activates C4. Products of the fibrinolytic and kinin systems can also activate complement.

There are many functional consequences of complement activation (Box 4, Figure 12). Formation of the membrane attack complex is the final common pathway of the different limbs of the cascade; it makes a pore in the membrane of the target cell that leads to cell lysis. The anaphylatoxins are fragments of activated complement components that have cytokine-like effects, activating inflammatory cells and acting as chemoattractants for them. They can also degranulate mast cells. Fragments that remain attached to the target, such as C3b, promote phagocytosis, i.e. they are opsonins.

Complement activation can lead to extensive tissue damage and plays an important part in hypersensitivity reactions (see Ch. 8).

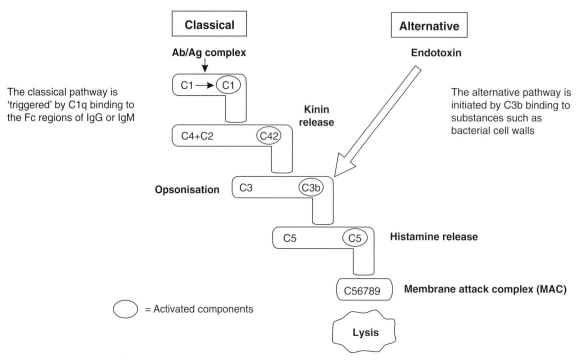

The classical pathway is 'triggered' by C1q binding to the Fc regions of IgG or IgM

The alternative pathway is initiated by C3b binding to substances such as bacterial cell walls

Figure 12 Complement cascade. Ab/Ag, antibody–antigen complex; complement components have C numbers, e.g. C1.

5.3 Haemostasis

Learning objectives

You should:
- give an account of how the blood vessel wall, platelets and the clotting cascade contribute to haemostasis
- distinguish the intrinsic from the extrinsic pathway
- state the role of the fibrinolytic pathway
- discuss the pathophysiology of disseminated intravascular coagulation.

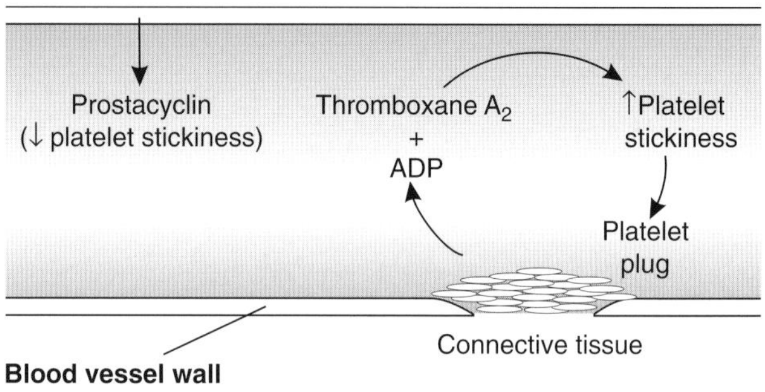

Prostacyclin (↓ platelet stickiness)

Thromboxane A_2 + ADP

↑Platelet stickiness

Platelet plug

Connective tissue

Blood vessel wall

Figure 13 The platelet plug.

Blood clotting

The blood vessel wall, platelets and the clotting cascade are the three major components of normal blood clotting (haemostasis). A clot that forms in the vascular spaces during life is called a thrombus.

Blood vessel wall

Normal continuous endothelium inhibits intravascular clotting by preventing blood platelets and clotting factors from coming into contact with the collagen of the vessel wall. Endothelial cells also produce substances such as prostaglandins (PGI_2), nitric oxide and plasminogen activator which inhibit platelet aggregation and promote fibrinolysis. When the endothelium is damaged and collagen is exposed to the blood, thrombogenic tissue factors will trigger the clotting cascade, and platelets will adhere to the exposed collagen. The aggregated platelets and strands of fibrin, together with entrapped blood cells, form a thrombus.

Platelets

Platelets have a central role in clotting and form the initial plug at an area of endothelial damage. To do this they have to adhere to collagen exposed at the site of injury and then release stored products from granules rich in adenosine diphosphate (ADP), platelet-derived growth factor (PDGF), serotonin, calcium and fibrinogen, which trigger further platelet aggregation and the clotting cascade. Thromboxane A_2 (TXA_2), synthesised and released by activated platelets, plays a key role in platelet aggregation (Figure 13). The platelet plug is not a robust structure and fibrin is required to stabilise it.

The clotting (coagulation) cascade

The clotting cascade is triggered by:

- exposure of blood to collagen (intrinsic pathway), activating factor XII; this pathway is also triggered if blood is placed in a glass test tube

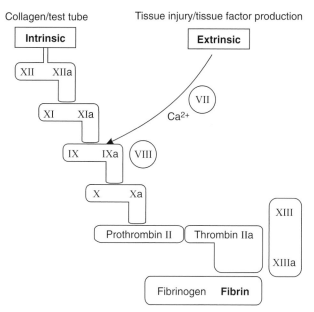

Figure 14 The clotting cascade.

- exposure to factors derived from injured cells (extrinsic pathway), activating factor VII.

In either case, the pathway leads to thrombin formation. Thrombin converts soluble fibrinogen to insoluble fibrin, the protein which ultimately stabilises the clot. The overall process is summarised in Figure 14.

Fibrinolysis

The fibrinolytic system is activated alongside the clotting system and results in the production of plasmin, which degrades fibrin and fibrin clots. Fibrinolysis counteracts and balances the haemostatic mechanisms; without fibrinolysis uncontrolled extension of a clot could occur. One of the 'triggers' involved in the activation of the fibrinolytic system is factor XII. Thus, factor XII initiates fibrinolysis at the same time as it promotes thrombosis. This is an example of the way in which these pathways are tightly interlinked in a complex web of relationships.

Disseminated intravascular coagulation (DIC)

This is an important condition where both clotting and haemorrhage occur together. The patient is usually very ill because of underlying diseases, such as:

- severe overwhelming infection (septicaemia)
- severe trauma or burns
- post-partum haemorrhage (massive bleeding after birth).

In all these conditions, there is activation of the coagulation system, either by the extrinsic or intrinsic pathways. Thus, endothelial cells may be damaged in burns and by immune complexes. Tissue factors may be released by the placenta. This mass activation of the clotting cascade leads to the consumption of vast amounts of platelets and fibrin.

The formation of multiple platelet thrombi occurs in the microvasculature, causing small areas of infarction in many organs.

At the same time the fibrinolytic system is activated and thrombi are rapidly dissolved, producing large amounts of fibrin degradation products (FDPs). Supplies of clotting factors and platelets may become exhausted (consumption coagulopathy) so that a paradoxical situation occurs, where there is disseminated thrombosis with multi-organ infarcts together with uncontrolled haemorrhage. Disseminated intravascular coagulation is a serious life-threatening illness which needs to be managed by treating the underlying cause, such as antibiotics for infection, and by anticoagulants and replacement of clotting factors.

5.4 Shock

Learning objectives

You should:
- define shock
- identify the main types of shock
- describe the main clinical features of shock.

Shock is systemic hypoperfusion due to a reduction in either cardiac output or the effective circulating blood volume. It is associated with hypotension.

In response to the systemic hypoperfusion, the body reacts to preserve an adequate blood supply to essential organs such as the brain. In consequence, the effects of shock are usually manifested in other organs initially. The hypoxia causes reversible cell injury if relatively mild, but severe hypoperfusion will cause irreversible cell injury. Examples include subendocardial necrosis of the heart, acute tubular necrosis of the kidneys, and infarction of the intestine. When widespread tissue damage has occurred, the patient will continue to deteriorate despite therapy; this is irreversible or refractory shock.

Shock can be subdivided into various types depending on the pathogenesis. Hypovolaemic and cardiogenic shock are associated with a reduction in cardiac output. In contrast, the cardiac output in anaphylactic and neurogenic shock may be increased, but there is widespread vascular dilatation so the vessels cannot be adequately filled by the circulating blood volume; the consequence is hypotension and tissue hypoperfusion. In septic shock, there is both widespread vascular dilatation and a reduction in cardiac output.

Hypovolaemic shock

This occurs after severe haemorrhage, e.g. traumatic severing of a major artery, or loss of body fluids such as water from the colon in cholera or from the skin in burns cases. To preserve blood flow to the heart and brain, major vasoconstriction in other organs occurs. This vasoconstriction accounts for the cold, pale skin of patients in hypovolaemic shock.

Cardiogenic shock

This usually occurs secondary to myocardial infarction, rupture of a cardiac valve cusp or arrhythmia, but it can also occur through any cause of 'pump' failure. The responses of the body mimic those of hypovolaemic shock.

Septic (endotoxic) shock

Circulatory failure occurs as the result of major bacterial infection, usually with Gram-negative bacteria such as *Escherichia coli*, *Klebsiella* or *Pseudomonas* spp. These bacteria release endotoxin (bacterial wall lipopolysaccharide), which activates macrophages and neutrophils and initiates the alternative complement pathway. In large amounts, endotoxin causes systemic vasodilatation and reduced myocardial contractility, resulting in shock. In addition, endotoxin has other effects, such as activation of the extrinsic coagulation pathway, which can complicate the clinical picture.

Anaphylactic shock

This occurs as a result of an acute systemic type 1 hypersensitivity reaction in individuals who are sensitised to the relevant antigen, e.g. penicillin or peanut allergy. It is a severe rapid reaction with bronchospasm, laryngeal oedema and hypotension. The hypotension is due to vasodilatation; severe hypotension causes shock.

Neurogenic shock

Damage to the spinal cord can cause loss of vascular tone, causing peripheral vasodilatation and pooling of blood. The blood volume cannot adequately fill the dilated vasculature and shock results.

Clinical features

In general, hypotension and tachycardia (fast heart rate) are common to all varieties of shock. In hypovolaemic and cardiogenic shock, there will also be a weak, thready pulse and cold, clammy skin due to peripheral vasoconstriction. In septic shock, the skin may be warm due to peripheral vasodilatation.

There is retention of salt and water by the kidneys, which acts to increase the circulating blood volume. Oliguria (reduced urine output) is thus a typical feature of shock. Ischaemic damage to the kidneys may reduce urine output further.

Self-assessment: questions

One best answer questions

1. A 22-year-old woman falls from a ladder. The paramedics who attend the scene find she appears to have broken her pelvis but movement and sensation in the lower limbs are normal. Prior to the accident she was well and had no symptoms. However, while performing their initial assessment the paramedics note her blood pressure is falling to dangerously low levels. The most likely cause of the falling blood pressure is:
   a. anaphylactic shock
   b. cardiogenic shock
   c. hypovolaemic shock
   d. septic shock
   e. neurogenic shock

2. A patient with extensive severe burns develops disseminated intravascular coagulation. Blood tests are performed. Which of the following is likely to be abnormally raised?
   a. antithrombin III
   b. blood volume
   c. fibrin degradation products
   d. fibrinogen
   e. platelets

3. Which of the following is insoluble in plasma?
   a. fibrin
   b. fibrinogen
   c. plasmin
   d. prothrombin
   e. thrombin

True-false questions

1. The following statements are true:
   a. factor VIII deficiency (haemophilia A) leads to defective haemostasis
   b. clotting factor VIII requires vitamin K for its synthesis
   c. the intrinsic coagulation pathway is triggered by exposed collagen
   d. platelet aggregation is promoted by thromboxane A_2
   e. activation of the kinin cascade in inflamed tissues is an important cause of pain

2. In the complement cascade:
   a. amplification of the response occurs at each step
   b. C5a causes lysis of cells
   c. C3b is an opsonin
   d. it takes at least 24 hours for the response to occur after the initial stimulus
   e. plasmin can activate complement via the classical pathway

Case history questions

Case history 1

A 59-year-old male lorry driver was involved in a road traffic accident in which he sustained severe injuries to the head and lower limbs. On admission to hospital, he was unconscious and hypotensive (blood pressure 60/30 mmHg). He was cold and clammy and had a pulse rate of 150 per minute.

1. What is the likely cause of shock in this patient?

The patient was transfused with 8 units of blood. Extensive surgery was required for bilateral fractured femurs and ruptured femoral blood vessels, after which his condition stabilised. Over the next few days, he regained consciousness, but it was noticed that he was not passing urine. Blood tests showed that he was in renal failure.

2. Why did the patient develop renal failure?
3. Is renal function likely to recover?

The patient then developed a wound infection and became pyrexial. Gram-negative bacteria were cultured from his blood, and he again became hypotensive, tachycardic and peripherally cyanosed.

4. Did this patient develop septicaemia or bacteraemia?
5. What is the pathogenesis of shock at this stage?

Self-assessment: answers

One best answer

1. c. Blood loss from the fractured pelvis may not be obvious if bleeding is occurring into the abdominal cavity, but this is the most likely cause in this scenario and the patient needs treatment to expand the blood volume urgently. Neurogenic shock is unlikely because the spinal cord appears intact (she has normal sensation and movement in the lower limbs). There are no clues in this vignette that might point towards heart disease, systemic sepsis or an anaphylactic reaction.

2. c. Fibrin degradation products (FDPs) are increased in disseminated intravascular coagulation because they are produced by fibrinolysis from the large amounts of fibrin in the intravascular thrombi. Laboratories often test for a specific type of cross-linked FDP called D-dimer. Fibrinogen and platelets are consumed at a rate faster than they can be produced and their levels are low, hence the tendency to haemorrhage in this condition. Antithrombin III inactivates thrombin and other coagulation factors; it is also consumed in the process and is a useful clinical indicator of disease severity. Blood volume is likely to be depleted because of fluid loss from the burnt skin in this case.

3. a. Fibrin is an insoluble fibrillary protein produced by the clotting cascade during haemostasis. It binds the blood clot and seals blood vessel defects. It is produced from the soluble circulating precursor, fibrinogen.

True-false answers

1. a. **True.** Haemophilia A is an X-linked genetic disorder, which means that it is mainly clinically apparent in males. Female carriers have approximately 50% of the normal levels of factor VIII and may occasionally show mild features of the condition. The lack of factor VIII causes inefficiency of the clotting cascade, and effective haemostasis cannot occur. Haemophilia B is caused by a genetic deficiency of factor IX; it is almost identical clinically to factor VIII deficiency. Individuals with haemophilia have haemorrhages into joints and tissues, often triggered by relatively minor trauma.
   b. **False.** Most of the clotting factors are synthesised in the liver, but only factors II, VII, IX and X are vitamin K dependent. Patients with liver disease commonly have problems with haemostasis as their diseased liver cannot produce adequate amounts of clotting factors.

   c. **True.** The intrinsic pathway is activated by exposed collagen, e.g. from vessel-wall trauma or atherosclerosis. It starts with factor XII and the cascade progresses quickly through to the formation of thrombin and fibrin.
   d. **True.** Thromboxane A_2 is a prostaglandin-like metabolite of arachidonic acid. It enhances platelet aggregation, which is an important step in the process of haemostasis.
   e. **True.** Bradykinin stimulates pain receptors.

2. a. **True.** This is a characteristic of cascades in general.
   b. **False.** It is the membrane attack complex (C5–C9) that causes cell lysis; C5a has other effects.
   c. **True.** When attached to bacteria, C3b promotes phagocytosis by binding to receptors on neutrophils and macrophages. Other opsonins include antibodies, lectins and C-reactive protein.
   d. **False.** The complement cascade can be activated very rapidly; clinical effects may be observed in minutes or hours.
   e. **True.** This is an important link between the clotting and complement systems.

Case history answers

Case history 1

1. This patient is in hypovolaemic shock as a result of massive blood loss from his fractured bones and torn blood vessels.

2. The patient has developed renal failure as a consequence of acute tubular necrosis. In severe shock with hypotension, the renal tubules become ischaemic, die and cease to function, leading to acute renal failure. The glomeruli are less susceptible to ischaemia and, therefore, would not be affected.

3. The epithelial cells of the renal tubules can regenerate from stem cells, provided that the basement membrane and matrix components of the tubules are intact. In clinical practice, as long as the condition is recognised and the patient can be supported with control of fluid, salt and acid–base balance, full recovery can occur.

4. *Comment*: distinction should be made between septicaemia, which is a life-threatening condition in which pathogenic organisms multiply and circulate in the bloodstream, and bacteraemia, in which non-harmful non-proliferating bacteria circulate in the blood but are easily removed by the body's phagocytic cells. Bacteraemia can occur whenever there is potential for bacteria to enter the blood-

stream, e.g. after a visit to the dentist, or after any invasive surgical procedure. In this case, the patient has septicaemia.

5. This patient now has septic shock associated with Gram-negative septicaemia. Endotoxin (bacterial wall lipopolysaccharides) in large amounts can directly trigger the alternative complement pathway and induce the production of excessive amounts of various cytokines by binding to toll-like receptors (see page 57, Pattern-recognition receptors). Consequences include fever, systemic vasodilatation, reduced contractility of the heart, and stimulation of inflammatory cells that release more pro-inflammatory cytokines. If the coagulation cascade is inappropriately triggered, disseminated intravascular coagulation may follow.

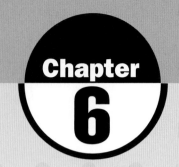

Atherosclerosis and thrombosis

Chapter 6

Chapter overview

Atherosclerosis, a common degenerative disease of arteries characterised by thickening of the intima as a result of deposition of lipids, is a common cause of illness in industrialised countries and is the main pathological process that leads to cardiovascular disease. Infarction can result from atherosclerosis, and also from the intravascular events of thrombosis and embolism.

6.1 Atherosclerosis

Learning objectives

You should:
- recognise risk factors for atherosclerosis
- describe the pathogenesis of atherosclerosis
- list the complications of atherosclerosis and discuss their possible consequences.

Atherosclerosis causes narrowing and/or weakening of arteries, and is the pathological process underlying many common diseases such as myocardial infarction (heart attacks), strokes and aneurysms. It is an acquired, degenerative condition which affects large- and medium-sized arteries, e.g. aorta, carotid and coronary arteries, where it begins in the innermost intimal layer. It is characterised by lipid deposition with consequent inflammation and fibrosis. Atheroma (from the Greek word for porridge that describes the necrotic material in the core of the lesions) is a term which is often used synonymously with atherosclerosis.

Epidemiology and risk factors

Atherosclerosis is common in industrialised countries but less common elsewhere. If individuals from countries with a low incidence migrate to one with a high incidence, their risk of atherosclerosis increases, presumably as a result of adopting a 'Western' lifestyle.

The risk factors for atherosclerosis can be divided into those that are non-modifiable (e.g. age, sex) and those that are modifiable as a result of lifestyle changes or drug therapy. Important risk factors are:

- **Age.** Death rates from the complications of atherosclerosis increase with age.
- **Male sex.** Premenopausal women have a low rate of death from complications of atherosclerosis; the protective factor is thought to be high oestrogen levels. After the menopause, the incidence of complications increases and by old age it equals that of males.
- **Family history.** A family history of atherosclerotic-related disease confers an increased risk. This familial predisposition is probably polygenic in most cases, but in some patients there is a specific inherited abnormality of lipid metabolism causing hyperlipidaemia.
- **Hyperlipidaemia.** The cholesterol in low-density lipoprotein (LDL) is particularly important as a risk factor. The ratio of LDL to high-density lipoprotein (HDL) is also important, since a low LDL/HDL ratio appears to have a protective effect. The mechanism is thought to be related to their functions: LDL delivers lipids to tissues, whereas HDL transports it to the liver for metabolism; therefore, HDL could remove lipids from developing plaques. The LDL/HDL ratio is lowered by exercise, consumption of polyunsaturated fatty acids and moderate amounts of alcohol, whereas it is increased by smoking, obesity and a diet rich in saturated fats. Circulating cholesterol can also be reduced by drugs (the statins).
- **Hypertension.** Reduction of blood pressure in hypertensive patients reduces the risk of strokes and ischaemic heart disease.
- **Cigarette smoking.** Tobacco can be atherogenic through damage to endothelial cells by toxins and through the increase in LDL/HDL ratio.
- **Diabetes mellitus.** This important risk factor could act through hypercholesterolaemia or a direct toxic effect on endothelial cells.

- **Obesity.** The effects of being overweight are related to the increased incidence of hypertension, diabetes and increased LDL/HDL ratio.
- **Physical inactivity.** Lack of exercise promotes obesity and increases LDL/HDL ratios.

Pathogenesis

The earliest visible lesion of atherosclerosis is the fatty streak which results from accumulation of lipid-laden macrophages within the intima and which can be seen in the arteries of children. Fatty streaks are flat, pale yellow spots.

Atheromatous plaques occur later in life and contain macrophages intermingled with proliferating smooth muscle cells, capped by fibrous tissue. Lipid, particularly cholesterol, may be present within both macrophages and smooth muscle cells. Angiogenesis (proliferation of small blood vessels) is stimulated at the periphery of the lesions. A mature fibrolipid plaque is composed of:

- a core of necrotic lipid-rich material
- a chronic inflammatory infiltrate containing lymphocytes, macrophages, smooth muscle cells and myofibroblasts surrounding the core
- a fibrous cap
- small blood vessels entering the periphery of the plaque.

These plaques protrude into the vessel lumen and can cause significant narrowing. The underlying arterial wall is weakened by the chronic inflammation.

The response to injury hypothesis

Several different theories have been proposed to explain the initiation and evolution of atherosclerosis. The current favoured idea is the 'response to injury hypothesis', which brings some of these theories together. Damage to the arterial endothelium leads to increased permeability of the vessel wall and attachment of platelets and monocytes. The increased permeability allows lipid to enter the vessel wall. Meanwhile, the attached platelets and monocytes produce growth factors which stimulate smooth muscle cells of the arterial media to migrate into the intima and proliferate. One of these growth factors is platelet-derived growth factor (PDGF). This is a locally acting polypeptide which binds to cell surface receptors and triggers a chain of events which may enable genes to switch on and produce proteins which promote cell proliferation. Proliferating smooth muscle cells acquire some fibroblast-like characteristics and produce collagens and proteoglycans, which form the fibrotic cap and matrix of the atherosclerotic plaque. The monocytes transform into macrophages within the intima. These macrophages ingest the lipid that has entered the intima through the leaky endothelium (Figure 15). Macrophages with lipid in their cytoplasm have a foamy appearance and are called foam cells. The macrophages oxidise the lipids they have ingested, and these oxidised lipids have a number of effects that seem to be important in the development of the plaque. In particular, oxidised lipids:

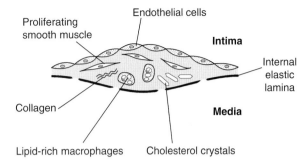

Figure 15 The fibrolipid plaque in atherosclerosis.

- are chemotactic for circulating monocytes
- inhibit motility of macrophages already in the plaque
- stimulate the macrophages to release growth factors and cytokines which attract inflammatory cells into and around the plaque
- upregulate endothelial cell adhesion molecules, thus promoting adherence of inflammatory cells (see Ch. 9)
- are cytotoxic and cause further endothelial damage.

Lipids and atherosclerosis

Low-density lipoproteins (LDL) are rich in cholesterol and raised blood levels of LDL are an important factor in plaque genesis. Both genetic and environmental dietary factors can determine the LDL levels, but the precise mechanism of this relationship with plaque development is not known. Genetic abnormalities can lead to increased blood levels in very young people, who may suffer heart attacks and strokes in their late teens or early twenties. There is a strong epidemiological correlation between cardiovascular disease and high LDL blood levels. In contrast, there is a reduced risk of atherosclerosis with high levels of high-density lipoproteins (HDL).

Fish oils

Populations which have a high dietary intake of fish oil containing omega-3 fatty acids (a special type of polyunsaturated fatty acid) seem to be protected from developing complicated atherosclerosis. Fish oils may have a lipid-lowering effect in the blood, resulting in reduced levels of LDL and raised levels of HDL. Fish oils may also reduce levels of thromboxane A_2, which is metabolised from arachidonic acid in platelets and increases their capacity to aggregate. Reducing thromboxane A_2 levels may reduce the risk of thrombosis.

Complications of atherosclerotic plaques

Atherosclerotic plaques are prone to a number of possible complications, namely:

- ulceration and thrombosis
- haemorrhage
- aneurysm
- calcification.

The reason atherosclerosis is a serious condition is that some of the above listed complications can produce potentially fatal diseases. Since the plaque is intimal and pro-

Six

47

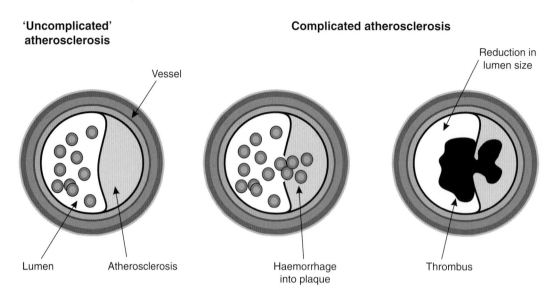

Figure 16 Complications occurring on or in the atherosclerotic plaque.

Box 5 Arterial supply

Some tissues receive blood from several different arteries via a collateral circulation. Obstruction of one of these arteries, whether by embolism, thrombosis, atherosclerosis or other cause, is unlikely to cause critical ischaemia because the blood supply can be maintained from the other arteries. However, in some tissues only one artery supplies any particular area, and obstruction of such a vessel is likely to cause an infarct; these arteries are called **end-arteries**. Organs with end-arteries include the heart and brain.

---

trudes into the lumen of the vessel, haemorrhage or thrombosis can cause narrowing (stenosis) or complete blockage (occlusion) of the artery (Figure 16). If the artery is an end-artery (see Box 5), the tissue supplied by the artery cannot get blood from elsewhere, and it will die, causing infarction. Alternatively, weakening of the wall by the inflammation associated with the atherosclerotic plaque can lead to aneurysm formation.

Ulceration and thrombosis

The atherosclerotic plaque usually bulges into the lumen of the artery. Fast-flowing blood may ulcerate the plaque, exposing the fibrous cap beneath the endothelium or even the necrotic core of the lesion, thus triggering thrombosis. The thrombus may occlude the already narrowed lumen. In an end-artery this may prove lethal; occurring in a coronary artery it could cause myocardial infarction and in a cerebral artery it could cause a stroke. Note that stenosis and occlusion generally do not affect the aorta, because its wide lumen is not significantly narrowed by atherosclerotic events.

Haemorrhage

Blood can be forced into the plaque from the lumen of the vessel or bleeding can occur from the vessels vascularising the base and edges of the plaque. The sudden increase in size of the plaque can cause critical ischaemia in the territory supplied by the artery.

Aneurysm formation

The presence of an intimal plaque leads to atrophy and weakening of the underlying media. The weakened vessel wall may dilate and eventually a large sac is formed. This is called an aneurysm (the definition of aneurysm is a permanent abnormal dilatation of an artery). Aneurysms can rupture, with consequent life-threatening haemorrhage. In addition, they commonly contain thrombus, fragments of which can become dislodged and embolise (see Section 6.3 Embolism).

Calcification

Old atherosclerotic plaques often undergo dystrophic calcification. Hence atherosclerotic arteries can sometimes be seen on radiographs. This complication, unlike the three mentioned previously, does not have lethal effects.

6.2 Thrombosis

Learning objectives

You should:
- define thrombosis
- use Virchow's triad to analyse the mechanism of thrombosis in clinical conditions
- state the possible outcomes of thrombus formation.

Thrombosis is the formation of a blood clot within vascular spaces during life, and the resulting clot is called a thrombus. This is in contrast to the term clotting, which can also be applied after death or to blood in a test tube.

Table 6 Predisposing factors for thrombosis

	Examples
Endothelial damage	Trauma, atherosclerosis, smoking, bacterial toxins
Stasis/turbulence	Postoperative immobility (inactive legs) and blood pooling; post-myocardial infarction (sluggish blood flow around body); turbulence around atherosclerotic plaques or within aneurysms
Increased coagulability	Pregnancy; oral contraceptives; leukaemia; cancer

There are three main predisposing factors for thrombus formation, known as Virchow's triad:

- damage to the endothelial lining of a blood vessel
- changes in blood flow (turbulence or stasis)
- increased coagulability of blood.

These predisposing factors are associated with particular conditions or lifestyles (see Table 6).

How does a thrombus form?

Any of the components of Virchow's triad, alone or in combination, may predispose to the formation of a thrombus. Thrombi build up from the initial platelet plug. The clotting cascade is triggered by endothelial damage and factors released by the aggregation of platelets. As the blood flows past, red cells become trapped in the fibrin mesh which is thus formed. The thrombus grows in layers in the direction of the blood flow, a process known as propagation. To the naked eye, a thrombus is a dark-red mass of blood in which delicate white lines of fibrin called lines of Zahn can be seen. When a pathologist finds clotted blood at autopsy, it is necessary to determine whether the clot occurred during life (i.e. is a thrombus) or after death. If lines of Zahn are present, they show the clot formed in flowing blood and are a useful indicator that the clot is, in fact, a thrombus; other distinguishing features are the granularity of the thrombus and the fact that it may be attached to the vessel wall.

Thrombi can occur in arteries, veins or within the heart chambers (mural thrombus). The outcome of thrombus formation can be:

- propagation leading to complete occlusion of vessel lumen
- removal by fibrinolysis with restoration of normal blood flow
- organisation, i.e. ingrowth of granulation tissue converting the thrombus into a fibrous scar; sometimes this process can recanalise an occlusive thrombus, i.e. capillary channels through the thrombus are produced, allowing some blood to flow through it
- embolism, i.e. carriage of thrombus through the circulation to lodge in a distant vessel.

6.3 Embolism

Learning objectives

You should:
- define embolism and name the common types of emboli
- distinguish between systemic, pulmonary and paradoxical emboli
- discuss the risk factors for pulmonary thrombo-embolism.

An embolus is a mass of material which is carried in the bloodstream and becomes lodged within a blood vessel, thus blocking it. The material may be a solid, liquid or gas. The effects of an embolus follow from the obstruction of blood flow to the tissues and depend on the precise site at which this occurs and whether or not there is an alternative tissue blood supply (see Box 5). Emboli travel through the circulatory system and obstruct the vessel lumen when the diameter prevents further passage. Table 7 gives the sources and types and of embolism; by far the most common in general clinical practice is thrombo-embolism.

Pulmonary embolism

Pulmonary emboli arise in the systemic veins or the right side of the heart and lodge in the pulmonary circulation. The vast majority arise from a thrombus in the deep leg or pelvic veins, i.e. a deep venous thrombosis (DVT). Small thrombo-emboli may go unnoticed and dissolve by fibrinolysis, whereas a large embolus which lodges in a main pulmonary artery may cause sudden death. Other emboli may cause severe respiratory and cardiac symptoms, relating to either infarction of the lung or right-sided heart strain.

Risk factors for DVT can be understood in terms of Virchow's triad.

- Change in blood flow, i.e. poor flow through the veins, as seen in:
  - *immobile or bedridden patients*
  - *heart failure.*
- Damage to endothelium, i.e. inflammation of the vein wall due to:
  - *trauma or surgery*
  - *vascular stasis.*
- Hypercoagulability of the blood, due to:
  - *release of pro-coagulant factors following trauma or surgery*
  - *inherited hypercoagulability (e.g. deficiency in antithrombin III, protein C or protein S)*
  - *increased oestrogen (pregnancy, contraceptive pill)*
  - *polycythaemia*
  - *cancer.*

DVT and consequent pulmonary thrombo-embolism are feared complications of major surgery, since postoperatively patients exhibit many of these predisposing factors. All postoperative patients should receive prophylaxis to reduce the risk of DVT.

Six

Table 7 Types of emboli and their sources

Type	Source
Thrombus (thrombo-embolus)	Commonly arise in deep veins of leg/pelvis (deep venous thrombosis, DVT), or in the heart (mural thrombus, e.g. over a myocardial infarct or within a fibrillating atrium)
Atherosclerotic plaque debris (cholesterol or atheromatous embolus)	Exposure of the necrotic core in an ulcerated plaque can release debris that embolises to distant sites downstream
Vegetations	Cardiac vegetations can embolise to lungs (right heart valves) or systemic circulation (left heart valves). In infective endocarditis, the bacteria-laden emboli can cause infection where they lodge, e.g. brain abscess
Amniotic fluid	Uterus at delivery: embolism to lungs via torn uterine veins
Nitrogen	Inadequate decompression in deep-sea divers: nitrogen bubbles can cause problems in joints, lungs, brain and spinal cord, bones, skin and elsewhere
Air	Typically introduced into the large veins of the neck or chest through trauma or surgery
Fat	Occurs after serious trauma, especially bone fractures and widespread burns. Although fragments of fatty marrow can embolise from fractured bones, most cases of fat embolism are due to coalescence of serum lipid into globules. Organs affected by emboli include lungs, central nervous system and skin
Foreign body	Occasionally, foreign bodies introduced into vessels can embolise, e.g. catheter tips

Systemic embolism

Systemic emboli arise in the left side of the heart or in the arterial system and lodge in the systemic circulation. For example, multiple small embolic showers of atherosclerotic debris from the carotid arteries may lead to temporary loss of blood flow to parts of the brain (transient ischaemic attack). A large piece of mural thrombus detaching from a myocardial infarction could lead to gut, splenic or renal ischaemia by blocking the appropriate artery. Aortic aneurysms can be a source of systemic thrombo-emboli.

Paradoxical embolism

On rare occasions, an embolus can pass between the left and right sides of the circulation through an atrial or ventricular septal defect or through a patent ductus arteriosus. In these circumstances, a systemic embolism can result from material originating in the systemic veins. This is called paradoxical embolism.

6.4 Infarction

Learning objectives

You should:
- define infarction
- discuss the pathogenesis of arterial and venous infarction
- interpret the morphological appearances of an infarct.

Infarction is defined as death of tissue caused by ischaemia, i.e. lack of oxygen. It may result from a partial or complete reduction of the blood supply (arterial infarction) or diminished drainage of blood from the tissue (venous infarction). The shape and size of the infarct depends on the territory normally supplied or drained by the occluded blood vessel. The appearance of an infarct

Table 8 Appearances of myocardial infarction

Time after infarct	Naked eye	Light microscope
8 hours	No visible changes	Cytoplasm looks more pink (eosinophilic) than normal
12 hours	No visible changes, or possible slight pallor or redness	Neutrophils start to appear at junction with surrounding viable tissue
24 hours	Pallor or redness	Features of coagulative necrosis, i.e. loss of nuclei and cross-striations
48 hours	Pallor or redness with a yellow rim, representing neutrophilic infiltrate	Macrophages start to ingest necrotic myocytes; increasing numbers of neutrophils
3–10 days	Brown, soft; yellow or red rim representing granulation tissue	Granulation tissue forms around the infarct
2–6 weeks	Brown, soft, with fibrosis developing at periphery	Granulation tissue grows into the infarct, organising it into a fibrous scar
After 6–8 weeks	Mature fibrous scar	Mature fibrous scar

varies, depending on how long the process has been going on, and on the nature of the tissue affected. The majority of infarcts are arterial in nature and are caused by thrombosis or embolism.

Most arterial infarcts are red because blood leaks into the damaged tissue from surrounding vessels; some infarcts are pale because of absence of leakage of blood. Examples of arterial infarction include coronary artery thrombosis leading to myocardial infarction, pulmonary embolism from a DVT causing pulmonary infarction, and clamping of an artery during surgery.

Obstruction of venous outflow causes intensely congested (haemorrhagic) infarcts. It occurs as a result of:

- twisting of an organ or other structure on its pedicle (e.g. torsion of testis, volvulus of sigmoid colon)
- constriction of an organ or structure by the neck of a hernia (e.g. entrapment of a loop of bowel in an inguinal or femoral hernia sac)
- compression of a vein by a tumour mass.

The appearances of an infarct change with time. The macroscopic (visible to the naked eye) and microscopic features of the resulting necrosis take time to develop. The morphological changes in a myocardial infarct are given in Table 8.

Self-assessment: questions

One best answer questions

1. A 75-year-old woman trips in her garden and is admitted to hospital with a fractured neck of femur. Hip replacement surgery is performed. Seven days after surgery she experiences haemoptysis and breathlessness. Which of the following events is most likely to have led to these symptoms?

   a. air embolism
   b. aortic aneurysm
   c. deep venous thrombosis
   d. fat embolism
   e. infective endocarditis

2. A pathologist performing an autopsy finds clotted blood in the pulmonary artery. Which one of the following features of the clot is likely to indicate that it formed during life rather than after death?

   a. 'chicken fat' appearance
   b. lines of Zahn
   c. presence of fibrin in the clot
   d. presence of platelets in the clot
   e. 'redcurrant jelly' appearance

3. Which of the following is most likely to form a significant component of an atheromatous plaque?

   a. adipocytes
   b. chondrocytes
   c. germ cells
   d. mesothelial cells
   e. smooth muscle cells

4. Which one of the following lesions is the precursor of atherosclerosis?

   a. aneurysm
   b. fatty streak
   c. squamous metaplasia
   d. thrombo-embolus
   e. vegetation

5. A 70-year-old man collapses suddenly while walking his dog. In hospital, a diagnosis of stroke is made. Radiological investigations reveal a brain infarct. He also has an abdominal aortic aneurysm. Which of the following pathological processes is most likely to be the cause of the stroke?

   a. calcification of the wall of the basilar artery
   b. deep venous thrombosis
   c. nitrogen bubbles in cerebral vessels
   d. thrombo-embolism from the abdominal aortic aneurysm
   e. ulcerated atherosclerotic plaque of the left carotid artery

True-false questions

1. The following statements are true:

   a. mural thrombus in the left ventricle may embolise to the brain
   b. dietary cholesterol levels are the most important determinant of plasma cholesterol levels
   c. vascular endothelium produces prothrombin
   d. atherosclerosis only occurs in large arteries with turbulent blood flow
   e. thrombus commonly develops on atherosclerotic plaques

2. The following are correctly paired:

   a. raised plasma high-density lipoprotein (HDL) – atherosclerosis
   b. atherosclerosis – aneurysm formation
   c. abdominal aortic aneurysm – leg ischaemia
   d. myocardial infarction – ventricular mural thrombus
   e. foamy macrophages – oxidised LDL

Case history questions

Case history 1

A 35-year-old woman gave birth to healthy twin babies. She went home after 5 days but was readmitted to hospital 2 days later complaining of feeling breathless with pleuritic chest pain (a sharp stabbing pain in the side of her chest which was worse on breathing in). Her left leg was slightly swollen and she was tender over the calf. Investigations showed that she had a small infarct in the left lower lung lobe. She was treated with the antifibrinolytic agent streptokinase and the anticoagulant heparin and made a good recovery. On discharge she was prescribed a course of warfarin.

1. What has caused the infarct in her lung (i.e. what is the diagnosis)?
2. State three ways in which pregnancy could have contributed to the development of this condition.
3. Describe the rationale for treatment with streptokinase, heparin and warfarin.

Case history 2

A 68-year-old man presented to his doctor with a painful, black big toe. This was gangrenous on examination and he was admitted to hospital urgently for treatment and surgical amputation. He made a good recovery and was well for a year. He then started to develop pain in the lower back which came and went but was not severe enough for him to go to his doctor. On one occasion, however, he experienced excruciating pain in the lower right back and rapidly became shocked and collapsed with a pulse rate of 120 per minute and a systolic blood pressure of 60 mmHg. He was rushed to hospital but died in the ambulance.

A post mortem was performed at which a large abdominal aneurysm was found which had ruptured. There were 3 L of fresh blood clot in the retroperitoneum, tracking up behind the right kidney. The aorta showed severe atherosclerosis elsewhere.

1. How might you connect the episode of gangrene in the toe with the autopsy findings in this man?

2. List four modifiable risk factors for atherosclerosis.

3. State three complications of aortic aneurysm.

Essay question

1. What is an infarct? Discuss the different pathological processes within vessels that can cause an infarct.

Self-assessment: answers

One best answer

1. c. This patient has a pulmonary infarct due to pulmonary thrombo-embolism resulting from a DVT. Postoperatively, patients have hypercoagulable blood; if they are also immobile and/or have suffered damage to veins of their leg or pelvis they are at great risk of DVT. Air embolism is only likely if trauma involves the neck or chest. Fat embolism typically follows severe trauma or extensive burns, not a simple fracture, and it affects many organs rather than just the lungs. There are no clues pointing towards infective endocarditis or aortic aneurysm in this vignette; in any case they would cause systemic emboli.

2. b. Lines of Zahn are produced in flowing blood. In contrast, post-mortem clots often resemble either redcurrant jelly or chicken fat, and pathologists sometimes use these terms descriptively. Both post-mortem and ante-mortem clots would be expected to contain platelets and fibrin.

3. e. Smooth muscle cells proliferate in the lesion. They take part in production of matrix materials like collagen and mucopolysaccharides. They may also acquire phagocytic properties and, along with macrophages, ingest lipid.

4. b. The fatty streak is the earliest visible lesion in the evolution of atherosclerosis.

5. e. Ulceration of a plaque in a carotid artery could cause thrombosis with consequent occlusion of the artery or thrombo-embolism to a cerebral vessel. Alternatively, the exposed necrotic core might produce cholesterol emboli. Either way, there would be occlusion of an end-artery supplying brain tissue. Calcification of arterial walls can complicate atherosclerosis or occur as an ageing phenomenon, but does not cause clinical problems. Deep venous thrombosis would be expected to cause pulmonary embolism (except for the very rare phenomenon of paradoxical embolism). Nitrogen bubbles occur in decompression sickness. Embolism of thrombus in aortic aneurysms is not uncommon, but the emboli would pass downstream, e.g. into the mesenteric or iliac arteries, but not the cerebral circulation.

True-false answers

1. a. **True.** Mural thrombus in the left ventricle may develop after myocardial infarction. If pieces break off and embolise then they can end up anywhere in the systemic circulation. The brain is a common site for this and an embolus travelling through the carotid arteries and then into a cerebral artery will cause ischaemic infarction of the brain (stroke). Cardiac mural thrombus can also embolise and cause infarcts in, for example, the spleen, gut or kidney.

    b. **False.** Although there is a relationship between high blood cholesterol levels and a high risk of coronary heart disease in Western countries and this is associated with diets which are high in saturated fat, dietary cholesterol consumption has only a modest influence on plasma cholesterol levels.

    c. **False.** Prothrombin is produced by the liver and is the inactive precursor of thrombin, the protein which causes fibrin to be formed and hence coagulation to occur. Vascular endothelium does produce plasminogen, which tends to counteract any tendency to coagulate.

    d. **False.** Atherosclerosis can occur in arteries of large or medium calibre. The presence of turbulent blood flow, smoking and high circulating LDL levels will all predispose to atherosclerosis.

    e. **True.** Superimposed thrombus is an important complication of atherosclerosis. It develops as a result of activation of the clotting cascade when plaque contents or blood vessel collagen are exposed to the blood. Platelet aggregation also occurs and triggers clotting. The resulting thrombus may propagate and cause occlusion of the vessel, for example in a coronary artery causing coronary thrombosis and myocardial infarction. Alternatively, the thrombus may break off and embolise to a distant vessel and cause occlusion there.

2. a. **False.** In fact, the opposite is true. HDL is involved in the transport of cholesterol from peripheral tissues to the liver. There is strong epidemiological evidence that high levels of HDL-cholesterol are associated with a reduced risk of heart disease and coronary artery atherosclerosis. High levels of LDLs are associated with heart disease.

    b. **True.** The atherosclerotic plaque is a proliferative and destructive lesion. The arterial wall becomes progressively less elastic and weaker as atherosclerosis progresses. Aneurysms commonly form as a result of this weakening. The most common site is the distal abdominal aorta.

    c. **True.** As the aneurysm enlarges because of the weakening of the aortic wall, there will be stasis of blood flow and thrombus forming in layers, gradually filling the sac. This thrombus may cause occlusion of blood flow to the legs via the iliac arteries or bits may break off and embolise to leg arteries, causing ischaemia of the foot.

d. **True.** Thrombi commonly form over the surface of a myocardial infarction where the blood flow is abnormal and the wall of the heart is inflamed. A thrombus may propagate and build up within the ventricle.

e. **True.** Macrophages in atherosclerotic plaques ingest lipid derived from circulating LDL and become foam cells. The lipid is oxidised principally by reactive oxygen species produced by the macrophages.

Case history answers

Case history 1

1. The diagnosis is pulmonary thrombo-embolism. The leg swelling and tenderness are features of DVT, the source of the embolism in this case. A thrombus has detached itself and embolised to a branch of the pulmonary artery. The segment of infarcted lung has become necrotic and haemorrhagic. The pleural surface of the lung will be involved and give rise to the sharp pain that the patient experiences. Sometimes patients with pulmonary embolus and infarction develop haemoptysis (coughing up of blood) from the bleeding into the dead lung segment. Because the lung has a dual blood supply from the pulmonary and bronchial arterial trees, infarction of the lung does not always occur with pulmonary embolism, and is more likely if the circulation is otherwise compromised, e.g. heart failure.

2. Three ways in which pregnancy could have contributed to the development of this condition are:

   - Pregnancy, especially with twins, may have led to stasis of blood in the pelvic veins.

   - Pregnancy is associated with an increase in the tendency of the blood to clot.

   - Immobility is another possible cause, since the patient spent 5 days in hospital just before the event.

3. Streptokinase is a fibrinolytic drug which dissolves the thrombo-embolus and restores blood flow to the infarcted area of tissue. Heparin and warfarin are anticoagulant drugs that prevent new thrombus

forming. Heparin is quick acting and inhibits factors IX and X. It is given subcutaneously or intravenously. Warfarin is taken orally and takes about 24 hours to work. It inhibits the synthesis of vitamin-K-dependent clotting factors (II, VII, IX and X).

Case history 2

1. Occlusion of a digital artery would have caused ischaemic infarction with subsequent infection by anaerobic organisms, leading to gangrene. In this case, it is most likely that atheromatous or thrombotic emboli from the abdominal aortic aneurysm were responsible.

2. Four modifiable risk factors for atherosclerosis are: smoking, lack of exercise, hyperlipidaemia, diabetes mellitus.

3. Atherosclerotic or thrombotic embolism to the lower limbs or abdominal organs. Rupture with massive haemorrhage into the retroperitoneum and peritoneal cavity. Atrophy of the lumbar vertebrae (this is thought to cause the backache experienced by many of these patients and is due to pressure from the expanding aneurysm).

Essay answer

Comment: To answer the first part of the question, define infarct as an area of tissue death due to a reduction in blood supply or venous drainage causing hypoxic cell death. In general, the changes in vessels relate to occlusion of an end-artery or to obstruction of venous drainage. You could discuss each of these under its own heading. Arterial obstruction can be caused by a number of different processes. One way of organising the answer is to divide the causes into changes within the vessel lumen, changes in the wall of the vessel, and changes outside the wall, again using headings: within the lumen you should mention emboli; important lesions of the arterial wall include atherosclerosis, arteritis and spasm; and lesions outside the wall include tumours and cysts. You could give examples of each. Obstruction of venous drainage is typically caused by torsion or by strangulation in a hernia. Make sure you are selective in what you write so you have time to discuss all these factors. It would be easy to get carried away writing about, for example, atherosclerosis, leaving no time to mention anything else. Note that the question does not ask for a discussion of infarcts themselves or the cellular changes that occur in hypoxic tissue, so inclusion of this material would not attract any marks.

The immune system 1

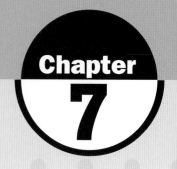

Chapter overview

The study of the immune system, immunology, is one of the most rapidly expanding and important areas of medicine. Immune mechanisms are involved in a wide range of processes, from inflammation to neoplasia. Diseases due to abnormalities of the immune system, e.g. acquired immune deficiency syndrome (AIDS) and autoimmune diseases, are encountered in virtually every branch of medicine.

7.1 Natural defences and immunity

Learning objectives

You should:

* distinguish innate from adaptive immunity
* name the cells important in innate and adaptive immunity and their main properties
* describe the morphological organisation of the immune system
* discuss the principles of specificity, memory, diversity and self-recognition.

The human body is constantly bombarded from the outside world by potentially harmful substances and microorganisms. To protect ourselves against these insults, we have evolved a sophisticated defence system composed of a complex web of cells and chemical mediators that interact to produce an integrated response. The defences can be divided into two main types:

* innate immunity – which has a general protective effect against a wide range of potential insults
* adaptive immunity – which is specific for particular foreign substances and microorganisms.

Together, the two arms of the immune system use a wide variety of different methods to distinguish between the components of the body, or 'self', from foreign invaders, or 'non-self'. Non-self includes unacceptable changes within the body, such as a normal cell becoming neoplastic.

Many different cells take part in host defence; some are involved only in adaptive immune reactions whereas others play a part in innate immunity as well. The characteristics of some of these cells are discussed further in Chapter 9.

Innate immunity

Natural (innate) immunity arose early in evolution. It is conferred by physical barriers and cellular responses that are not specific against any one particular insult, but provide an effective first line of defence. The most important types are give below.

Mechanical barriers

The intact skin and mucosal surfaces provide a physical barrier to microorganisms and foreign substances. Tight junctions between the cells and the continuous basement membrane are important components. The keratinised surface of the skin is particularly tough; only a minority of microorganisms can breach intact skin.

Secretion

The acidity of the gastric and vaginal secretions creates a hostile microenvironment which kills many organisms. Lysozyme, found in tears, has an antibacterial action. Paneth cells in the intestine secrete antibacterial proteins called defensins when stimulated by the presence of bacteria. Activation of the complement cascade by the alternative and mannose-binding lectin (MBL) pathways are also part of innate immunity (see Ch. 5).

Secretion and excretion currents

The flow of urine regularly flushes away any bacteria that ascend the urethra, helping to keep the bladder sterile. Bronchial mucus is constantly swept towards the pharynx, carrying with it any contaminating bacteria; when it reaches the pharynx it is coughed out or swallowed into the acid environment of the stomach. Tears have an analogous effect. Stasis of the normal flow of secretions or excretions is a potent cause of infection.

Commensal bacteria

The normal bacterial flora which colonises the skin, mouth, intestines, etc., inhibits the growth of pathogenic organisms by competing for nutrients and by secretion of toxins. In the vagina, the commensal lactobacilli help keep the pH acidic.

Phagocytes

Although neutrophils and macrophages participate in adaptive immune reactions and their activity is greatly enhanced when stimulated by specific immune responses, they have phagocytic and antimicrobial properties independent of the adaptive immune system. Thus, neutrophils and macrophages also contribute to innate immunity.

Mast cells and eosinophils

Like neutrophils and macrophages, mast cells and eosinophils participate in adaptive immune responses. However, they can also act independently of adaptive immunity. Mast cells (and the closely related basophils) release histamine, cytokines and other substances from their granules when stimulated, promoting inflammation (see Table 13, Ch. 8). Eosinophils secrete a range of substances that are toxic to microorganisms. The actions of mast cells and eosinophils seem to be particularly involved in defence against parasites, but they have other defensive roles and are also involved in allergic reactions.

Natural killer cells

Natural killer (NK) cells are lymphocytes that have the ability to lyse host cells, in particular virally infected cells and neoplastic cells. In this respect, they form part of innate immunity. In addition, NK cells take part in adaptive immunity by their ability to lyse cells opsonised with IgG (antibody-dependent cell-mediated cytotoxicity, see Section 7.4).

Pattern-recognition receptors

These receptors are found on many cells of the immune system and recognise a wide range of molecules found on bacteria, viruses and fungi. They represent a type of host defence found not only in animals but also in bacteria and plants. Binding of a pattern-recognition receptor triggers a response in an effector cell. An important group of pattern-recognition receptors comprises the toll-like receptors. For example, toll-like receptor 1 (TLR1) is expressed on macrophages, dendritic cells and B cells, and recognises a kind of lipopeptide found in bacteria.

Adaptive immunity

Adaptive immunity is specific to the foreign substance which invokes it and becomes quicker and more intense with subsequent exposure to it. Thus the adaptive immune response 'remembers' previous challenges with the same substance and can mount a heightened and more rapid response. Adaptive immunity is only seen in higher vertebrates such as mammals.

Cells of the adaptive immune system

Central to the adaptive immune response are two types of lymphocyte, called B cells and T cells. Both these cell types possess membrane receptors which can bind to foreign material (antigen). This triggers a series of intracellular events in the lymphocyte which leads to its activation, multiplication and enhanced ability to destroy or neutralise the antigen. By definition, adaptive immunity (as opposed to innate immunity) involves the antigen-specific receptors on B cells and T cells.

Both types of lymphocyte are derived from precursor cells in the bone marrow. B cell maturation occurs in the bone marrow itself, whereas T cells migrate to the thymus for maturation. B and T cells have distinct functions, but they are interdependent and rely on cooperation with each other and other cells of the immune system.

B cells

The B cell surface receptor is a type of antibody molecule, namely monomeric IgM. When the appropriate antigen binds to the receptor, the B cell is activated. It multiplies and the offspring ultimately mature into plasma cells, which synthesise and secrete large amounts of antibody into the extracellular fluid; this antibody has the same specificity as the B cell receptor, allowing disposal of the antigen that stimulated it. This process is known as humoral immunity; it is especially important in defence against extracellular bacteria.

T cells

These have a surface antigen recognition system known as the T cell receptor, which is similar to the antibody molecule. There are discrete subsets of T cells which, when triggered by antigen-receptor binding, have functions as diverse as killing cells, coordinating B and T cell responses and stopping the immune response. T cells are particularly involved with the immune response to intracellular organisms (e.g. viruses and certain bacteria such as *Mycobacterium tuberculosis*). This process is known as cellular immunity.

Organisation of the adaptive immune system

In order to optimise the combined functions of surveillance of the body's tissues for antigen and production of a coordinated immune response, the cells of the adaptive immune response are organised into structured lymphoid tissues, namely lymph nodes, thymus, mucosa-associated lymphoid tissue and spleen. Lymphocytes are also found in the bone marrow.

The bone marrow and the thymus are sometimes known as primary lymphoid organs, where lymphocytes are produced and mature (B cells in bone marrow, T cells in thymus), whereas the peripheral lymph nodes and other lymphoid sites are called secondary organs, where lymphocytes live and recognise antigens and initiate the immune response. The spleen is primarily involved in clearing the blood of unwanted antigens, while the lymph nodes are responsible for clearing the lymphatic fluid. The mucosal surfaces represent potential portals of entry for microbes, and the mucosa-associated lymphoid tissue

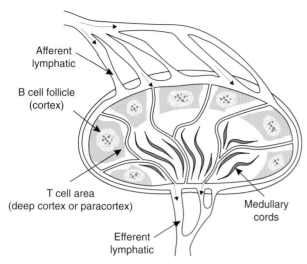

Seven

Figure 17 Structure of a lymph node.

forms an important part of the body's defences. This lymphoid tissue is often concentrated into distinct structures such as the tonsils in the throat, the Peyer patches in the intestine, and the lymphoid tissue of the appendix.

There are similarities in the structure of many of the lymphoid tissues. In general, B cells are found in the discrete nodular structures known as lymphoid follicles. These follicles are surrounded by a sea of T lymphocytes admixed with other cells of the immune response and small blood or lymphatic channels. A lymph node is shown in Figure 17. Lymphocytes can circulate via the lymphatics and bloodstream between the lymphoid organs.

Properties of the immune response
Specificity
The response is specific. Most antigens are foreign macromolecules or microbes that are made up of large numbers of differently shaped structural components (usually proteins or carbohydrates). Some of these components will be recognised by a receptor on the membrane of a restricted number of lymphocytes. Only these few lymphocytes can, therefore, initially respond to the foreign substance. The smallest components recognisable by B cell and T cell receptors are called epitopes or determinants. Some molecules (haptens) are too small to be recognised by themselves, but will be recognised if they are bound to a larger molecule.

Memory
The immune response has memory. Exposure to a previously encountered antigen results in a quicker and larger response. This is, at least in part, through the generation of memory cells during the first challenge with antigen. Memory cells are long-lived cells that have the antigen receptor on their surface and on a subsequent occasion can proliferate quickly to mount a response.

Diversity
The response is diverse. The number of different antigen-specific lymphocytes is vast. We have millions of lymphocytes, each bearing a receptor recognising a slightly different shaped or structured antigenic determinant. When exposed to a particular antigen, e.g. a bacterium, the lymphocyte with the appropriate receptor is selected from this vast available pool and stimulated to multiply. This process is called clonal selection.

The diversity of the system results from the variability in the structure of the lymphocyte surface receptor. The basic structure of the T cell receptor and the immunoglobulin molecule are similar, both being members of the immunoglobulin 'superfamily'. The enormous diversity of B cell and T cell receptors is due to random rearrangement of a small number of genes within the cell allowing the generation of many different receptors. The result is considerable diversity in the variable region of the antibody molecules and T cell receptors. Molecular techniques such as Southern blot analysis (see Ch. 2) have shown that the portions of DNA containing the immunoglobulin gene are of a different size in B cells and cells that do not produce antibody. This can be explained by the genes being far apart in 'ordinary' cells, but close together in B cells. Therefore, B cells must be able to rearrange these genes during their development. This is done in a precise order (e.g. the first rearrangement involves the heavy chains).

Recognition of self
The immune system can distinguish between self and non-self. Thus, under normal circumstances, lymphocytes recognise and respond to molecules that they perceive as foreign but apparently ignore the millions of potential antigens present in normal human tissues and organs. This non-response to our own tissues by our own lymphocytes is known as tolerance and is partly achieved by the early deletion (by apoptosis) of potentially self-reacting cells. If cells reacting with self escape from these control measures, autoimmune disease occurs and our own tissues are damaged and destroyed (see Ch. 8).

7.2 Humoral immunity

Learning objectives
You should:
- describe the humoral immune reaction and the role of antigen-presenting cells
- describe the structure and function of immunoglobulin
- name the classes of immunoglobulin and state their distinguishing properties.

The B cell response

Antibodies are synthesised by B cells; they are then either secreted into the tissue fluids for combination with antigen or are inserted into the B cell membrane to act as receptors. If a human is exposed to an antigen, a number of B cells may each recognise a different epitope of the antigen by means of their surface antibody (immunoglobulin) receptors. The proliferation of different B cells with different antibodies being produced by the resultant plasma cells is called a polyclonal response.

Occasionally, a monoclonal response may occur. The classic example of this is an abnormal proliferation of a single B cell (in effect a cancer of the B cell), resulting in the production of millions of only one type of plasma cell and thus one single type of antibody. This malignant proliferation of plasma cells is known as multiple myeloma.

Antibody structure

The basic structure of an antibody is shown in Figure 18. In its simplest form, an antibody is composed of two identical light chains and two identical heavy chains. The molecular weight is about 150 000. The light chains are joined to the heavy chains and the heavy chains to each other by covalent disulphide bonds. Overall, the antibody molecule has a 'Y' shape, with movement of the arms possible at the hinge. Light chains and heavy chains can be further subdivided into domains, each approximately 110 amino acid residues long. There are four domains per heavy chain and two per light chain. The amino acid sequence in the N-terminal domain of both the light and heavy chains is very variable – the so-called variable region – and it is here that antigen binding occurs. The remaining domains are relatively constant. The different types of immunoglobulin are classified according the Fc region, which is responsible for the actions of the antibody. For example, IgG and IgM opsonise bacteria to which they are bound (because phagocytes have receptors for IgG and IgM Fc regions), and IgE uses its Fc portion to attach to the surface of mast cells and basophils. There are different classes of antibody, which have different functions (Table 9), but they all are based on the simple prototype.

Antibodies have a number of functions. They agglutinate particles by binding them together, and can thus inhibit the movement of motile bacteria. By attaching to molecules they can neutralise the function of those molecules, e.g. microbial cell surface receptors or bacterial toxins. IgG and IgM can activate complement via the classical pathway by interacting with C1. Bound antibody can activate other cells of the immune system such as macrophages, neutrophils and NK cells. In addition, antibodies are opsonins, i.e. when bound to bacteria they facilitate phagocytosis.

Fate of antigen–antibody immune complexes

An antigen–antibody (immune) complex is formed when soluble antigen combines with antibody to form a particle. We are constantly being challenged by antigens, and the formation of small numbers of immune complexes is a normal event. When we mount an antibody response to a significant infection, vast numbers of immune complexes

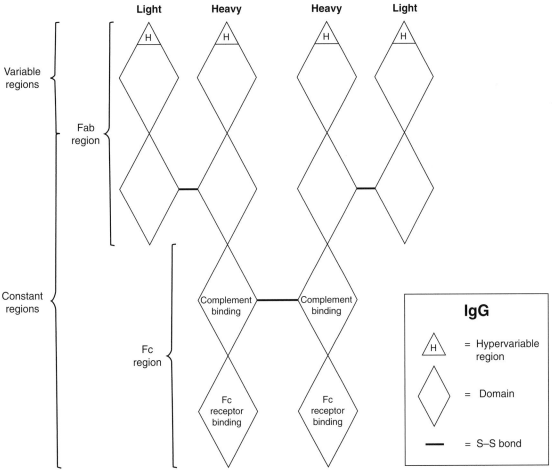

Figure 18 The basic structure of an antibody (immunoglobulin).

Table 9 Classes and functions of antibodies

Antibody class	Functions
IgM	First class of antibody, produced before IgG supervenes
	Pentamer with 10 antigen-binding sites
	Intravascular: cannot cross placenta
	Activates complement and agglutinates foreign substances
IgG	Four subclasses
	Can attach to phagocytic cells via Fc fragment (opsonisation)
	Found in tissues and can cross placenta
	Activates complement
IgA	Main antibody in secretions and excretions and in urine and gut contents
	Two subclasses: can dimerise (molecular weight 320 000) and has an additional secretory piece – this prevents digestion
	Stops microbes entering tissues from external surfaces
IgE	Involved in acute allergic reaction (type 1 hypersensitivity)
	Involved in defence against parasites
IgD	Found on the surface of B cells, but not expressed in activated cells
	Function unclear, possibly a receptor

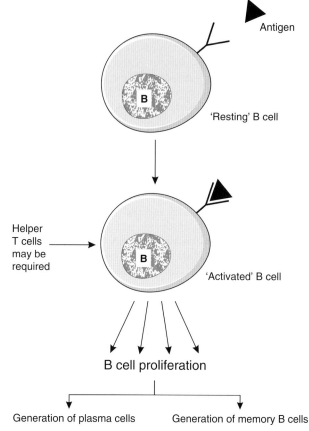

Figure 19 The antibody response.

are formed as antibodies bind to and neutralise microbial antigens.

The disposal of immune complexes is important since, potentially, they can lodge in blood vessel walls and cause damage by activating complement and initiating an inflammatory reaction, i.e. type III hypersensitivity (Ch. 8). The macrophages of the liver and spleen perform a large part of this disposal function.

Antigen-presenting cells

'Professional' antigen-presenting cells take antigens into their cytoplasm, process them and then present them to T cells and B cells on their cell surface in association with class II major histocompatibility complex (MHC) molecules (see Section 7.4). They also produce cytokines and other factors which coordinate and amplify the immune response. Antigen-presenting cells are of two main types:

- Cells derived from monocytes produced in the bone marrow. These cells are of two main types:
  - *macrophages: some are freely mobile, others are fixed at certain sites (e.g. Kupffer cells in the liver)*
  - *dendritic cells: examples include Langerhans' cells of the skin and follicular dendritic cells of the lymph nodes.*
- B cells. B lymphocytes also present antigen with class II molecules.

The antibody response

Certain antigens, e.g. large polysaccharides, can trigger antibody production directly. Others, including most proteins, require T cells – in particular T helper cells – to assist in triggering antibody production. The B cell presents antigen with class II human leucocyte antigen (HLA) molecules to T helper cells which then secrete cytokines that drive the differentiation of B cells into antibody-secreting plasma cells. Helper T cells can be divided broadly into two types called Th1 and Th2, depending on the cytokines they secrete (see Section 7.3).

There is a significant difference between the response to antigen of previously unstimulated B cells (the primary antibody response) and the response of memory B cells that have been produced during a previous encounter with the same antigen (the secondary antibody response). The primary response takes longer to develop. Typically, IgM is produced first, followed by IgG. The secondary response is faster; IgM is again produced first but the amount of IgG produced is greatly increased compared to the primary response. The secondary reaction requires helper T cells that recognise the antigen and activate B cells that react to the same antigen. The processes occurring in the B cell to achieve a response to antigen are shown in Figures 19 and 20. Note that free antigen can initiate a B cell response; this is in contrast with the T cell response

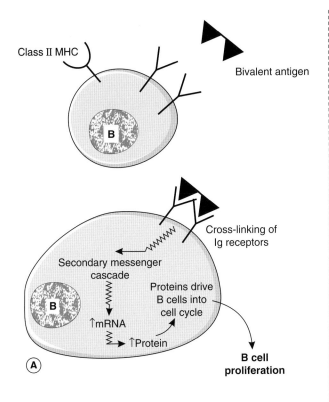

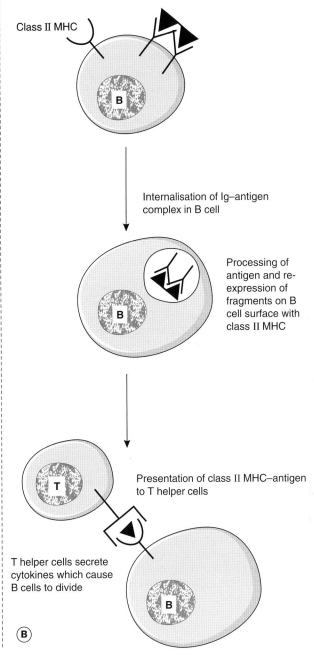

Figure 20 How antigens trigger B cells to produce antibody.

which always requires processing of antigen by antigen-presenting cells.

7.3 Cellular immunity

Learning objectives

You should:
- discuss the functions of Th, Tc and Ts cells
- distinguish between the Th1 and Th2 response.

T cell-mediated immunity

T cells, which mediate the cellular immune response, have two major functions:

- recognition and attack of cell-surface antigens
- regulation of the T and B cells in the immune response.

There are several subclasses of T cells with different functional characteristics (Table 10). These characteristics are reflected in the cell surface receptor molecules they express. In general, these molecules are named using the CD system

Table 10 T lymphocyte subsets

T cell subset	Function	CD status	MHC requirement
Helper (Th)	Two main types: Th1 promote cell-mediated immunity and delayed hypersensitivity; Th2 promote humoral immunity	CD4+ CD8–	II
Cytotoxic (Tc)	Kill cells with abnormal surface antigens, e.g. virus-infected cells, transplants	CD4– CD8+	I
Suppressor (Ts)	Suppress immune response, including against self-antigens	CD4– CD8+	I

Box 6 CD nomenclature

The CD (cluster of differentiation) system is a way of categorising surface molecules of different types with a variety of different functions. The nomenclature was originally designed for cells of the haemopoietic system, but many other cells also express CD molecules. For example, all mature T cells have CD2 and CD3 on their surface, and are described as CD2+ CD3+. Mature helper T cells express CD4 in addition but, unlike cytotoxic cells, do not express CD8; they are thus CD4+ CD8–. The CD antigens can be recognised in tissue samples using immunohistochemistry or flow cytometry.

(Box 6). CD4+ T helper cells (Th), which represent about 60% of the total T cell population, can only recognise antigen when it is presented together with MHC (see Section 7.4) class II antigen. CD8+ cells can only recognise antigen when presented with class I MHC antigen. This is known as restriction: a response can only be mounted against an antigen that is presented with the correct MHC molecule. The post-stimulus response of the T cell depends on various surface molecules such as CD3.

Class II antigens display a sample of extracellular proteins that have been endocytosed. With a few exceptions, class II antigens are only found on antigen-presenting cells. Class I antigens are found on virtually all nucleated cells and platelets. Class I antigens display a sample of the intracellular protein content; this can stimulate the CD8+ cytotoxic T cells (Tc) to destroy such cells if they display a foreign protein, e.g. as a result of viral infection.

How do T cells attack antigen?

T cell attack on antigen is seen in many circumstances, e.g. infection with intracellular microorganisms (such as viruses and mycobacteria), fungi and protozoans.

Cytotoxic T cells

Cytotoxic T cells express CD8. They kill cells infected with intracellular organisms, which are inaccessible to antibodies. Microbial antigens are displayed on the host cell surface in association with class I antigen. The infected cell is in effect alerting the cytotoxic T cell, which kills the cell by one of two mechanisms:

1. Insertion of a doughnut-shaped protein (perforin) into the cell membrane. The cell cytoplasm then leaks out through the hole and the cell dies.
2. Expression of Fas ligand (see Ch. 4) or release of granzymes that enter through the perforin pores; these events initiate apoptosis by triggering the caspase cascade. One advantage of apoptosis over oncosis in this context is that the endonucleases activated during apoptosis degrade the DNA not only of the cell but also of any infective organisms within the cell.

Helper T cells

Helper T cells express CD4 and mediate their effects via cytokines. There are two main types: Th1 and Th2.

Th1 cells promote cell-mediated immunity by stimulating macrophages and NK cells. This reaction is often called delayed hypersensitivity; a classic example is mycobacterial infections, e.g. tuberculosis (caused by *Mycobacterium tuberculosis*). Th1 cells with receptors for antigens of *M. tuberculosis* are activated and release cytokines which attract macrophages to the site of infection and activate them. The activation of macrophages promotes intracellular killing of infecting organisms. Th1 cells also inhibit the Th2 response.

Th2 cells secrete cytokines that promote humoral immune reactions, especially the IgE response, and activate eosinophils. They also inhibit the Th1 response. One hypothesis that is based on the Th1/Th2 concept is that allergic reactions represent an inflammatory response overly weighted towards Th2.

Suppressor T cells

Suppressor (Ts) cells express CD8 and function to inhibit (deactivate) the immune response. Relatively little is known about how they do this. They may not require processing and display of antigen by antigen-presenting cells and, therefore, may not be MHC restricted, despite being CD8+. They probably perform their suppressor functions by secreting cytokines which stop cell activation or proliferation or directly cause cell death.

7.4 Other components of the immune response

Cytokines

Cytokines are soluble polypeptide or glycoprotein molecules of low molecular weight, produced by cells involved in the immune response at sites of injury or inflammation. They bind to specific cell surface receptors, and thus act as messengers between the cells, allowing communication between them and coordination of the complex chain of events which occurs in response to antigen. Their effects can be autocrine, paracrine or endocrine.

Cytokines include interleukins, which are involved in lymphocyte proliferation and differentiation, interferons, which protect against viral infection, and colony-stimulating factors, which regulate the production of bone marrow blood cells (Box 7). The role of cytokines in inflammation is considered in more depth in Chapter 9.

The major histocompatibility complex

The MHC system occurs in all vertebrates and is the major system that distinguishes self from non-self. The human MHC system is known as the human leucocyte antigen (HLA) system. The HLA genes are found on the short arm of chromosome 6. They code for cell surface glycoproteins and are important in many cell-mediated immunological reactions.

The six loci that code for these cell surface glycoproteins are known as DP, DQ, DR (class II genes producing class II antigens) and A, B and C (class I) (Table 11). At each of these loci, there are several possible alleles (versions of the gene). Therefore, the number of possible combinations on both chromosomes is astronomical.

Class I HLA antigens are transmembrane glycoproteins and consist of two polypeptide chains which grip peptide fragments to be presented to cytotoxic T cells (CD8+). If the peptide is not a normal part of the cell, such as a viral protein, it is recognised and the cell destroyed. Almost all nucleated cells display class I antigens.

Class II HLA molecules are also composed of two polypeptide chains spanning the cell membrane. The main function of these molecules is to present foreign antigens to CD4+ T helper cells; they are potent stimulators of T cell proliferation. Generally, class II molecules are expressed only by a few specialised cells, the 'professional' antigen-presenting cells, namely dendritic cells, macrophages and B cells.

Since the advent of tissue typing, it has been found that some diseases are commoner in people with a particular type, or combination of types, of HLA. An example is the arthritic disease ankylosing spondylitis: the HLA B27 allele is found about 20 times more commonly in people with ankylosing spondylitis than in those without the disease.

Complement

The complement system is an enzymatic cascade which can be activated by antibody (classical pathway) or antigen (alternative and MBL pathways). Complement proteins are made in the liver and are numbered 1–9 (see Ch. 5).

Natural killer cells

This special type of non-B, non-T lymphocyte does not have immunoglobulin or T cell receptors and does not require prior exposure to antigen for its activity; therefore it is classified as part of innate immunity. The main function of NK cells is to destroy cells that are damaged or

---

Box 7 TNF-α: an example of a cytokine

Although it was originally named 'tumour necrosis factor' because of its effects on tumour cells, TNF alpha (TNF-α) (like most cytokines) has a wide variety of different actions, all of which are modulated by other cytokines. TNF-α is secreted by several different cell types, but macrophages are particularly important. Examples of its effects include, among others:

- activation of neutrophils and macrophages to promote microbial killing
- stimulation of T cells and B cells
- stimulation of endothelial cells to promote leucocyte adhesion
- raising the thermoregulatory set point of the hypothalamus, i.e. it produces fever
- stimulation of the liver to produce acute phase reactants such as C-reactive protein.

Thus, a macrophage secreting TNF-α can have autocrine actions on itself, paracrine actions on neighbouring inflammatory cells and endothelial cells, and endocrine actions on the liver and hypothalamus.

Table 11 Major histocompatibility antigens

Class	Chromosome location	Number of molecules	Cell location
I	6	3(HLA A, B, C)	All nucleated cells
II	6	3(HLA DP, DQ, DR)	Antigen-presenting cells

Each of the class I and class II molecules is polymorphic (has many variants). One person can have only two variants of each molecule, one coded by each parent.

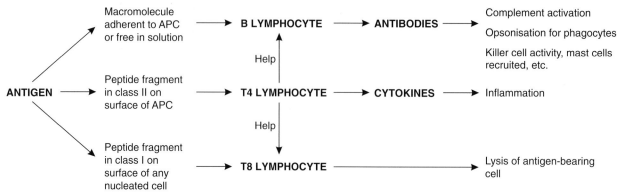

Figure 21 Overview of the immune response. APC, antigen-presenting cell.

Table 12 The immune response: principal players and their functions

Component	Function
B lymphocytes	Recognition of antigen
	Presentation of antigenic peptides to CD4 T cells
	Secretion of antibody
CD4 T helper lymphocytes	Recognition of antigens on MHC class II cells after endocytosis and processing
	Promoting local inflammation by recruitment and activation of macrophages
	Helping T and/or B cell responses
CD8 cytotoxic T lymphocytes	Recognition of intracellular antigens presented on MHC class I after cytosolic processing
	Killing cells which present abnormal proteins in class I MHC
Macrophages	Phagocytosis and destruction of microbes, dead cells and tissue debris, promoted by coatings of antibody and complement
	Walling off infection in granulomas
	Presentation of antigens to CD4 cells
Antibodies	Acting as receptors on the surface of B cells
	Neutralising toxins and microbial invaders
	Marking microbes and abnormal body cells for destruction by complement and effector cells
Cytokines	Control of cellular activities

infected. NK cells can do this by recognising cells with reduced levels of MHC I expression, which occurs in neoplastic and virally infected cells. The NK cell then destroys the cell by insertion of perforin channels. In addition, NK cells express CD16, a receptor for the Fc portion of IgG, on their surface. Therefore, they can bind to IgG-coated cells and destroy them; this type of killing is called antibody-dependent cell-mediated cytotoxicity. Other ways in which NK cells recognise target cells include receptors for complement component C3b, and for heat shock proteins that are upregulated in injured cells.

Summary

All the components discussed in this chapter are inter-linked in their functions and requirements for activation (Table 12 and Figure 21).

Self-assessment: questions

One best answer questions

1. What name is given to a small molecule that by itself cannot stimulate an immune response, but does so when coupled to a larger molecule?
   a. epitope
   b. hapten
   c. immunoglobulin
   d. secretory component
   e. tolerogen

2. Binding of a toll-like receptor on a macrophage to its ligand is most likely to cause the macrophage to:
   a. become activated
   b. die by apoptosis
   c. die by oncosis
   d. secrete immunoglobulin
   e. secrete eosinophil major basic protein

3. Immunoglobulins that act as efficient opsonins are:
   a. IgA and IgE
   b. IgA and IgG
   c. IgE and IgG
   d. IgG and IgM
   e. IgM and IgE

4. Which one of the following is most effective at clearing extracellular bacteria?
   a. apoptosis induced by CD8+ T cells
   b. apoptosis induced by NK cells
   c. complement and antibody action
   d. fibrin deposition
   e. suppressor T cell activity

5. In the saliva, the immunoglobulin with the highest concentration is:
   a. IgA
   b. IgD
   c. IgE
   d. IgG
   e. IgM

True-false questions

1. The following are correctly paired:
   a. IgG – cannot cross placenta
   b. CD8 – class II MHC
   c. IgM – complement activation
   d. B cells – cell-mediated immunity
   e. Interleukin-1 – fever

2. The following statements are true:
   a. dendritic cells and Langerhans' cells can present antigen
   b. Th1 cells promote cell-mediated immunity
   c. CD3 is found on T cells
   d. proliferation of cytotoxic (CD8+) T cells usually requires the presence of helper (CD4+) cells
   e. in humans, the genes for the MHC system are found on chromosome 7

Extended matching items questions (EMIs)

EMI 1

Theme: Antigen binding and processing

A. antigen-T cell receptor binding
B. binding to IgE Fc
C. binding to IgE variable region
D. binding to IgG Fc
E. binding to IgG variable region
F. binding to IgM Fc
G. binding to IgM variable region
H. insertion of perforin channels
I. presentation of ingested antigens
J. presentation of peptides derived from the cell cytoplasm

For each of the following statements, select the most appropriate action from the list.

1. The principal function of the HLA class I molecule.
2. The principal function of the HLA class II molecule.
3. The means by which mast cells attach antibody to their membranes.
4. A means of cell execution shared by CD8+ T lymphocytes and NK cells.
5. The way IgG molecules recognise antigen.

Case history questions

Case history 1

A 10-year-old girl has a sore throat. A throat swab is taken and the culture grows *Streptococcus* bacteria. During the course of her illness, her general practitioner notes that her neck lymph nodes are enlarged.

1. What changes would you expect to see in this girl's lymph nodes?
2. How would it differ if the infection was viral?

The girl is treated with antibiotics and after a few days her symptoms resolve. Two weeks later, she notices that her urine is blood-stained and she begins to feel generally unwell.

3. How might the second bout of illness relate to her sore throat?

4. Name an autoimmune condition affecting the heart that is associated with streptococcal sore throat and describe its pathogenesis.

Self-assessment: answers

One best answer

1. b. A hapten is too small to be recognised by B cells and T cells, but if it is bound to a larger carrier molecule it can be recognised and initiate an immune response. An example of a hapten is the toxic chemical in poison ivy. This chemical binds to proteins in the skin that act as carriers. As a result, the immune system becomes sensitised to the toxin and mounts an immune response on subsequent exposure to poison ivy (a type IV hypersensitivity reaction, see Ch. 8), causing the blistering rash. An epitope is defined as the smallest identifiable part of an antigenic molecule that can be recognised by a B cell or T cell receptor. An immunoglobulin is an antibody molecule. Secretory component is a molecule produced by epithelial cells that combines with IgA when it is secreted. A tolerogen is a substance that is recognised by B cells and T cells but induces tolerance (i.e. a failure to respond immunologically to the tolerogen) rather than an immune reaction.

2. a. Pattern-recognition receptors such as the toll-like receptors represent a type of host defence that is ancient in evolutionary terms. Immunoglobulin is not secreted by macrophages but by plasma cells, which are derived from B lymphocytes. Eosinophil major basic protein is highly toxic to parasites; it is stored by eosinophils in their granules and released when they are activated.

3. d. IgG and IgM are opsonins. Neutrophils and macrophages have receptors for the Fc portions of these types of antibody.

4. c. Extracellular bacteria are accessible to serum antibody and complement. IgG, IgM and complement components all act as opsonins. In addition, the complement membrane attack complex can cause lysis of bacteria. Cellular immunity, in which cytotoxic T cells and NK cells participate, is more important in defence against viruses, fungi, intracellular bacteria and protozoa. Fibrin deposition occurs in inflammation (Ch. 9) but does not clear bacteria. Suppressor T cells damp down the immune reaction.

5. a. IgA is secreted as a dimer into the fluids produced by mucous membranes, e.g. saliva, tears, gastrointestinal juice, sweat and breast milk.

True-false answers

1. a. **False.** IgG can cross the placenta, the other types of immunoglobulins cannot. If IgM antibodies to a particular organism are present within the fetal circulation, this indicates that it is the fetus itself which is infected and mounting an immune response; IgG antibodies could be maternal in origin. The half-life in the circulation of IgG is about 3–4 weeks, so IgG of maternal origin that enters the fetus persists after birth and provides useful defence against infection in the first few months of extrauterine life.

   b. **False.** CD4+ (helper) T cells recognise antigen in association with class II MHC molecules, and then secrete cytokines to activate other cells of the immune system. CD8+ (cytotoxic) T cells use class I molecules, and may then kill the cell if they recognise the antigen as foreign.

   c. **True.** IgM is very efficient at complement activation.

   d. **False.** Cell-mediated immunity involves responses by cytotoxic T cells in association with macrophages.

   e. **True.** Fever (pyrexia) is caused by a number of cytokines, including interleukin-1, which raise the thermoregulatory set point of the hypothalamus so that the homeostatic mechanisms of temperature control maintain body temperature higher than normal. A substance that does this is called a pyrogen. Endotoxin (bacterial lipopolysaccharide) is also a pyrogen. The function of fever is unclear, but it may assist in the defence against infection: for example, raising the body temperature seems to inhibit viral replication.

2. a. **True.** Dendritic cells and Langerhans' cells load antigen into class II HLA molecules and present it to T helper cells.

   b. **True.** The cytokines produced by Th1 cells, e.g. interleukin-2, TNF-α and interferon gamma, promote cell-mediated immunity to a greater extent than humoral immunity.

   c. **True.** There are numerous CD molecules on the surface of lymphocytes, macrophages and antigen-presenting cells. The structure and function of many of these protein molecules are now well characterised. CD3 is found on all T cells and is associated with the T cell receptor. It is a useful marker of T cell differentiation in the diagnostic laboratory.

   d. **True.** An important function of the cytotoxic T cell is to destroy viral-infected cells, recognised by the association of class I MHC molecules with viral antigens on the surface of the infected cell. In order to proliferate, the CD8+ Tc cell requires stimulation by cytokines from CD4+ Th cells.

e. **False.** The genes of the human MHC (known as the HLA) are found on the short arm of chromosome 6. There are two sets of genes (class I and class II) and each contains three loci. Each locus has a large number of alleles coding for MHC molecules. The HLA molecules can themselves act as antigens when organs are transplanted from one individual to another.

EMI answers

EMI 1

Theme: Antigen binding and processing

1. J. Proteins degraded in proteasomes are presented on the cell surface by being loaded into MHC class I molecules. In this way, potential immunogens such as virus components that might otherwise evade immune surveillance can be shown to cells of the immune system. This procedure is different from the one used by antigen-presenting cells to ingest antigen and process it for display (see next answer).

2. I. The class II molecules are found on antigen-presenting cells, which take up antigen from outside the cell. The antigen is processed in a phagolysosome and is ultimately bound to an MHC class II molecule, which is then transported to the cell surface where it displays the antigen.

3. B. IgE binds to mast cells and basophils before it encounters its specific antigen. When antigen cross-links IgE molecules on the cell surface, the result is degranulation with release of the various mediators (histamine etc.).

4. H. Perforin creates a hole in the target cell membrane. The contents leak out and the cell dies by lysis. Alternatively, the perforin channel allows granzyme molecules to enter the target cell and initiate apoptosis.

5. E. The variable region of an immunoglobulin molecule binds to the antigen. It is the great variety of shapes exhibited by variable regions that accounts for the huge range of antigens specifically recognised by antibodies.

Case history answers

Case history 1

1. Bacterial infections tend to elicit a strong humoral (antibody) immune response. The local lymph nodes draining the site of infection will be stimulated to produce plasma cells. In a normal lymph node, B cell areas are found in the outer cortex in areas known as follicles – densely packed aggregates of cells. When B cell production is stimulated, these follicles acquire a germinal centre. Transformation of B cells occurs in germinal centres with the production of numerous memory cells. B cells differentiate into plasma cells in the cortical areas deep to and between the follicles – the paracortex. Plasma cells then enter the medullary vascular system (medullary cords) and produce antibody as they leave in the efferent lymphatics, draining the site of infection. The local lymph nodes will have large cortical follicles with prominent germinal centres. (See Ch. 24.)

2. Viral infections generally stimulate a T cell response – cytotoxic T cells (CD8+) can recognise and destroy infected cells if the viral antigen is displayed on the cell's surface by a class I MHC molecule. The T cell areas of the lymph node are found in the paracortex and massive expansion of this region can occur during viral infections. The B cell follicles will be relatively inconspicuous.

3. Soluble antigen from the streptococci has combined with antibody to form complexes that have deposited in the girl's kidneys causing them to function abnormally (see Section 23.3 in Ch. 23). In particular, they have lodged in the glomeruli, evoking an inflammatory reaction which causes the glomerular capillaries to become leaky. Blood can then be found in the urine (haematuria). Other organs that may be damaged by immune complex deposition are the joints and skin. Fortunately, in most cases, once the inflammatory response has died down, normal kidney function is restored. The delay in onset of the problem is a result of the time taken to produce large amounts of antibody.

4. One important autoimmune disease which occurs after a streptococcal infection is rheumatic fever. In this disease, now rare in industrialised countries, antibodies produced against streptococcal antigens cross-react with antigens in the patient's own tissues. The heart is often affected and the inflammatory damage may lead to fibrosis and distortion of the valves. This can lead to heart failure and death if the valve is not replaced. (See Ch. 14.)

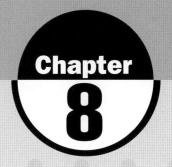

The immune system 2

Chapter overview

The immune system deals with foreign invaders and abnormal host cells (such as neoplastic cells), and its normal function is essential to health, as explained in the previous chapter. There are four main ways in which the immune system contributes to disease.

- A defective (insufficient) immune response will compromise the host defences against microorganisms and predispose to infection. In severe cases, there is also a predisposition to certain neoplasms.
- In hypersensitivity reactions, host tissue is secondarily destroyed during an immune response.
- If the immune system fails to distinguish between self and non-self antigens, the immune system will attack normal tissues. This is autoimmunity.
- Undesirable immune responses are also seen in patients in whom there is rejection of tissue transplants.

8.1 Hypersensitivity

Learning objectives

You should:
- define the four types of hypersensitivity
- explain their pathogenesis.

Hypersensitivity is a process whereby the host's tissue is injured during an immune response to a foreign antigen. When this process is inappropriate 'hypersensitivity diseases' occur. They are divided into four types; types I–III are mediated by antibodies (humoral immunity), whereas type IV is mediated by cellular immunity.

Type I hypersensitivity

Type I hypersensitivity is commonly called allergy. It is due to the interaction of antigen with IgE antibody previously bound to the surfaces of mast cells and basophils. In this context, the antigen is referred to as an allergen. Type I hypersensitivity is rapid (hence its alternative name, immediate hypersensitivity) and triggers mast cells and/or basophils to release substances that cause blood vessels to dilate and become leaky and cause smooth muscle contraction in bronchial walls and elsewhere. Later, eosinophils and other inflammatory cells infiltrate the tissue, causing further damage. The reaction can be localised or generalised.

Localised reactions

Common examples of localised type I hypersensitivity reactions are asthma, hay fever and urticaria. In susceptible, sensitised individuals, exposure to antigen (allergen) results in an immediate and acute immune response mediated by IgE. The reaction can be triggered by substances which are commonly found all around us. For example, asthma can be triggered by house dust or animal proteins, and hay fever can be caused by pollen.

Generalised reactions

Rarely, antigen enters the bloodstream of a sensitised individual and binds to IgE on circulating basophils. This can lead to a severe reaction known as anaphylaxis in which there is acute bronchospasm, shock (circulatory collapse as a result of peripheral vasodilatation), and even death. This may happen to people who are sensitised to penicillin or bee stings, for example.

Sequence of events

This is the same in both localised and generalised type I hypersensitivity reactions. In sensitised people, IgE is bound to the surface of tissue mast cells (and also their circulating counterparts, basophils), which have specific receptors for the Fc portion of the antibody, leaving the antigen-binding sites free to link with antigen. This binding has high affinity. After antigen and IgE have linked together, there follows an increase in membrane permeability to calcium with activation of a cascade of intracellular signals. This leads to degranulation of mast cells, which release histamine, a powerful vasodilator and constrictor of smooth muscle, and an eosinophil chemotactic factor (Table 13). Degranulation of mast cells can also be caused by substances other than IgE, e.g. drugs such as morphine, activated complement components C3a and C5a, and by physical stimuli such as heat, cold and trauma.

Table 13 Properties of mast cells

Substances found in mast cell granules	Action
Eosinophil and neutrophil chemotactic factors	Chemotaxis
Histamine	Vasodilatation, increased permeability
Heparin	Late phase reactions
Trypsin	Late phase reactions
Substances made by mast cells during response	
Leukotrienes	Chemotaxis, smooth muscle contraction
Prostaglandins	Vasodilatation, smooth muscle contraction
Platelet-activating factor	Platelet aggregation, smooth muscle contraction, increased permeability

Independent of the granule system, there is local release of bioactive lipids, which are produced by macrophages and mast cells in the vicinity. These substances include leukotrienes and prostaglandins. These also cause smooth muscle constriction and may be important in the pathogenesis of asthma.

Type II hypersensitivity

In type II hypersensitivity reactions, antibody binds directly to tissues: antibodies are directed against and bind with normal or altered components on the cell surface which they recognise as non-self. The presence of bound antibody induces damage by three main mechanisms:

- complement-mediated cytotoxicity: fixation of complement to the cell surface produces lysis via the membrane attack complex
- opsonisation: cells coated with antibody and complement C3b fragments are susceptible to phagocytosis
- antibody-dependent cell-mediated cytotoxicity: target cells are coated with IgG (or occasionally IgE); the cells are attacked by cells which have receptors for Fc that enable them to recognise and kill cells that have immunoglobulin bound to them. Such cells are the natural killer (NK) cells, neutrophils, macrophages, and (in the case of IgE) eosinophils. However, NK cells appear to be most important in this process.

Examples of such reactions are transfusion reactions, haemolytic disease of the newborn and Goodpasture's syndrome.

Incompatible blood transfusion reaction

Antibodies against a blood group antigen, e.g. rhesus or ABO, bind directly to the surface of the blood cells, causing haemolysis. Thus, a patient who has antibodies to blood group B but is inadvertently given type B blood will experience massive intravascular haemolysis.

Haemolytic disease of the newborn

Rhesus (Rh) blood group antigens are present in about 85% of people (rhesus positive); the remainder of the population are rhesus negative. Rhesus antigen is inherited through a dominant gene (D) so that rhesus-positive individuals can be homozygous (DD) or heterozygous (Dd). Haemolytic disease of the newborn may arise if a rhesus-negative mother carries a rhesus-positive fetus. When fetal red cells enter the maternal circulation, usually at delivery, maternal antibodies against fetal rhesus antigen will be produced. The first rhesus-positive baby from a rhesus-negative mother is usually normal, but the mother will have become sensitised to the rhesus antigen during delivery of this pregnancy. The next time she carries a rhesus-positive fetus, she will be able to mount a secondary immune response to the rhesus antigen, causing haemolysis of the red cells in the developing fetus. Therefore, subsequent babies from a sensitised mother will tend to develop progressively more severe haemolysis. The disease can be prevented by injecting the mother with IgG rhesus antibody immediately after delivery to 'mop up' any fetal cells and prevent her producing natural antibody.

Goodpasture's syndrome

Goodpasture's syndrome is an autoimmune disease. Autoantibodies to type IV collagen develop and bind to the type IV collagen in the basement membrane of the glomeruli and the lungs. Consequently, complement is fixed and antibody-dependent cell-mediated cytotoxicity is activated, causing glomerulonephritis (see Ch. 23, Section 23.3) and inflammation of the lung.

Type III hypersensitivity

Type III hypersensitivity is caused by antigen–antibody complexes. When antibody reacts with antigen in certain proportions, complexes form that can be deposited either locally or at a distant site. The antigen–antibody (immune) complexes cause tissue damage where they are deposited, usually in blood vessel walls, where they induce an inflammatory reaction as a result of complement activation and infiltration by neutrophils.

Localised immune complex disease (Arthus reaction)

The Arthus reaction is an example of immune complex damage following injection of an antigen into the skin of an individual with high levels of preformed antibody. Within 2–8 hours, a haemorrhagic oedematous reaction occurs. After 12–24 hours, skin necrosis occurs as a result of localised vasculitis (inflammation of vessels causing necrosis of the wall) from local immune complex deposition. Histologically there is an acute inflammatory reaction with numerous neutrophils.

Systemic immune complex disease

When an antigen first stimulates the formation of antibody, there is antigen excess. As levels of antibody rise, antigen/antibody equivalence occurs and as antigen is

Definition. Chronic autoimmune illness with fluctuating activity. Multisystem involvement, especially skin, joints, kidneys and serosal surfaces.

Age/sex. Young to middle-aged females typically.

Cause. Most cases are spontaneous and probably mediated by polyclonal B cell hyperactivity with autoantibody production and immune complex formation. The autoantibodies are antinuclear (anti-double-stranded DNA antibodies); this is diagnostic of the disease. Some cases occur in patients on drugs (hydralazine). The tissue injury is caused by a type III hypersensitivity reaction.

Pathological processes. The main pathological changes and their resulting symptoms are:

- vasculitis (inflammation of vessels) with necrosis: rashes, muscle weakness
- glomerulonephritis: haematuria, proteinuria, renal failure
- synovitis: arthritis
- pleuritis, lung inflammation: chest pain, breathlessness
- pericarditis, endocarditis: chest pain, heart failure.

Clinical course. Very varied. A few patients die rapidly with heart/renal failure. Most have a chronic illness requiring repeated courses of immunosuppressive drugs.

tuberculosis (TB) or been immunised with BCG (bacille Calmette–Guérin derived from TB) and therefore have primed T cells, an area of reddening develops in 12 hours. The reaction is maximal at 1 week and histologically the tissue at the reaction site shows granulomas, which are accumulations of lymphocytes and macrophages. The macrophages are typically transformed into epithelioid cells, and some fuse together to form giant cells (see Ch. 9).

At the first encounter with the tubercle bacillus, CD4+ T cells recognise antigen when it is presented with class II MHC molecules on antigen-presenting cells. Memory T cells are then formed. On re-encountering the antigen, sensitised T cells react with antigen on the antigen-presenting cell surface, become stimulated to produce cytokines (e.g. interleukin-2) which in turn activate CD8+ T cells and recruit macrophages into the area. Interleukin-1 from macrophages increases T cell proliferation and promotes the release of acute phase reactants, which have a number of effects including fever production.

8.2 Autoimmune disease

removed, there is a relative excess of antibody in the circulation. Small soluble immune complexes are formed when there is antigen excess. They are not easily phagocytosed and may be deposited in the walls of blood vessels in the kidney (glomerulus), heart, joints and skin. Here they activate complement and cause tissue damage. Large immune complexes are formed when there is antigen/antibody equivalence or antibody excess and these are readily cleared from the circulation by macrophage phagocytosis.

There are various clinical situations in which systemic immune complexes can form and cause disease:

- infection, e.g. post-streptococcal glomerulonephritis
- autoimmune disease, e.g. systemic lupus erythematosus (see Box 8).

Type IV hypersensitivity

Type IV hypersensitivity is a reaction mediated by sensitised T cells rather than antibodies. It characterises the host response to a variety of microorganisms, including viruses, fungi, protozoans and mycobacteria, but it is also seen in many other circumstances, e.g. transplanted organs, inflammatory drug reactions, and contact sensitivities (such as poison ivy reaction). It takes time for primed T cells to react and hence there is a delay of at least 12 hours before the reaction can be seen. For this reason, type IV hypersensitivity is sometimes called 'delayed hypersensitivity'.

The prototype of this reaction is the tuberculin test. If a small amount of protein derived from tubercle bacilli is injected into the skin of a non-immune person, there will be no reaction. However, in people who have already had

Patients with autoimmune disease mount an immune response against their own tissues. They typically have antibodies directed against components of their own tissues (autoantibodies) in their blood; autoantibodies can be detected serologically and serve as a clinical test for autoimmune diseases. In many cases, a hypersensitivity reaction of type II, III or IV is responsible. In some diseases, however, there is antibody-mediated cellular dysfunction, in which antibodies against cell surface receptor molecules impair their function. For example, in Graves' disease the autoantibodies bind to the receptor for thyroid-stimulating hormone and activate it, causing the thyroid cells to secrete excessive amounts of thyroxine. Autoimmune disease can affect one particular cell type, one organ system or many systems of the body (multisystem disease).

Normally, the immune system recognises the body's own antigens as being 'friendly' and does not attack them, i.e. the immune system normally exhibits tolerance to self-antigens. In essence, autoimmunity is a failure of the mechanisms of self-tolerance. The processes by which the body's immune system is triggered to attack itself are only partially understood. It is possible that cross-reaction of an antibody produced against a foreign antigen (e.g. bacterium) with a normal tissue antigen occurs (e.g. rheumatic heart disease), or that tissue antigens can be altered by drugs. Sometimes, marked changes in major histocompatibility complex (MHC) expression occur with both increased expression and de novo expression of class II in previously negative cell types (see Table 14). In addition,

Table 14 Autoimmune diseases with changed MHC expression

Disease	Cells affected
Graves' disease	Thyroid epithelium
Type 1 diabetes mellitus	Pancreatic β cells
Primary biliary cirrhosis	Bile duct epithelium
Sjögren's syndrome	Salivary ducts

Box 9 Rheumatoid disease

Definition. Systemic, chronic inflammatory autoimmune disease. Erroneously called rheumatoid arthritis, since blood vessels, kidneys, heart, skin and lungs may also be affected.

Age/sex. Young to middle-aged females. About 1–2% of the adult population are affected worldwide.

Cause. Unknown. However, most patients (~80%) with rheumatoid disease (and particularly joint problems) have circulating rheumatoid factors, which are autoantibodies, usually IgM, against the Fc region of IgG. It is thought that the disease is initiated by an infectious agent, e.g. virus or bacterium. Rheumatoid disease can be complicated by amyloid deposition (see Ch. 13).

Clinicopathological features:

- joints – the synovium is initially targeted leading to destruction of cartilage and bone and damage to tendons and ligaments
- skin – firm 'rheumatoid nodules' are found in about a quarter of patients, especially on the elbows. These are seen down the microscope as large necrotic areas surrounded by macrophages
- blood vessels – vasculitis
- lungs, heart, kidney – non-specific inflammation and/or vasculitis.

Clinical course. Variable. There may be sudden onset of debilitating arthritis or slow, inexorable loss of joint movements. Rarely, patients die from systemic complications (e.g. vasculitis, amyloidosis). Often a variety of powerful anti-inflammatory drug therapies are required to slow disease progression.

---

abnormalities in the regulation of T and B lymphocyte function have been implicated. Two classic examples of multisystem autoimmune diseases are systemic lupus erythematosus (Box 8) and rheumatoid disease (Box 9).

8.3 Transplantation

Learning objectives

You should:
- Analyse transplant rejection in terms of the underlying pathology.

Organ transplantation is an important part of medicine that over the years has become relatively commonplace. A working knowledge of basic immune mechanisms is needed to understand the phenomenon of rejection. The target antigens are called histocompatibility antigens; the human leucocyte antigen (HLA) (MHC) antigens are the target of the most destructive reactions, hence the importance of HLA typing in transplantation. Both the cell-mediated and humoral arms of the immune response are involved in rejection reactions, which can be classified according to:

- whether the response is cell and/or antibody mediated
- the speed of evolution of the response.

Hyperacute rejection

Hyperacute rejection is antibody mediated and occurs when a donated organ is placed in a patient who has preformed, circulating antibodies to donor antigens (e.g. multiparous women, patients undergoing multiple transfusions). The rejection occurs within minutes of the new organ having its blood supply established as antibodies target HLA on the vascular endothelium. Inflammation of vessels, thrombosis and necrosis occur.

Acute rejection

Acute rejection typically appears a week or two after transplantation. It is due to cellular immunity and is initiated by the generation of CD8+ (cytotoxic) T cells which, through various effector mechanisms, destroy the donor organ. An important component of some acute rejection reactions is vasculitis causing intimal proliferation and stenosis or obliteration of graft vessels. This process, called acute vascular rejection, causes necrosis and scarring.

Chronic rejection

Chronic rejection is due to cellular immunity and takes the form of a slow diminution in organ function over time. Characteristically, plasma cells, lymphocytes and eosinophils are seen within the tissue; intimal fibrosis is also prominent.

Rejection of grafts can now be prevented, or at least slowed, by a variety of drugs (see Box 10).

Box 10 Prevention and treatment of allograft rejection

- Reduce graft immunogenicity by:
  - ensuring ABO compatibility
  - 'matching' class I and class II MHC in donor and recipient.
- Immunosuppression of recipient. The drugs used and their actions include:
  - corticosteroids: cytokine gene transcription blocker
  - azathioprine: metabolic toxin
  - cyclosporin A: interleukin-2 gene transcription blocker
  - FK506: cytokine gene transcription blocker; less nephrotoxic than cyclosporin A.

Most drugs act by inhibiting T cell function.

8.4 Immunodeficiency

Learning objectives

You should:
- distinguish primary from secondary immunodeficiency and give examples of each
- describe the pathology of AIDS.

Immunodeficiency can be classified as congenital (primary) (see Box 11) and acquired (secondary) types. The human immunodeficiency virus (HIV) is responsible for the acquired immunodeficiency syndrome (AIDS) and worldwide is the most important cause of secondary immunodeficiency. Other infections can also adversely affect the immune system, although not to the same extent as encountered in AIDS. The use of drugs also gives rise to secondary immunodeficiencies. For example, cytotoxics damage or kill replicating cells (including replicating cells of the immune system), whereas corticosteroids and immunosuppressive drugs interfere with cytokine production. Patients who are malnourished or elderly also have diminished immune responses.

Immunodeficiency can also be associated with the development of cancer. Presumably, the lack of normal immune reactions to abnormal cells (see Ch. 7) allows neoplastic cells to survive and multiply. For example, some high-grade B cell lymphomas arise in the setting of severely compromised T cell function, as seen in AIDS or in patients with transplants who are taking immunosuppressive medication.

AIDS

Aetiology

AIDS follows, after a varying time interval, infection with human immunodeficiency virus (HIV).

Box 11 Primary immunodeficiencies

- Bruton's agammaglobulinaemia:
  - X linked
  - no mature B cells, T cells normal
  - recurrent bacterial infections.
- DiGeorge syndrome:
  - maldevelopment of thymus gland
  - no cell-mediated response; reduced T cell levels, but normal antibody levels
  - recurrent viral and fungal infections.
- Severe combined immunodeficiency disease (SCID):
  - autosomal recessive and X linked forms
  - defect is at the stem cell level; defective T and B cell responses; virtually absent lymphoid tissue
  - early death from opportunistic infections.

Pathogenesis

The CD4 molecule of CD4+ T cells acts as a receptor for HIV allowing it to enter the cell. The virus then uses reverse transcriptase to produce DNA from its own RNA. The viral DNA produced is inserted into the lymphocyte's chromosomes. The DNA may be transcribed to form more HIV or lie dormant. Tissue macrophages (CD4+) can also be infected. By insertion of viral DNA into the host genome, irreversible and permanent infection of the cell occurs. Direct lysis of CD4+ T cells, the cytopathic effects of viral RNA, DNA and protein, and inhibition of CD4+ T cell maturation as well as autoimmune destruction all contribute to the immunodeficiency. Severe immunosuppression occurs in AIDS patients, leaving them susceptible to a variety of infections and tumours.

Clinical features

Opportunistic infections

The following organisms do not affect individuals with normal immunity, or cause only mild disease, but they can cause debilitating and fatal illness in patients with AIDS (or immunodeficiency from other causes):

- *Pneumocystis carinii*
- atypical mycobacteria e.g. *Mycobacterium avium-intracellulare*
- Epstein–Barr virus (EBV)
- herpes simplex virus (HSV)
- Cryptosporidiosis
- Cryptococcosis
- Toxoplasmosis
- cytomegalovirus (CMV).

Tumours

AIDS is associated with the development of Kaposi's sarcoma, high-grade B cell lymphomas, primary brain lymphomas and cervical carcinoma.

Brain

This is a major site of HIV infection. Most patients develop some form of encephalitis or dementia.

At-risk populations

These include:

- homosexual/bisexual men
- intravenous substance users
- recipients of blood products prior to the introduction of screening blood donations for HIV
- heterosexual contacts of members of other high-risk groups.

Transmission

Transmission is via:

- sexual intercourse (vaginal or anal)
- direct inoculation of the virus through the bloodstream, e.g. needle stick injury
- placenta (mother-to-child).

Self-assessment: questions

One best answer questions

1. The cell predominantly responsible for antibody-dependent cell-mediated cytotoxicity is the:
   a. B cell
   b. mast cell
   c. neutrophil
   d. NK cell
   e. T cell

2. Which of the following generally produces the fastest response after exposure to an antigen?
   a. type I hypersensitivity
   b. type II hypersensitivity
   c. type III hypersensitivity
   d. type IV hypersensitivity

3. A 22-year-old woman complains of pain and swelling in several joints. She also says she has been lacking in energy recently. On examination she has a facial rash and a pleural effusion. Urinalysis shows haematuria and proteinuria. Which one of the following mechanisms is most likely to be responsible?
   a. anaphylactic reaction
   b. immune complex disease
   c. neoplastic proliferation of B cells
   d. primary immunodeficiency
   e. steroid-induced immunodeficiency

True-false questions

1. The following statements are true:
   a. asthma is primarily a T cell-mediated immune disease
   b. skin prick tests are a useful way of predicting immediate hypersensitivity reactions
   c. rheumatic fever is thought to be immune complex mediated
   d. Goodpasture's syndrome is due to immune complex deposition
   e. the complement product C3a can cause non-IgE-mediated mast cell degranulation

2. Immune complexes:
   a. are made up of antigen and antibody
   b. contain antibody of the IgG class
   c. are usually insoluble
   d. combine with complement, which initiates an inflammatory reaction
   e. are responsible for post-streptococcal glomerulonephritis

3. Type II (antibody-mediated) reactions:
   a. may involve opsonisation
   b. may involve complement-mediated cytotoxicity
   c. are characterised histologically by large numbers of eosinophils
   d. are responsible for transfusion reactions
   e. are responsible for granuloma formation in tuberculosis

Case history questions

Case history 1

A 26-year-old rhesus-negative woman with a 20-week pregnancy was admitted to an obstetric observation unit. She had not felt the baby move for 3 days. An ultrasound scan confirmed the fetus was dead and a stillbirth occurred the following day. At post-mortem examination, the fetus was swollen and had massive pleural effusions and ascites. A high level of anti-D antibodies was detected in the mother's blood. The father had a blood test which showed him to be O rhesus-positive. The woman had had three previous pregnancies by the same man; the babies were completely normal.

1. What was the underlying immunological process which led to the death of the baby? Why were there no problems with the first baby?

2. Give two other examples of this type of hypersensitivity reaction.

Self-assessment: answers

One best answer

1. d. The NK cell is the main cell effecting this reaction.

2. a. Type I hypersensitivity can cause clinical effects in minutes or hours, because IgE-mediated mast cell degranulation occurs very rapidly.

3. b. The woman has systemic lupus erythematosus, which is a type III hypersensitivity disease. Even if you did not know the diagnosis, the involvement of multiple organs suggests a systemic autoimmune disease caused by immune complex deposition: in particular, the renal glomeruli, blood vessel walls, synovial membranes of joints and the skin seem particularly prone to accumulate immune complexes. She does not have an immune deficiency; the disease is rather caused by over-activity of the immune system. A neoplastic proliferation of B cells is multiple myeloma. This condition can cause proteinuria due to excretion of excess light chains, but it does not commonly present with the other features of this case; furthermore, it tends to cause immunodeficiency as the patient's B cells are gradually replaced with the monoclonal proliferation. Anaphylaxis is a systemic type I reaction.

True-false answers

1. a. **False.** Asthma is a disease caused by an immediate (type I) hypersensitivity reaction, mediated by IgE. The intense bronchoconstriction which causes the breathlessness and wheezing results from the action of smooth muscle contractors released by mast cells.

   b. **True.** If a small amount of allergen such as house dust or pollen is injected into the skin of a person already sensitised to the substance, i.e. who already has IgE antibodies against the substance, an immediate wheal and flare reaction will occur. This clinical test is a useful way of predicting hypersensitivity reactions and also for determining which antigens are likely to trigger them.

   c. **False.** Rheumatic fever is an autoimmune disease due to cross-reactive antibodies produced during an infection with the group A streptococci. The disease often affects children and usually follows a few weeks after a group A streptococcal sore throat. During the course of the immune response to the streptococci, antibodies are produced which cross-react with the body's own tissues. There is a breakdown in the principle of self-tolerance, and the antibodies attack tissues of the heart, joints and brain, causing an acute febrile illness. This is different from post-streptococcal glomerulonephritis, which is a type III reaction.

   d. **False.** Goodpasture's syndrome is an autoimmune disease mediated by type II hypersensitivity; immune complexes are not a significant component of the pathogenesis.

   e. **True.** A variety of substances cause degranulation of mast cells independent of IgE. These include the complement components C3a and C5a (the anaphylatoxins, see Ch. 5) and drugs such as morphine and physical stimuli.

2. a. **True.** Classical experiments in the 1960s and 1970s showed that if rabbits are injected with bovine serum albumin (BSA), they quickly produce anti-BSA antibodies, and immune complexes of BSA-anti-BSA form. These initially circulate in the bloodstream and are then deposited in tissues (e.g. glomerulus).

   b. **True.** IgG is nearly always the antibody involved in complex formation.

   c. **False.** Small soluble complexes are the ones which deposit in blood vessel walls and cause damage. Large insoluble complexes are easily phagocytosed and removed by tissue macrophages.

   d. **True.** Tissue damage occurs following the classical pathway of complement activation (see Ch. 5).

   e. **True.** Soluble immune complexes composed of IgG and streptococcal antigen deposit in the glomerular capillary loops and initiate a complement-mediated inflammatory reaction. Alternatively, if some streptococcal antigens are positively charged they may 'stick' in the negatively charged matrix of the glomerulus and in situ immune complex formation occurs. There is damage to the glomerular basement membrane via a type III hypersensitivity reaction and neutrophils and macrophages are recruited to the site. Immune complexes can be demonstrated in tissue sections of the glomerulus by immunofluorescent or immunohistochemical techniques.

3. a. **True.** Opsonisation is the coating of a target structure by immunoglobulin, encouraging phagocytosis.

   b. **True.** Complement is activated by immunoglobulin.

   c. **False.** Eosinophils characterise type I reactions. Antibody is produced by plasma cells.

d. **True.** Antibody attacks the red cells perceived as foreign by the immune system.

e. **False.** Granulomas are part of the type IV response.

Case history answers

Case history 1

1. The baby died of haemolytic disease of the newborn (HDN), in this case caused by rhesus incompatibility. If a fetus inherits paternal red cell rhesus antigens that are foreign to the mother's immune system, reaction to these antigens may occur. In this case, the father is rhesus-positive so he must have at least one copy of the D allele to pass on to his offspring. At the time of birth, leakage of the baby's red cells into the maternal circulation occurs. If these blood cells express the rhesus antigen, the mother will recognise it as foreign and become immunologically sensitised. Although there will be no effect on the first baby, who will be a week or two old by this time, subsequent rhesus-positive fetuses will be at risk. If fetal blood crosses into the mother's circulation during a subsequent pregnancy, maternal IgG anti-D antibodies will be produced quickly. IgG antibodies can cross the placenta and fix to the antigen on fetal red cells, causing them to be rapidly destroyed (haemolysed). In severe cases, there is hypoxic injury to the heart and liver. Liver failure results in reduced production of albumin with consequent reduced oncotic pressure and thus oedema, ascites and pleural effusions, leading to the swollen appearance of the baby. The destruction of red cells produces high levels of circulating unconjugated bilirubin, which can deposit in and damage the brain, causing fits and death if untreated. As a reaction to the loss of red cells, a phenomenon known as extramedullary haemopoiesis (EMH) occurs. Bone marrow elements producing red cells, white cells and platelets are present in sites other than the medullary cavities of bones. In severe HDN, there are red cell precursors in the liver, spleen, skin and many other organs, in an attempt to maintain red cell numbers and circulating and tissue oxygen levels. Normally, EMH is only seen in the first and second trimester when the fetus cannot fully depend on bone marrow precursors for blood formation. Sites of EMH are mainly the liver, spleen and yolk sac. Some EMH is seen in full-term infants, but the bone marrow takes over soon after birth. Not all cases of HDN are caused by rhesus incompatibility. In fact, ABO incompatibility is more common but rarely causes clinical problems, partly because the antibodies are IgM and cannot cross the placenta. The routine administration of anti-D immunoglobulin to women soon after birth means that rhesus incompatibility is now an unusual clinical problem where this prophylaxis is available.

2. Rhesus incompatibility is an example of a type II hypersensitivity reaction. Other examples include incompatible blood transfusion reactions (blood group ABO antigens), Goodpasture's syndrome, and some autoimmune haemolytic anaemias.

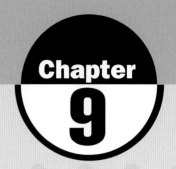

Inflammation

Chapter 9

Chapter overview

Inflammatory processes are part of the body's natural defence and repair mechanisms. However, their beneficial effects can be accompanied by significant tissue damage. Inflammation involves the coordination of many different functions by a wide variety of cells. Soluble molecules called inflammatory mediators (e.g. cytokines) are important in this process, as are cell–cell and cell–matrix interactions. To help conceptualise this complex web of activity, it is helpful to think about these processes as vascular events (changes in blood vessels) and cellular events (the activities of inflammatory cells).

9.1 General principles

Learning objectives

You should:
- define inflammation and state the four 'cardinal signs'
- recognise clinical features of inflammation and describe their pathogenesis
- use the suffix '-itis' to designate inflammation
- distinguish acute inflammation from chronic inflammation.

Inflammation is the local response to injury in living, vascularised tissues. Its purpose is to localise and eliminate the injurious agent, such as infecting organisms, and then, as far as possible, to restore the tissue to normal structure and function. However, inflammation may be seen as a two-edged sword. On the one hand, it has beneficial effects by localising and eliminating an injurious agent; on the other, the consequent tissue damage may be detrimental to the host. Inflamed tissues are named with the suffix '-itis'; thus appendicitis is inflammation of the appendix and hepatitis is inflammation of the liver.

Chemical inflammatory mediators

Chemical inflammatory mediators have an important role in orchestrating the inflammatory response. They are widely distributed throughout the body (Table 15). Some circulate as plasma proteins (the clotting factors, fibrinolytic factors, kinin system and complement proteins); the others are released, synthesised or activated locally. Inactivation occurs rapidly after release, which is important for the control and localisation of inflammation.

Clinical features of inflammation

There are four clinical features that have been known to be associated with inflammation since antiquity. They are known as the 'cardinal signs':

- redness (from dilatation of blood vessels)
- pain (from oedema and inflammatory mediators)
- heat (from vasodilatation)
- swelling (from oedema).

In addition, patients with inflammation frequently experience systemic effects due to circulating cytokines such as tumour necrosis factor alpha (TNF-α) and interleukin 1 (IL-1) released from the inflamed tissue. Malaise and loss of appetite are common, and fever is due to re-setting of the set-point of the thermostat in the hypothalamus to a higher temperature. The liver releases a variety of proteins called acute-phase reactants that can have a role in the inflammatory response, e.g. C-reactive protein and serum amyloid-A protein (SAA), which have antibacterial effects, and clotting factors such as fibrinogen. The numbers of circulating leucocytes increase as leucocytes are released from the bone marrow. When neutrophils are released from the bone marrow in this way, the proportion of less mature forms in the blood increases; haematologists describe this as a 'shift to the left' in neutrophil morphology. Weight loss is common in long-standing inflammation due to a negative nitrogen balance caused by a combination of increased metabolic activity and loss of appetite.

Acute inflammation

Acute inflammation is defined as the early inflammatory response to an injurious agent, and is characterised by the presence of neutrophil polymorphs and later macrophages. Acute inflammation usually lasts for a few hours or days.

Table 15 Chemical mediators involved in inflammation

Mediator	Common sources	Important functions
Histamine and serotonin	Mast cells and basophils, platelets	Vasodilatation and early increase in vascular permeability
Cytokines	Lymphocytes, macrophages, many other cells	Activation and modulation of inflammatory cell activity, chemotaxis of inflammatory cells (chemotactic cytokines are called chemokines)
Platelet activating factor (PAF)	Most white cells, vascular endothelium	Increases vascular permeability, increases adhesion of white cells to endothelium and induces platelet aggregation
Prostaglandins (PG) and PG-like substances	Mast cells, endothelium, platelets	PGE_2 causes pain, PGE_2 and PGI_2 cause vasodilatation, thromboxane A_2 (produced by platelets) causes vasoconstriction
Leukotrienes	Neutrophils	Neutrophil chemotaxis, increased vascular permeability, vasoconstriction
Nitric oxide	Vascular endothelium, macrophages	Vasodilatation, toxic to bacteria
Lysosomal compounds (proteases, acid hydrolases)	Neutrophils, macrophages	Increased vascular permeability, activation of complement, increased tissue damage
Coagulation factors	Plasma proteins	Thrombin activates many cells, including platelets, endothelial cells and smooth muscle cells; fibrin forms a clot-like mesh in the inflammatory exudate
Fibrinolytic system	Plasma proteins	Plasmin dissolves fibrin but also activates C3
Kinin system	Plasma proteins	Pain, vasodilatation, increased vascular permeability
Complement cascade	Plasma proteins	See Chapter 5

Causes of acute inflammation

- Microbial infections: the pyogenic bacteria and some fungi are particularly prone to cause acute inflammation
- Hypersensitivity reactions: types I–IV
- Physical agents: physical trauma, burns, UV light, radiation
- Chemicals: acids, alkalis, oxidising agents
- Tissue necrosis: e.g. infarction

The acute inflammatory response is characterised by increased blood flow, exudation of protein-rich fluid, and the accumulation of neutrophils (Figure 22). The mechanisms responsible are discussed later in this chapter. Within tissues, the exudate accumulates as oedema fluid, but exudate from inflamed serous membranes can accumulate in body cavities such as the pleural, pericardial and peritoneal cavities. The exudate contains large amounts of fibrin that can cause clots to form. Histologically, the presence of neutrophils is an important feature indicating the presence of acute inflammation to the pathologist.

Outcomes of acute inflammation

Healing by resolution

Acute inflammation may disappear after a few days and the tissue returns to normal. Fluid and degraded proteins are drained by the lymphatic channels and the exudate, cell debris and fibrin are removed by neutrophils and monocytes. To prevent further acute inflammation, the inflammatory cells are finally removed by apoptosis. The end result is that the tissue returns to normal and normal

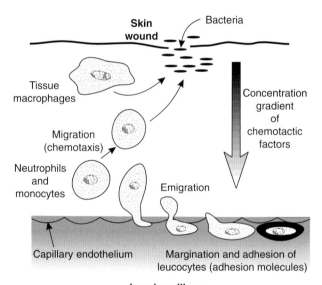

Figure 22 Acute inflammation.

anatomy is restored. Resolution is only possible if there is minimal destruction of the extracellular matrix and the tissue has cells capable of dividing by mitosis to replace cells lost in the inflammatory process.

Healing by fibrosis

This is the process of organisation by granulation tissue (see Ch. 10).

Progression to chronic inflammation

If the cause of the acute inflammation is not eliminated, the inflammatory process can become chronic.

Chronic inflammation

Chronic inflammation is an inflammatory response lasting more than a few days and is characterised by the presence of lymphocytes, plasma cells and macrophages. It is generally associated with significant tissue damage and so healing occurs by granulation tissue formation and fibrosis (see Ch. 10).

Clinically, chronic inflammation may occur as a result of:

- progression from acute inflammation due to persistence of the inflammatory stimulus, such as a foreign body or persistent microorganisms
- chronic inflammation ab initio (i.e. without preceding acute inflammation): typically seen as the response to intracellular organisms (e.g. mycobacteria, viruses), in many autoimmune diseases (e.g. rheumatoid arthritis, contact dermatitis), and in cases of chronic rejection of transplants.

9.2 Vascular events in inflammation

Learning objectives

You should:
- analyse inflammatory processes in terms of the vascular changes involved.

Vasodilatation

This occurs rapidly in the early acute inflammatory response and leads to increased blood flow into the damaged tissue. It is principally due to relaxation of arterioles.

Increased vascular permeability

Venules and capillaries are lined by a continuous layer of endothelium which keeps blood cells and large proteins within the vessel; water, oxygen and carbon dioxide pass freely through the vessel wall. In inflamed tissue, there is an increase in hydrostatic pressure due to the relaxation of arterioles. There is also an increase in the permeability ('leakiness') of the blood vessel to proteins, which can occur in a number of ways:

- gaps between endothelial cells induced by histamine, leukotrienes, etc.
- direct injury to the endothelial cells by the injurious agent (toxins, ischaemia, burns, etc.)
- increased transport of proteins across cell membranes stimulated by cytokines.

The increased intravascular hydrostatic pressure and increased permeability allow fluid and proteins to leak into the extracellular tissues. This protein-rich fluid is called exudate and is responsible for the oedema of inflammation. Within the dilated vascular beds, blood flow will slow dramatically as exudate is lost from the vascular space into tissues. Many of the proteins in the exudate are important in the inflammatory reaction, e.g. antibodies and acute-phase reactants.

9.3 Cellular processes of inflammation

Learning objectives

You should:
- name the principal inflammatory cells and give an account of their functions.
- analyse inflammatory processes in terms of the cellular processes involved.

Cells of the inflammatory response

Neutrophil polymorphs

Neutrophils are the first cells to appear at the site of acute inflammation. They are phagocytes, and their function is to degrade cell debris and to ingest and kill microbes. Neutrophils originate in the bone marrow and have a short tissue lifespan of only 3–4 days.

They kill microorganisms by two main mechanisms: digestive enzymes in lysosomes and oxygen-dependent production of free radicals (see Box 12 and Figure 23). Neutrophils are an important component of pus (Box 13).

Eosinophils

These phagocytic cells originate in the bone marrow and have striking red/pink intracytoplasmic granules when

---

Box 12 Microbial killing by phagocytes

Neutrophils and macrophages both kill microorganisms by two main methods:

- Their lysosomes contain bactericidal intracellular enzymes:
  - myeloperoxidase
  - lysozyme
  - acid hydrolase.

The lysosomes fuse with the vacuole containing the ingested material, releasing the enzymes which can destroy the contents. The resulting structure is called a phagolysosome.

- Highly reactive oxygen species and other free radicals that are toxic to microorganisms are produced in the wall of the phagolysosome. This process requires a burst of oxidative phosphorylation, and so it is called the oxygen-dependent mechanism.

Neutrophils, macrophages and eosinophils can all release their antimicrobial products into the extracellular space. This process occurs if the antigen cannot be ingested. Although of potential benefit, for example by attacking parasites that are too big for phagocytosis, there is also the potential for considerable damage to adjacent tissues.

Nine

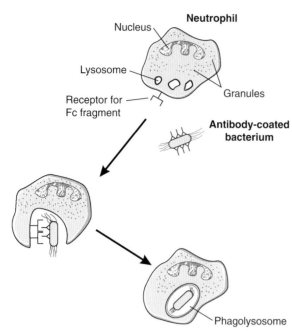

Nucleus

Lysosome

Receptor for
Fc fragment

Neutrophil

Granules

**Antibody-coated
bacterium**

Phagolysosome

Figure 23 Phagocytosis: phagocytic cells ingest cell debris and microbes, which are digested in vacuoles by lysosomal enzymes.

Box 13 Pus

Pus is thick, sticky fluid, white, yellow or greenish, formed from neutrophils (both alive and dead), cell debris from necrotic tissue, bacteria (both alive and dead) and inflammatory fluid exudate. Although it occurs under a wide variety of different circumstances, it is particularly characteristic of inflammation caused by pyogenic bacteria (see Glossary). Inflammation characterised by pus is called suppurative inflammation.

A collection of pus within the tissues is called an abscess. Unless drained, abscesses become surrounded by granulation tissue and fibrosis. The pressure inside abscesses tends to increase due to osmotic influx of water into the abscess cavity from the surrounding tissues. Abscesses may discharge their contents via a sinus tract, which is defined as an abnormal connection, lined by granulation tissue or epithelium, connecting an abscess with a mucosal surface or the skin. Sometimes, this process leads to an abnormal passage between two mucosal surfaces or a mucosal surface and the skin, called a fistula. If pus accumulates in a pre-existing body cavity, e.g. the gall bladder or pleural cavity, the term empyema is used.

---

visualised using a haematoxylin and eosin stain. They are associated with type I hypersensitivity responses and parasitic infestations. Their granules contain substances such as major basic protein which are toxic to parasites. Large numbers of eosinophils may alert the pathologist to the possibility of an allergic reaction or the presence of a parasite.

Basophils and mast cells

Mast cells have cytoplasmic granules which contain heparin and histamine and enzymes such as tryptase and acid hydrolase. They release these substances rapidly by degranulation in response to a variety of stimuli. An important cause of mast cell degranulation is the type I hypersensitivity reaction mediated by IgE. They have IgE Fc receptors on their cell membranes, and binding of IgE to the Fc receptors leads to release of the granule contents into the tissues. Other causes of degranulation include physical agents (heat, cold, trauma), various cytokines, and complement components C3a and C5a.

Basophils resemble mast cells but are found circulating in the blood rather than in tissues.

Macrophages

Macrophages are the major scavenger cells of the body. They are derived from blood monocytes and are attracted to sites of inflammation by chemotactic factors, appearing 12–24 hours later than neutrophils. A term sometimes used for macrophages by pathologists is 'histiocytes'. Macrophages are long-lived phagocytic cells and contain powerful intracellular enzymes which degrade particulate matter including dead neutrophils and microorganisms (see Box 12 and Figure 23). In addition to their phagocytic function they orchestrate many of the cellular, vascular and reparative responses of inflammation by releasing cytokines (e.g. interleukins, interferons, TNF-α, transforming growth factor beta (TGF-β) and neutrophil chemotactic factor). They also produce coagulation factors such as factor VIII. The role of macrophages in antigen presentation is discussed in Chapters 7 and 8.

Lymphocytes and plasma cells

These cells are seen in a wide variety of different inflammatory reactions. They are discussed in Chapters 7 and 8.

Recruitment of inflammatory cells to sites of inflammation

The recruitment of inflammatory cells involves a number of steps, all of which are controlled by a variety of mechanisms. The overall process is called extravasation or emigration.

Margination

In inflammation, blood flow slows as vessels dilate and fluid enters the interstitium, as described previously. Consequently, leucocytes move out of the central (axial) column of blood, where they usually flow, and accumulate at the periphery of the vessels, where they can interact with endothelial cells. This process, the first step in extravasation, is called margination and occurs particularly in the post-capillary venules.

Rolling and adhesion

Both endothelial cells and leucocytes can display a number of cell adhesion molecules on their surface membranes. In inflammation, under the influence of cytokines, cell adhesion molecules are up-regulated. For example, vascular endothelial cells can display adhesion molecules which will bind to neutrophils and monocytes; some are already present within the endothelial cell and are redistributed to the surface, others are newly produced. The neutrophils and monocytes also have surface adhesion molecules (integrins) that can bind to their ligands on the endothelial surface.

The interactions between leucocytes and endothelial cells result in the former rolling along the endothelial surface. Finally, the leucocytes become firmly stuck (adhesion; see Box 14).

Emigration

The leucocytes are able to move into the tissues through the endothelium, mainly by passing between endothelial cells and then degrading the basement membrane with collagenases. This process is called emigration. The cells move in an amoeboid fashion.

Chemotaxis

After extravasation, the leucocytes are attracted by substances produced in the inflamed tissue. To be precise, the leucocytes move through the tissues along a concentration gradient (chemotaxis), serving to bring them to the site of inflammation. Substances that may be chemotactic for leucocytes include bacterial products, complement components (especially C5a) and cytokines.

Box 14 Cell adhesion molecules

Interactions between different cells and between cells and connective tissue are mediated by cell adhesion molecules, which are transmembrane molecules with extracellular and intracellular domains. The latter may attach to the cytoskeleton. The interactions are essentially those of receptor and ligand, i.e. they link to one another in a similar manner to a lock and key. Cell adhesion molecules are involved in a wide variety of cellular processes. In normal tissues, they are the mechanism whereby cells adhere to each other and the interstitial matrix. Furthermore, this binding is not simply a passive process – the intracellular domain can act a the first step in a signal transduction sequence. Thus, the differentiation of a cell depends in part on the nature of the underlying matrix. When cells move through tissues (whether during tissue remodelling or inflammation), cell adhesion molecules are involved. Malignant cells show abnormalities of cell adhesion molecule expression, allowing them to detach from adjacent cells and then move abnormally through the tissues (i.e. invade). In addition, cell adhesion molecules can be a component of immune reactions.

Nine

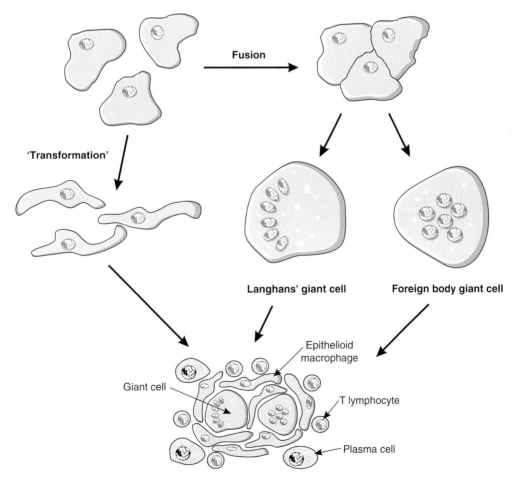

Langhans' giant cell

Foreign body giant cell

Epithelioid macrophage

Giant cell

T lymphocyte

Plasma cell

Epithelioid granuloma

Figure 24 Giant cells and the granuloma.

Red cell extravasation

In severe inflammation, red blood cells pass passively through damaged endothelium into the tissues, where they are eventually broken down. Their iron may accumulate as haemosiderin in the inflamed tissues.

9.4 Granulomatous inflammation

Learning objectives

You should:
- state the characteristics of epithelioid cells and giant cells
- define granuloma and state the significance of granulomatous inflammation.

Under some circumstances, macrophages may transform into epithelioid macrophages or fuse to form giant cells. Epithelioid macrophages have developed into cells that specialise in secreting cytokines and other products; they have a secretory morphology, i.e. abundant ribosomes and endoplasmic reticulum, and only limited phagocytic capabilities. Giant cells are large multinucleated cells, sometimes with dozens of nuclei. They form when multiple macrophages attempt to engulf indigestible material such as foreign substances or certain microorganisms, and the macrophages fuse together producing a multinucleated giant cell. Giant cells in which the nuclei are arranged in a peripheral rim are known as Langhans' giant cells; they are often (though not always) associated with tuberculosis.

A granuloma is an aggregate of epithelioid macrophages, often with giant cells as well. Thus, granulomatous inflammation is a special type of chronic inflammation in which granulomas are present (Figure 24). The identification of granulomas in a specimen may suggest the diagnosis of one of the specific causes of granulomatous inflammation, for example:

- indigestible organisms, e.g. mycobacteria, some fungi, parasites
- exogenous foreign materials, e.g. silica, talc, suture material, beryllium
- endogenous foreign materials, e.g. cholesterol crystals, uric acid crystals, free keratin
- unknown mechanisms, as seen in conditions such as rheumatoid arthritis, Crohn's disease and sarcoidosis.

The presence of caseating necrosis in the centre of a granuloma is particularly associated with mycobacterial infection (see Ch. 4). Note that granulation tissue is different from a granuloma – the two are sometimes confused by students.

Self-assessment: questions

One best answer questions

1. Which one of the following substances in the inflammatory exudate is a substrate for thrombin?

   a. arachidonic acid

   b. fibrinogen

   c. kallikrein

   d. PGE$_2$

   e. serotonin

2. Which of the following is *not* a 'cardinal sign' of inflammation?

   a. atrophy

   b. heat

   c. pain

   d. redness

   e. swelling

3. A 46-year-old man presents with a painful nodule on the skin of his neck. The nodule is inflamed and tender. When incised, it drains sticky yellow fluid that contains large numbers of neutrophils. Which organism is most likely to be responsible?

   a. *Clostridium perfringens*

   b. Guinea worm (*Dracunculus medinensis*)

   c. Louse (*Pediculus* sp.)

   d. *Mycobacterium tuberculosis*

   e. *Staphylococcus aureus*

4. Which of the following cells is specific for acute inflammation when observed in tissue sections?

   a. eosinophil

   b. myofibroblast

   c. neutrophil

   d. plasma cell

   e. T lymphocyte

True-false questions

1. During the acute inflammatory response:

   a. histamine causes vasodilatation

   b. the exuded fibrin is formed by local fibroblasts

   c. there is upregulation of cell adhesion molecules on endothelial cells

   d. red cell extravasation is a passive phenomenon

   e. complement components may act as chemoattractants

2. The following are correctly paired:

   a. granulomatous inflammation – *Mycobacterium tuberculosis*

   b. plasma cells – phagocytosis

   c. pus – collection of neutrophils

   d. eosinophils – parasitic infection

   e. Langerhans' cells – *Mycobacterium tuberculosis*

Extended matching items questions (EMIs)

EMI 1

Theme: Inflammatory mediators

A. C-reactive protein

B. histamine

C. immunoglobulin

D. IL-1

E. neutrophil acid hydrolase

F. nitric oxide

For each of the following, select the most appropriate response from the list:

1. An acute-phase reactant.

2. A cytokine.

3. A principal product of mast cells.

Case history questions

Case history 1

A 10-year-old girl is admitted to hospital with a 3-day history of right iliac fossa pain and fever. On examination there is severe abdominal tenderness. Appendicectomy is performed. At operation, the tip of the appendix is swollen and the serosal surface covered in a purulent exudate.

1. State the most likely diagnosis.

2. The appendix is submitted to the histopathology laboratory for examination. What are the likely histological features of the tip of the appendix?

3. Explain the likely pathogenesis of the raised temperature.

4. What are the possible outcomes of acute appendicitis?

5. What is the difference between an exudate and a transudate?

Case history 2

A 63-year-old man has part of his large bowel removed through an abdominal incision. Five days after operation, the wound is red, hot and painful and pus is seen coming out from one end.

1. Briefly describe the likely pathogenesis.

2. The patient's doctor wishes to identify the organism responsible. What sample should be taken and where should it be sent?

After appropriate treatment, the wound heals and a scar forms. However, a small, firm area within the scar causes the man some discomfort and this is removed about 2 years after his original operation. The histology report states 'a foreign body giant cell reaction to suture (stitch) material is present'.

3. What is the nature of the giant cells in this case?

4. Name three other types of pathological giant cell and briefly state their main characteristics.

Self-assessment: answers

One best answer

1. **b.** The inflammatory exudate is rich in fibrinogen (an acute-phase reactant), which becomes converted to a fibrin meshwork by thrombin. This inhibits the movement of organisms and gives phagocytes a supporting structure.

2. **a.** It is worth knowing the cardinal signs, if only because they are a favoured question for medical students!

3. **e.** The clinical description is of a skin abscess called a boil; the fluid that was drained was pus. Such lesions are typically due to pyogenic organisms such as *Staph. aureus*. These organisms cause suppurative inflammation. Pus may form diffusely in tissue planes, or collect in discrete foci that may become walled-off by fibrin, granulation tissue and eventually fibrous scarring (i.e. an abscess). An abscess wall effectively isolates the infected locus, but this can prevent the body's inflammatory cells reaching it and also prevent antibiotics from being effective. This is why surgical intervention to drain the abscess is the most effective treatment. In this case, incision and drainage (sometimes called lancing the boil) was performed. *Clostridium perfringens* causes gas gangrene (see Ch. 4) and not discrete abscesses. Guinea worm is a parasite, so eosinophil-rich inflammation would be expected rather than an abscess (unless there is secondary infection with a skin organism such as *Staph. aureus*). Lice cause an itchy rash, although they may also be a vector for various systemic infections such as typhus. Mycobacteria cause caseous inflammation, not suppuration.

4. **c.** Neutrophils characterise acute inflammation. Plasma cells, lymphocytes and eosinophils are found in chronic inflammatory reactions (although some neutrophils may be present also).

True-false answers

1. a. **True.** Histamine is a vasoactive amine secreted by mast cells. It acts via receptors on post-capillary venules during the early phase of acute inflammation to increase permeability of the vessel.

   b. **False.** This is a common examiner's trick. Fibroblasts secrete procollagen, which is converted to collagen outside the cell. In fact no cells produce fibrin; fibrin is derived from fibrinogen, a hepatocyte-derived clotting factor.

   c. **True.** Upregulation of adhesion molecules promotes adherence by circulating neutrophils.

   d. **True.** Whereas the process of inflammatory cell emigration is an active, 'purposeful' phenomenon, red cells leave the vessel as a result of the combined effects of raised intravascular hydrostatic pressure and vascular leakiness. This passive emigration of red cells is called diapedesis.

   e. **True.** Chemotaxis is the unidirectional, purposeful flow of neutrophils or macrophages towards a chemoattractant. The cells typically have receptors for the molecule on their surfaces. Components of the complement pathway such as C5a can attract inflammatory cells such as neutrophils into the inflamed area.

2. a. **True.** Tuberculosis is a classic example of a chronic granulomatous inflammatory disease.

   b. **False.** Phagocytosis is the process by which neutrophils and macrophages engulf and then dispose of particulate material. Plasma cells have no such ability; their function is to produce antibody.

   c. **True.** Pus is a collection of viable and dead or dying neutrophils, admixed with exudate and the non-viable tissue in which the acute inflammatory reaction has occurred.

   d. **True.** Eosinophils are often the dominant inflammatory cell involved in parasitic infections. Eosinophil products make the microenvironment around the parasites unsuitable for their continuing survival.

   e. **False.** This is a common misconception. The giant cells in a tuberculosis granuloma are known as Langhans' giant cells *not* Langerhans' cells, which are dendritic antigen-presenting cells in the epidermis.

EMI answers

EMI 1

Theme: Inflammatory mediators

1. **A.** C-reactive protein is one of the acute-phase proteins released from the liver as part of the systemic inflammatory response. Its function seems to be to act as an opsonin, promoting phagocytosis of bacteria.

2. **D.** IL-1 is an important cytokine with local and systemic effects. A useful way of thinking about cytokines is to divide them into pro-inflammatory cytokines that upregulate inflammatory responses, and anti-inflammatory cytokines that inhibit inflammation and damp down the process. IL-1 is a pro-inflammatory cytokine (others are TNF-α, IL-2 and IL-6). Anti-inflammatory cytokines include IL-4, IL-10 and TGF-β.

3. B. Histamine is stored in mast cell granules, ready for instant action when released on degranulation.

Case history answers

Case history 1

1. Acute appendicitis.

2. Likely findings include: infiltration of the wall by neutrophils, oedema, and congestion and dilatation of vessels. The exudate of the outer surface (peritoneum) will be characterised by pus and fibrin deposition (a fibrinopurulent exudate). Other possible findings include small aggregates of neutrophils (micro-abscesses), pus in the appendiceal lumen, and ulceration of mucosa. In severe cases, there is necrosis of the wall, producing gangrenous appendicitis.

3. In general, chemicals that cause a rise in body temperature are called pyrogens. They act on the hypothalamus to raise the set-point of the temperature receptors, which has the same effect as raising the setting on a thermostat. The temperature control mechanisms of the body act to raise the core temperature until the new set-point is reached. Pyrogens produced by inflammatory tissues include IL-1 and TNF-α.

4. Mild inflammation could heal by resolution, provided that there is minimal damage to the interstitial matrix. More severe damage could cause healing by fibrosis producing scarring. Persistence of the cause of the inflammation could result in the development of chronic inflammation, although this is unusual in the appendix and tends to be associated with specific infections such as yersiniosis. Gangrenous appendicitis is associated with weakening of the appendiceal wall; rupture may occur with the spread of infection into the peritoneal cavity. This can result in a periappendiceal abscess formed by omentum and other periappendiceal tissues, or occasionally diffuse peritonitis. These conditions can lead to septicaemia. Occasionally, a fistula between the appendix and an adjacent organ can form. A rare complication is spread along the portal vein to produce a hepatic abscess.

5. Inflammatory exudates result from the process of increased vascular permeability where plasma proteins and inflammatory cells move out into the injured tissues. In contrast, a transudate is composed of oedema fluid which leaks out of capillaries as a result of an increase in hydrostatic pressure relative to oncotic pressure; there is no increase in the permeability of the capillary to proteins. Therefore, transudates are low in protein, whereas exudates are protein-rich.

Case history 2

1. The patient's wound site exhibits features of inflammation with pus formation. The probable cause is acute suppurative inflammation due to infection of the wound. The causative bacteria could derive from the skin or bowel.

2. Swabs of the pus and wound edges should be taken and submitted to the microbiology laboratory for microscopy and culture.

3. Foreign body giant cells are derived from macrophages. They have multiple nuclei and contain indigestible foreign material in their cytoplasm.

4. • Langhans' giant cells: often found in granulomas; have nuclei disposed in a rim (Figure 24).
   • Touton giant cells: found in lipid-containing lesions such as xanthelasma and areas of fat necrosis; they have a central, ring-like arrangement of nuclei and peripheral fat droplets in their cytoplasm.
   • Multinucleated tumour giant cell: seen in some neoplasms.

Comment: You might have thought of other types of giant cell, but note that not all large, multinucleated cells are pathological: examples include bone-resorbing osteoclasts and platelet-producing megakaryocytes.

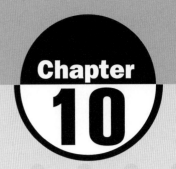
Healing and repair

Chapter overview

Healing is the replacement of dead or injured tissue by healthy tissue; this can be accomplished either by regeneration, when the damage is mild and cells can multiply to replace lost tissue, or by repair, which involves the formation of granulation tissue and then a scar. Repair occurs if there is extensive tissue injury or in permanent cell populations.

10.1 The healing process

Learning objectives

You should:
- distinguish regeneration from repair
- state the components of granulation tissue and describe its production
- describe the healing process in skin and in bone
- state the consequences of fibrosis.

Healing is a general term for the processes involved in the replacement of dead and injured tissue by healthy tissue. Regeneration and repair are the two mechanisms whereby this is accomplished. Regeneration is the replacement of dead cells by an exactly similar cell population, so that the anatomy returns to normal. In contrast, repair involves the production of scar tissue to replace dead cells.

For regeneration to occur two conditions must be fulfilled. First, there must be little or no disruption to the intercellular matrix, because the matrix provides the 'scaffolding' for new cells. Second, the damage must involve cell populations capable of dividing (i.e. labile or stable cell populations). Repair by scar tissue formation occurs if:

- there is significant disruption of the connective tissue matrix
- cells cannot divide to replace lost cells (this occurs in permanent cell populations such as the heart).

When does healing occur?

Healing occurs in damaged tissues. It begins early in the inflammatory reaction, when phagocytes clear dead cells and other debris. If the injury is mild then healing may take place by regeneration; there is replacement of injured tissue with cells of the same type and normal anatomy is restored, leaving no trace of damage. An example is resolution following lobar pneumonia; there is acute inflammation associated with extensive loss of alveolar cells, but there is typically no significant destruction of lung tissue matrix and thus healing by regeneration can take place.

If regeneration is not possible, there is repair by granulation tissue formation and subsequent fibrosis (scarring). This results in loss of specialised cells and hence loss of function. The anatomy is altered, although structural integrity is preserved.

Skin healing has been extensively studied and much of our understanding of the healing process comes from observation of surgical skin wounds. The central pathological process in healing by repair is the formation of granulation tissue.

What is granulation tissue?

This bright pink, granular tissue is seen, for example, in the base of a healing skin wound, and denotes the process of repair. Granulation tissue is composed of:

- small blood vessels (capillary-sized channels)
- proliferating fibroblasts and myofibroblasts
- inflammatory cells.

The development of new blood vessels is called angiogenesis or neovascularisation. Endothelial cells initially form solid cords, but they soon open into capillary loops at the edges of the lesion accompanied by new lymphatic channels. The endothelial cells derive firstly from sprouts produced by adjacent capillaries and secondly from endothelial precursor cells (EPCs) produced in the bone marrow. EPCs are mobilised from the marrow and circulate to the site of injury where they migrate into the tissues. New arterioles and venules are formed as the proliferating capillaries become surrounded by pericytes and smooth muscle cells.

Fibroblasts migrate to the area and produce collagen and other components of the extracellular matrix, such as fibronectin and proteoglycans. Type III collagen tends to be produced first; it is gradually replaced by type I collagen, which is stronger. Many fibroblasts also have significant contractile abilities due to the presence of muscle-type intracytoplasmic filaments; such cells are called myofibroblasts and contract to reduce the wound size. Consequently, the volume of a scar is generally less than the volume of the original tissue damage.

Granulation tissue also contains a variety of inflammatory cells, the types and proportions of which depend on the cause of the tissue damage. For example, granulation tissue surrounding an abscess is rich in neutrophils.

The transformation of necrotic material or fibrin to a fibrous scar by granulation tissue is called **organisation**. The granulation tissue grows into the dead tissue and eventually replaces it.

The cellular events in healing are orchestrated by a large number of cytokines. For example, epidermal growth factor (EGF), produced by epidermal cells around the damaged area, is important in stimulating regeneration of epithelial cells. Neovascularisation is triggered by fibroblast growth factor (FGF) and various endothelial growth factors, which are produced by macrophages. FGF and transforming growth factor beta (TGF-β), again derived from macrophages, and platelet-derived growth factor (PDGF) from platelets in the clot in the wound, are important mediators of fibroblast activity.

Scarring

Over the course of a few weeks granulation tissue matures into a scar. This process is called **fibrosis**. The inflammatory cells gradually disappear and the amount of collagen in the matrix increases, with type III collagen being replaced by type I. The new blood vessels are remodelled and the (myo)fibroblasts reduce in number. The final result is a mature scar mainly composed of collagen-rich matrix and scattered residual fibroblasts supplied by a new circulation. After the scar has formed, its strength increases over subsequent months through increased cross-linking of collagen and increased collagen fibre diameter. The collagen fibres also align themselves along lines of stress. This remodelling of the scar requires the production of metalloproteinases, a family of enzymes that degrade collagen, by fibroblasts and other cells such as macrophages.

Scarring provides benefit by restoring the integrity of the damaged tissue but it may have significant complications. Scar tissue tends to contract with time and will not function in the same way as the original tissue. Examples of consequences arising from fibrosis include:

- cosmetic problems produced by unsightly scar tissue
- skin contractures following severe burns that can limit movement
- obstruction of tubular structures due to fibrous narrowing (stricture formation), e.g. duodenal obstruction following healing of a peptic ulcer
- heart failure due to impaired left ventricular function following myocardial infarction and scarring
- adhesion formation – adhesions are scars that stick serosal surfaces together; they can follow organisation of fibrinous exudates in serosal cavities (occasionally, peritoneal adhesions can cause bowel obstruction).

Examples of types of tissue healing

Skin wound healing

There are two pathways by which skin wounds are repaired, named primary and secondary union. Similar principles apply elsewhere in the body. A simple incised surgical wound will heal by primary union (also called healing by primary intention). This means that the clean edges of a wound once placed together (apposed) will heal quickly with minimal granulation tissue formation and thus minimal scarring (Figure 25A). There are several stages:

1. Blood escapes from damaged vessels and fills the gap.
2. Fibrin clot binds the edges together loosely and dries on the surface, forming a scab.
3. An acute inflammatory reaction develops around the wound in 24 hours and the exudate adds more fibrin, polymorphs and macrophages to the wound. These produce lytic enzymes which start to digest any clot and remove any debris from the wound site.
4. Epithelial cells start to regenerate and bridge the gap within 48 hours.
5. Fibrin in the wound provides stability so that blood vessels can regrow. Only a small amount of granulation tissue forms and the final scar will be thin and inconspicuous.

If the wound is large and gaping, infected, or there is substantial tissue loss, e.g. a large burn or ulcer, then

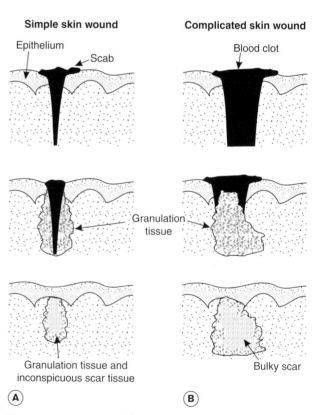

Figure 25 Wound healing. (A) Healing by primary intention. (B) Healing by secondary intention.

healing by secondary union (secondary intention) takes place (Figure 25B). Granulation tissue forms at the base of the wound and fills it up. Epithelial cells can then regenerate over this 'bridge'. Fibroblasts migrate into the wound and, by about day 4, begin producing type III collagen, which has a relatively low tensile strength but forms a scaffolding for other cells. Later, the stronger type I collagen is the dominant form. The resulting scar is broad and conspicuous since a large amount of granulation tissue was formed.

Bone fracture healing

When a bone breaks, haematoma (blood clot) forms around the broken ends of the bone. Healing occurs through organisation of this haematoma by granulation tissue. However, this process is modified because the granulation tissue contains proliferating cells derived from the periosteum and endosteum which differentiate into chondroblasts and osteoblasts that lay down new cartilage and immature (woven) bone. The result is hard tissue called callus surrounding and joining the broken ends of the bone. Bony union occurs when new bone produced in the callus links the bone fragments together. The cartilage and woven bone are gradually replaced by lamellar bone (the type found in mature bone). This new bone can be remodelled so that the anatomy can return close to normal. However, the fractured bone fragments must be aligned and placed together (apposed) for optimum healing to occur, otherwise the callus may not adequately bridge the gap between them, resulting in permanent deformity.

Note that normal fracture healing does not result in a fibrous scar, because of the modified nature of the granulation tissue.

Gastrointestinal tract

An ulcer is a defect in an epithelial surface. In the gastrointestinal tract, an ulcer confined to the mucosa is often called an erosion; such lesions can heal by regeneration. In contrast, an ulcer that extends beyond the mucosa will heal by granulation tissue formation and scarring with re-epithelialisation of the surface.

10.2 Factors affecting wound healing

> **Learning objectives**
>
> You should:
> * identify local and general factors that adversely affect healing.

Ideally, healing occurs quickly with resolution or the formation of a strong scar. However, a variety of factors will adversely affect this process.

Local factors

Tissue apposition

The edges of a wound or a broken bone need to be closely aligned for healing to be most effective. Otherwise, large amounts of granulation tissue are required to bridge the gap.

Infection

An infected wound or tissue will take longer to heal because the persistent inflammation associated with host defence will prevent regeneration and inhibit scar formation.

Dead tissue

This must be removed surgically (debridement) or naturally by phagocytosis (macrophages, neutrophils) before healing can be completed. Persistence of necrotic tissue inhibits healing.

Blood supply

Ischaemic tissues do not heal properly because blood brings the cells involved in healing to the site and provides oxygen for their high metabolic demands.

Foreign body

A foreign body, whether introduced accidentally at the time of injury or a prosthesis introduced surgically, can have an adverse effect on healing. In part, this is because the foreign object acts as a 'sanctuary site' where bacteria can grow partially protected from the host defence mechanisms.

General factors

Diet

An adequate diet is important to ensure healing processes can occur. For example, vitamin C deficiency (scurvy) leads to inadequate collagen formation and poor healing. Generalised starvation/malnutrition is associated with lack of dietary proteins and depression of immunity, causing poor wound healing.

Therapy

Many modern therapeutic treatments may adversely affect a particular stage of the healing process. Steroids inhibit the growth of new blood vessels and many macrophage functions. Immunosuppressive drugs prevent the natural immune response involved in healing. Many anti-cancer drugs inhibit stages in the cell cycle or kill cells involved in active proliferation – healing can be profoundly affected because it involves the multiplication of many different cells. Likewise, radiotherapy also destroys actively dividing cells.

Blood supply

Blood brings many of the vital ingredients of the healing process, e.g. inflammatory cells and EPCs, immunoglobulins and acute phase proteins, and oxygen and nutrients. Tissue that has a poor blood supply tends to heal poorly. Thus, severe atherosclerosis leads to an inadequate blood supply to wounded tissues (commonly seen in the distal lower limb), and heart failure can cause generalised poor perfusion.

Systemic disease

Many systemic diseases have secondary effects that adversely affect healing and repair. The immune system may be depressed by acquired disease processes such as acquired immune deficiency syndrome (AIDS), haematological malignancies, malnutrition and extremes of age, or by inherited abnormalities of the immune system. In Cushing's syndrome, excessive amounts of endogenous cortisone are produced and have a similar effect to steroid therapy on repair processes. Diabetes mellitus is also associated with poor healing.

Self-assessment: questions

One best answer questions

1. Which one of the following represents an essential component of granulation tissue?
   a. epithelioid macrophages and giant cells
   b. epithelial cells
   c. fibroblasts and endothelial cells
   d. lymphocytes and plasma cells
   e. mast cells and basophils

2. In which of the following circumstances is healing by resolution most likely?
   a. a 10 cm diameter full-thickness burn to the forearm
   b. a 5 cm ulcer of the ankle in a diabetic person
   c. myocardial infarction of the lateral wall of the left ventricle
   d. lobar pneumonia with consolidation of the left lower lobe
   e. a 3 cm diameter chronic abscess of the liver

3. Endothelial precursor cells are mainly produced in the:
   a. bone marrow
   b. liver
   c. lung
   d. skin
   e. thymus

4. A patient has skin damage due to trauma that heals by fibrosis. Which of the following is mainly responsible for contraction of the wound?
   a. endothelial cells
   b. fibroblasts
   c. macrophages
   d. myofibroblasts
   e. smooth muscle cells

5. A mature scar differs from granulation tissue in that it has more:
   a. blood vessels
   b. crossed-linked collagen
   c. fibroblasts
   d. inflammatory cells
   e. type III collagen

True-false questions

1. A deficiency of the following is known to impair wound healing:
   a. vitamin C
   b. lead
   c. vitamin B$_{12}$
   d. zinc
   e. corticosteroids

2. The following are characteristic of healing by primary union (healing by first intention) in the skin:
   a. large amounts of granulation tissue
   b. close apposition of skin edges
   c. relatively inconspicuous scarring
   d. production of type I and type III collagen
   e. proliferation of epidermal cells

Case history questions

Case history 1

A 37-year-old fireman suffers full-thickness burns to the skin of his hands, face and neck during the course of his duties.

1. What is a full-thickness skin burn and how might it heal?

Two weeks later, one of the burns is inflamed and exuding pus. A wound swab grows *Staphylococcus aureus*.

2. Will the presence of *Staph. aureus* have any effect on healing? Explain your answer.

Six months after this episode, he develops pain in his neck at the site of the burn scar. The scar and skin around it appear twisted and distorted.

3. What complication has occurred?

Case history 2

An 89-year-old woman falls in the street and suffers a compound fracture of her lower right forearm. She takes tolbutamide for diabetes and prednisolone for temporal arteritis. She is otherwise in good general health, although she takes vitamin C supplements she buys from the supermarket.

1. Identify local and systemic factors in the above vignette that might inhibit healing of the fracture.

The woman is treated with antibiotics and the fracture is surgically immobilised with the bone ends in close apposition.

2. Describe the stages of healing in fractures of this type.

Self-assessment: answers

One best answer

1. c. Although all these cells may be involved in healing and thus be found in granulation tissue, only fibroblasts and endothelial cells are essential components. Note that epithelioid macrophages and macrophage-derived giant cells are components of granulomas, not granulation tissue. This is a common exam 'catch'.

2. d. Lobar pneumonia typically resolves, unless there are complications that damage the alveolar walls. The burn, ankle ulcer and chronic abscess will be associated with severe tissue destruction, precluding healing by resolution. The myocardial infarct (no matter what its size) will not resolve either, because adult heart muscle cells do not regenerate. These conditions will heal by granulation tissue formation and fibrosis.

3. a. EPCs are produced in the bone marrow and circulate to sites of injury where they participate in angiogenesis.

4. d. Myofibroblasts have contractile filaments in their cytoplasm and are an important component of granulation tissue.

5. b. A mature scar is characterised by a predominance of type I collagen that shows increasing cross-linking as it remodels. The numbers of cells and blood vessels diminish as granulation tissue turns into a scar.

True-false answers

1. a. **True.** Vitamin C is required as a co-factor in collagen synthesis. A deficiency of this vitamin leads to scurvy.

   b. **False.** Lead is poisonous and even in small amounts is detrimental to humans.

   c. **False.** Vitamin B_{12} deficiency causes a macrocytic megaloblastic anaemia.

   d. **True.** Zinc, like vitamin C, is required for normal collagen synthesis. Zinc supplements can improve wound healing in zinc-deficient patients.

   e. **False.** It is an excess of corticosteroids that hinders wound healing. This is a side effect of steroid therapy, and is also seen in Cushing's syndrome.

2. a. **False.** Primary union involves minimal granulation tissue.

   b. **True.** Unless the skin edges are brought together, primary union cannot occur.

   c. **True.** In contrast, secondary union produces relatively large amounts of scar tissue.

   d. **True.** All healing by repair involves collagen production – type III predominates early in the process, type I later.

   e. **True.** Epidermal cells multiply and spread over the top of the defect. In primary union, this only takes a few days, whereas in secondary union it may take weeks or months, depending on the size of the defect and whether factors inhibiting healing are present.

Case history answers

Case history 1

1. A full-thickness burn extends deeper than the dermis, i.e. it involves subcutaneous tissue. Granulation tissue will form in the exposed subcutaneous tissue. Because the epithelial cells of the skin have all been destroyed, re-epithelialisation of the surface will take place from the edges of the burn where viable skin remains; this process may take a long time (hence, skin grafts are often used to treat burns of this sort).

2. The presence of infection in this case may delay healing, because infection inhibits the healing process. In addition, there may be larger amounts of granulation tissue production as a result of continuing tissue damage, so the final scar may be larger.

3. The scar has contracted (largely as a result of the contractile properties of myofibroblasts) causing the distortion. This phenomenon of distorted contraction of a scar is known as cicatrisation or contracture formation, and is particularly common in large, full-thickness burns.

Case history 2

1. Local and systemic factors in the above vignette that might inhibit healing of the fracture are:

   • Age – as an elderly person, her immune and healing responses may be diminished.

   • Compound fracture (i.e. there is a breach in the overlying skin) – may allow infection or foreign bodies into the fracture site.

   • Diabetes – inhibits the immune response. It also causes atherosclerosis and microangiopathy (see chapter on diabetes) that could cause poor blood supply, although this is more commonly a problem in the lower limbs.

   • Steroid therapy – inhibits healing through its effects on macrophage function and endothelial cell regeneration.

Comment: Note that the vitamin C will not have a deleterious effect – it is *lack* of vitamin C that is associated with poor healing.

2. In the few hours after the fracture, blood forms a haematoma at the fracture site. Within 1–2 days, neutrophils and macrophages begin to digest the haematoma. At around day 3, granulation tissue forms and begins to organise the haematoma. This granulation tissue also contains chondroblasts and osteoblasts that produce cartilage and woven bone.

In 1–2 weeks this modified granulation tissue becomes hard as the cartilage and bone are calcified, producing callus that seals the bone ends. The bone is remodelled over the subsequent weeks, until eventually the fractured fragments are linked by lamellar bone. Remodelling continues for several months: the strength of the bone increases, the cortex reappears and the contour of the bone approaches normal.

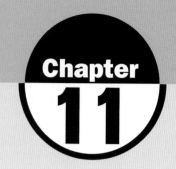

Neoplasia: general characteristics and carcinogenesis

Chapter 11

Chapter overview

Neoplasia is abnormal cell growth that does not respond normally to factors controlling growth and differentiation. It is due to genetic abnormalities in the neoplastic cells. The cells form masses (neoplasms or tumours) that may remain confined to the tissue of origin (benign neoplasms) or have the potential to spread to other tissues and organs (malignant neoplasms). Intraepithelial neoplasia is often referred to as dysplasia. Neoplastic transformation (carcinogenesis or oncogenesis) is a multistep process by which cells acquire neoplastic properties and produce tumours.

11.1 Dysplasia and neoplasia

Learning objectives

You should:
- define neoplasm
- distinguish benign from malignant neoplasia
- describe biological characteristics of neoplastic cells that are associated with excessive growth, invasion and metastasis
- discuss dysplasia (intraepithelial neoplasia) and give clinically relevant examples.

Neoplasia

Neoplasia literally means 'new growth'. A definition of neoplasm is given in Box 15. The term 'tumour' (which actually means a swelling) is usually used synonymously with 'neoplasm'.

Our current concept of oncogenesis (the process whereby cells become neoplastic) is that neoplasms are derived from stem cells whose normal control of growth and differentiation has been pathologically changed through genetic defects. Stem cells, which have the capacity to divide continuously as well as produce mature differentiated cells, are found throughout the body in labile and stable cell populations. Differentiated cells have specialised functions which are not present in the precursor stem cell. For example, mucin-secreting goblet cells are derived from epithelial stem cells, and mature lymphocytes are derived from lymphoid stem cells.

Although each somatic cell contains the whole human genome, groups of genes can be switched on or off, and this mechanism determines the differentiation of the cell by controlling which genes will be transcribed. This process is controlled by the genetic programming of the cell and the local environment in which it grows (systemic hormones, local growth factors and matrix proteins).

The normal cell signalling and cell division pathways that maintain normal differentiation and growth are subverted by the genetic abnormalities characteristic of neoplasia. Thus, neoplastic cells continue to multiply inappropriately and may show reduced or abnormal functional specialisation. The genetic events involved are considered in more detail in Section 11.2.

Neoplasms (tumours) consist of neoplastic cells together with the connective tissue framework called the stroma. The blood vessels in the stroma represent the blood supply to the neoplastic cells, and the growth of the neoplasm depends on the ability of the neoplastic cells to induce the growth of these new blood vessels. In malignant neoplasms, the stroma often has a characteristic appearance called 'desmoplasia' due to the presence of large numbers of active fibroblasts.

Neoplastic cells show morphological changes that allow them to be recognised by pathologists. Sometimes, pathologists refer to these changes as 'atypia' in pathology reports. The features may include one or more of:

- variation in cell shape and size (pleomorphism)
- large nuclei in relation to cytoplasm
- dark-staining nuclei (hyperchromatism)
- irregularities of nuclear contour and chromatin pattern
- loss of normal maturation
- increased mitotic figures – some may be atypical, i.e. of abnormal shape
- enlarged nucleoli.

> **Box 15** Definition of neoplasm
>
> A neoplasm is an abnormal mass of tissue, the growth of which exceeds and is uncoordinated with that of normal tissue. The proliferation is purposeless and continues without regard to its effects on the surrounding tissues or the requirements of the organism. The cells do not respond normally to biological constraints on cell growth. These characteristics are due to genetic changes in the cells.

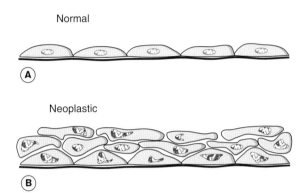

Normal

Neoplastic

Figure 26 Growth of normal versus neoplastic cells.

Some of these morphological changes are related to the increased number of chromosomes often found in neoplasms. Enlarged, hyperchromatic nuclei have an increased content of DNA.

Neoplastic cells may closely resemble their normal counterparts, in which case they are said to be well differentiated. In contrast, tumour cells that bear little resemblance to normal are poorly differentiated. Occasionally, the cells lose all their differentiating features and are called anaplastic or undifferentiated.

It is possible to grow neoplastic cells in culture in the laboratory. As a result of such work, several important differences in the behaviour of neoplastic cells compared with normal cells have been identified. In particular, neoplastic cells show:

- The transformed phenotype (Figure 26), which means that they:
  - *do not require extrinsic growth factors*
  - *proliferate to form a colony derived from a single parent stem cell (clone)*
  - *show reduced cell cohesiveness*
  - *show altered surface antigens*
  - *grow to higher cell densities in a haphazard way*
  - *do not show normal cell orientation.*
- Tumorigenicity, which means that they will grow into tumours when injected into immunosuppressed animals.
- Immortality, which means that they can undergo indefinite replication without showing senescence. In most cases, this is due to the expression of telomerase, an enzyme normally only found in stem cells that prevents the shortening of the telomeres on the ends of chromosomes. (In untransformed cells, the

shortening of the telomeres with each cell division limits the number of times a cell can divide.)
- The ability to evade the host defences against malignant cells. Immune cells, principally natural killer cells and T lymphocytes, are able to recognise neoplastic cells because of altered expression of cell surface antigens. If a neoplasm is to grow successfully, it must be able to avoid immune destruction.

The concepts of benign and malignant

Neoplasms are divided into two main types: benign and malignant. Benign tumours remain confined to their tissue of origin, but malignant neoplasms can spread to other tissues and organs. The term 'cancer' means 'malignant neoplasm'.

By definition, benign tumours do not spread beyond their site of origin. However, they may grow to be extremely large and may distort or disrupt local tissues. Thus, a benign tumour can, by virtue of its position and local effects, kill the patient. For example, a benign tumour in a vital area of the brain can be lethal. Benign neoplasms tend to be:

- well circumscribed or encapsulated
- slow growing (low mitotic rate)
- well differentiated, i.e. resemble the tissue of origin.

The defining characteristic of malignant neoplasms is their ability to invade from the site of origin into other tissues. They often (though not always) show the following features:

- poorly circumscribed
- rapid growth
- may be poorly differentiated
- can metastasise
- extensive disease may be associated with cachexia (generalised body wasting).

Spread of malignant neoplasms

Malignant tumours can show local and metastatic spread.

Local invasion

Local invasion is direct spread into tissues adjacent to the cancer. For example, cervical cancer can invade the uterine body, vagina, rectum, urinary bladder and ureters. A special form of local invasion is perineural spread, in which tumour cells acquire the ability to invade along nerves. Tumours showing this feature often spread rapidly into adjacent tissues, and so pathologists search for perineural invasion when examining malignancies under the microscope.

Metastasis

Metastasis is the spread of the tumour to distant sites away from the original tumour. The metastatic deposits are called secondary tumours, while the original tumour is the primary tumour. Metastases may arise from spread via the lymphatics, via the bloodstream, or across body cavities:

- Lymphatic spread: involvement of lymph nodes is common in many malignancies, e.g. axillary lymph node involvement in breast cancer and inguinal lymph node involvement in a malignant melanoma of the skin of the leg.
- Haematogenous spread: the most common sites for blood-borne metastases are bone, lung, brain and liver, e.g. liver involvement in gastric cancer and bone metastases from breast cancer.
- Direct seeding across cavities (transcoelomic spread), e.g. colorectal cancer can spread across the peritoneal cavity to produce metastases on the peritoneal surfaces of other organs.

Mechanisms of invasion and metastasis

Malignant neoplasms (cancers) can invade other tissues and spread to distant parts of the body. For invasion to occur, the tumour cells must possess these abilities:

- separation from adjacent cells
- attachment to matrix components
- degradation of extracellular matrix
- migration through extracellular matrix.

An important factor in the poor cohesiveness of cancer cells, allowing them to separate from each other, is abnormal expression of cell adhesion molecules. A cell adhesion molecule often down-regulated in epithelial cancers is E-cadherin. Once separated from their fellows, the cells need to attach to matrix components so they can start to move through the matrix; this is accomplished through expression of various receptors such as integrins. Degradation of matrix is performed by proteases which digest components of the extracellular matrix such as collagen; many of these enzymes are members of the matrix metalloproteinase family. These matrix-degrading enzymes produce corridors for invasion through the tissue. Normal tissues produce protease inhibitors but these may be neutralised by tumour cells.

The process of metastasis through blood or lymph to produce secondary tumours requires the tumour cells to exhibit a number of features:

- invasion through extracellular matrix
- passage through lymphatic or blood vessel into bloodstream (intravasation)
- survival in bloodstream or lymphatic fluid for transfer to a distant site
- passage from vessel lumen into adjacent tissue (extravasation)
- ability to multiply in new tissue
- ability to induce new blood vessel formation (angiogenesis) to supply the enlarging metastasis.

Conditions predisposing to neoplasia

Hyperplasia and metaplasia

In some circumstances, hyperplasia and metaplasia can predispose to the development of neoplasia. However, these conditions should not be confused with each other. Unlike neoplasia, hyperplasia and metaplasia are potentially reversible and are subject to normal constraints on cell growth.

Dysplasia

Dysplasia literally means disordered or abnormal growth. However, in general usage it specifically refers to the histological appearances of intraepithelial neoplasia, i.e. neoplastic change in epithelial cells that are still confined by the basement membrane. The dysplastic cells exhibit the morphological changes of neoplasia that were discussed earlier in this section. Dysplasia predisposes to malignancy, which by definition occurs when the neoplastic cells penetrate through the basement membrane and spread into other tissues. As such, dysplasia is a premalignant condition. If recognised, it can be treated before it progresses to cancer.

Dysplasia may arise de novo, or from tissues already showing pathological hyperplasia, metaplasia or chronic inflammation. Early dysplasia may be reversible under certain circumstances if the stimulus is removed. Severe dysplastic changes are sometimes termed 'carcinoma in situ'.

Clinical examples of the dysplasia to carcinoma sequence

Benign colorectal adenomas

Benign colorectal adenomas are polyps composed of dysplastic epithelial glands. If left in situ, without treatment, many of these will turn into malignant neoplasms over the course of several years (Figure 27). Familial adenomatous polyposis (FAP) is an inherited autosomal dominant disease in which thousands of adenomas develop in the colon. These all have malignant potential and the colon must be removed prophylactically, i.e. to prevent colon cancer occurring.

Cervical intraepithelial neoplasia

In the uterine cervix, squamous metaplasia associated with human papillomavirus infection may be followed by the development of dysplasia which, in the cervix, is called cervical intraepithelial neoplasia (CIN). If untreated, CIN can develop into cancer. This is the basis of the cervical smear test, designed to identify abnormal cells derived from CIN. Appropriate treatment can then be given to prevent the development of invasive cervical cancer, e.g. excision biopsy of the abnormal area.

Carcinoma in situ of the breast epithelium

Carcinoma in situ of the breast epithelium may be detected using mammography, which forms part of the breast screening programme. Such lesions are surgically excised to prevent the development of breast cancer.

11.2 Carcinogenesis

Learning objectives

You should:
- state the characteristics of a carcinogen
- use the terms oncogene, proto-oncogene and tumour suppressor gene, and discuss their role in carcinogenesis.

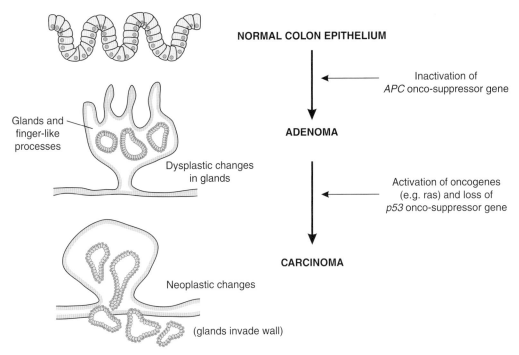

NORMAL COLON EPITHELIUM

Inactivation of
APC onco-suppressor gene

Glands and
finger-like
processes

Dysplastic changes
in glands

ADENOMA

Activation of oncogenes
(e.g. ras) and loss of
p53 onco-suppressor gene

CARCINOMA

Neoplastic changes

(glands invade wall)

Figure 27 The adenoma-carcinoma sequence.

The events that result in the development of a neoplasm are called oncogenesis, tumorigenesis or carcinogenesis (Figure 28). Molecular biology techniques have revolutionised our understanding of the role of genes in this process. The basic principle is that mutations in genes involved with cell growth and differentiation cause the neoplastic phenotype. The risk of a mutation increases with the number of mitotic divisions experienced by a cell, so that tissues with rapidly dividing stem cells (e.g. epithelia) tend to be more prone to neoplastic change.

Transformation is the term given to a cell that has undergone neoplastic change. A transformed cell is not subject to the normal constraints on cell growth, can divide indefinitely without ageing, and can sufficiently evade the process of apoptosis such that the rate of cell production exceeds the rate of cell loss. Thus, transformation is due to genetic changes (mutations) that interfere with the processes of cell division, apoptosis and differentiation. The genetic changes are inherited by the daughter cells, resulting in a clone of cells that forms the tumour mass.

A carcinogen is a substance which can cause neoplasia (Table 16). Most known carcinogens act directly on DNA, causing mutations. For example, polycyclic hydrocarbons can bind covalently to DNA producing molecules called adducts, while radiation damages DNA through its ionising effects. Viruses have a more complex range of effects as discussed in the section on oncogenes. In some circumstances, the effects of a carcinogen may be epigenetic, i.e. there is a change in DNA expression without mutation; anabolic steroids may act this way. However, it appears that epigenetic events alone are unable to produce the full neoplastic phenotype.

Since rapidly multiplying cells are more at risk of mutational events, factors that increase cell replication may also

Table 16 Examples of known carcinogens

Carcinogen group	Examples	Cancer
Chemicals	Polycyclic hydrocarbons	Lung cancer (smoking)
	Azo dyes	Bladder cancer
Viruses	Hepatitis B virus	Liver cancer
	Human papilloma virus	Cervical cancer
Radiation	X-rays, UV light	Skin cancer
	Uranium/radon	Lung cancer
	Radioactive iodine	Thyroid cancer
Hormones	Anabolic steroids	Liver cancer
Toxins	Aflatoxins	Liver cancer
Parasites	Liver fluke	Bile duct cancer
Industrial dust	Asbestos	Lung cancer, pleural cancer (mesothelioma)
	Wood dust	Nasal cancer

have a carcinogenetic effect. For example, some infections promote the multiplication of lymphocytes and may thus increase the risk of developing lymphoma.

There may be a long latent interval between exposure to the carcinogen and development of cancer. If more than one carcinogenetic factor is present, the effect is synergistic, i.e. the risk of developing cancer is much higher than with either factor alone.

Eleven

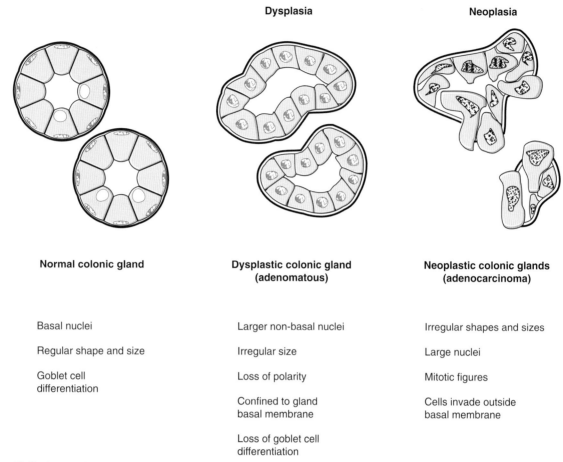

Dysplasia

Neoplasia

Normal colonic gland

Dysplastic colonic gland (adenomatous)

Neoplastic colonic glands (adenocarcinoma)

Basal nuclei

Regular shape and size

Goblet cell differentiation

Larger non-basal nuclei

Irregular size

Loss of polarity

Confined to gland basal membrane

Loss of goblet cell differentiation

Irregular shapes and sizes

Large nuclei

Mitotic figures

Cells invade outside basal membrane

Figure 28 Carcinogenesis.

Genetic changes in neoplasia

Genes involved in carcinogenesis can be divided into several types.

Oncogenes

Oncogenes are abnormal genes that are expressed in neoplastic cells. They are derived from proto-oncogenes, which are normal human genes. Proto-oncogenes typically promote growth or inhibit apoptosis under normal circumstances, whereas the oncogenes derived from them do so abnormally.

The genetic abnormalities include point mutations, deletions and translocations. In some cases, the proto-oncogene may be amplified, with multiple copies causing excessive production of gene product (e.g. growth factors). An example is the gene *HER2*; it encodes a cell surface growth receptor which is over-expressed in about 30% of breast carcinomas. These carcinomas can be treated with an inhibitor for this growth factor receptor.

Alternatively, chromosomal translocation may place the proto-oncogene next to a normally distant promotor DNA sequence which causes activation. Integration of tumorigenic viruses into human DNA may cause activation of proto-oncogenes in a similar way.

Viral oncogenes are derived from certain viruses and their expression causes transformation. Typically, part of the viral genome becomes incorporated into the DNA of human cell and produces proteins that affect the cell cycle or apoptosis. (This is not to be confused with the activation of proto-oncogenes by integrated viral DNA.) Interestingly, oncogenes in retroviruses appear to have arisen during evolution as copies of host proto-oncogenes.

Tumour suppressor genes

Tumour suppressor genes (onco-suppressor genes, anti-oncogenes) are normal genes which act to prevent neoplasia, e.g. by promoting apoptosis or inhibiting cell proliferation. The inactivation of these genes predisposes to cancer.

In human cancer families, where there is a familial tendency to develop cancer, the genetic abnormalities often involve an inherited inactivation of a normal tumour suppressor gene. The best described are the *RB-1* gene for familial retinoblastoma and *APC* in familial adenomatous polyposis (FAP).

Another important anti-oncogene is *TP53*. Its product, the protein p53, normally causes cell cycle arrest if DNA damage occurs, allowing time for DNA repair enzymes to correct the damage. If repair cannot be effected in reasonable time p53 induces apoptosis. Failure of these mechanisms due to loss of normal p53 function is an important factor in many neoplastic growths (Figure 29).

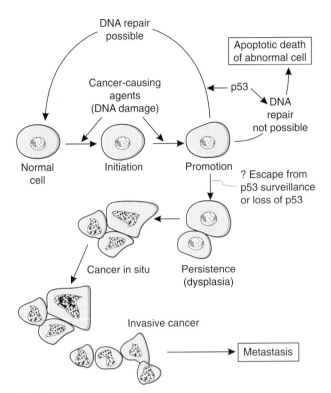

Figure 29 Control of DNA damage.

Epidemiological factors

There are many well-recognised epidemiological factors which are associated with the development of cancer:

- genetic and cultural factors: stomach cancer is very common in Japan, much less so in the UK
- diet: smoked and preserved foods are linked to gastric cancer
- lifestyle: smoking and lung cancer
- occupation: asbestos exposure and cancers of the lung and mesothelium
- gender: males are at greater risk of rectal cancer
- family history: breast and colon cancer in first-degree relatives
- premalignant conditions: ulcerative colitis, undescended testis
- fetal exposure: maternal stilboestrol treatment leading to vaginal cancer in female offspring.

Eleven

Self-assessment: questions

One best answer questions

1. Which one of the following is a neoplasm?
   a. Barrett's oesophagus (glandular metaplasia of the oesophagus)
   b. colonic adenoma
   c. hyperplasia of the endometrium
   d. hypertrophic cardiomyopathy
   e. squamous metaplasia of the cervix

2. Which one of the following is most likely to be found in a malignant neoplasm?
   a. abnormal p53 expression
   b. inability to spread beyond site of origin
   c. normal genome
   d. normal expression of cell surface antigens
   e. normal regulation of cell cycle

3. The DNA of an epithelial cell combines with a hydrocarbon to produce an adduct. What type of bond characterises this reaction?
   a. covalent bond
   b. hydrogen bond
   c. ionic bond
   d. metallic bond
   e. van der Waals bond

True-false questions

1. Dysplastic epithelium:
   a. rarely progresses to malignancy
   b. exhibits cytological abnormalities
   c. responds normally to hormonal stimuli
   d. may occur in metaplastic epithelium
   e. in the cervix may be detected by a smear

2. Oncogenes:
   a. are found in neoplastic cells
   b. are produced by activation of proto-oncogenes
   c. cannot be detected in histological preparations
   d. produce mutant oncoproteins
   e. may result from chromosomal translocation

3. Compared with normal tissue, malignant neoplastic cells are likely to exhibit:
   a. a reduction in the ratio of mitosis to apoptosis
   b. increased expression of E-cadherin
   c. increased expression of matrix metalloproteinases
   d. atypical mitotic figures
   e. reduced nuclear size

4. The following are correctly paired:
   a. metaplasia – irreversible
   b. hepatitis B virus – liver cancer
   c. cancer – reduced expression of telomerase
   d. asbestos bodies – mesothelioma
   e. UV light – skin cancer

Case history questions

Case history 1

A 74-year-old man is admitted to hospital with a cough, producing sputum which is sometimes bloodstained, breathlessness and weight loss. A chest X-ray shows a shadow in the upper part of the left lung. Sputum is sent to the pathology laboratory for examination of any cells coughed up. The pathologist's report says 'numerous severely atypical (dysplastic) squamous cells seen'.

1. What is meant by dysplasia? What microscopic features of the cells would lead the pathologist to this diagnosis?

A biopsy is taken from the area of lung shadowing and this shows a malignant neoplasm (carcinoma). The lung is removed surgically. When samples are taken from the bronchial epithelium adjacent to the cancer, squamous metaplasia is seen.

2. Define metaplasia. Give three examples.

3. How might the normal tissue–metaplastic tissue–neoplastic tissue sequence occur in this case?

Self-assessment: answers

One best answer

1. b. Adenomas of the colon are neoplasms characterised by intraepithelial neoplasia (dysplasia) of the intestinal epithelium. They are pre-malignant. In contrast, metaplasia, hyperplasia and hypertrophy are not neoplastic – although some examples do predispose to the development of neoplasia.

2. a. Abnormal p53 is common in malignancy. Cell surface antigen expression and regulation of cell cycle are also abnormal in neoplasia. Genetic abnormalities are found in all malignancies. Answer (b) is incorrect because by definition malignant tumours can spread beyond the tissue of origin.

3. a. Adducts are characterised by covalent bonds. This type of bond is strong and stable.

True-false answers

1. a. **False.** If it is untreated, the progression of dysplasia to malignancy is common.
    b. **True.** They include pleomorphism, hyperchromatism and other abnormalities in nuclear appearances, loss of polarity (the cells do not show a normal relationship to each other), and loss of normal cytoplasmic differentiation. These cytological changes become more pronounced as the dysplasia progresses towards malignancy.
    c. **False.** Dysplastic epithelium is neoplastic and does not respond normally to constraints on cell growth. That is, any response is only partial.
    d. **True.** Metaplasia may be complicated by dysplasia. For example, Barrett's metaplasia of the oesophagus is a condition in which the squamous lining of the oesophagus is replaced by intestinalised, glandular epithelium as a result of chronic inflammation due to reflux. Patients with this condition are at risk of developing dysplastic and then malignant changes if not treated.
    e. **True.** Detection of epithelial dysplasia (CIN) by cervical smears is the basis of the screening programme for cervical cancer.

2. a. **True.** Oncogenes are pieces of DNA which are present in neoplastic cells and promote the neoplastic phenotype through their effects on the cell cycle, cell signalling mechanisms, etc.
    b. **True.** The proto-oncogene or normal cellular oncogene is abnormally activated or amplified, and thus becomes an oncogene. MYC and RAS are good examples of oncogenes which have well-characterised effects in the early stages of tumorigenesis.
    c. **False.** Using molecular biology techniques, it is possible to apply DNA probes for various oncogenes to tissue sections of normal and neoplastic tissues. This enables the pathologist to visualise the distribution of the abnormal expression of oncogenes.
    d. **True.** When an oncogene is 'switched on' this may result in the production of an abnormal gene product or, alternatively, excessively increased amounts of a normal protein product. Oncoproteins are involved in the regulation of cell proliferation, growth factors, growth factor receptors and intracellular signalling mechanisms.
    e. **True.** For example, bcl-2 is a protein that prevents apoptosis by inhibiting caspases. Therefore, the gene BCL-2 that encodes this protein is a proto-oncogene because over-expression of bcl-2 will abnormally inhibit programmed cell death. In some lymphomas, the portion of chromosome 18 containing BCL-2 is translocated to the portion of chromosome 14 containing the antibody heavy chain locus. This t(14;18) translocation places BCL-2 close to the heavy chain gene enhancer. The consequent over-expression of bcl-2 protects the cell from apoptosis.

3. a. **False.** In order for neoplasms to grow faster than the surrounding tissues, the number of mitoses relative to the number of apoptoses must be increased. This may be due to an increase in the rate of cell division, a reduction in apoptosis, or (usually) both.
    b. **False.** The reduced cell-cell adhesiveness of malignant tumours is due to reduced expression of molecules responsible for cell-cell adhesion. E-cadherin is a common example.
    c. **True.** These enzymes break down matrix proteins, facilitating invasion by tumour cells.
    d. **True.** The abnormal DNA in malignant cells may show abnormally shaped mitoses.
    e. **False.** Neoplastic cells often have enlarged nuclei, and the nuclear-cytoplasmic ratio is typically increased.

4. a. **False.** Metaplasia is essentially a reversible process, although many metaplastic lesions carry the risk of progression to dysplasia.
    b. **True.** Hepatitis B virus is strongly associated with the development of liver cancer. The virus

inserts its DNA into the hepatocyte DNA. In the Far East, HBV infection is endemic and liver cancer is very common.

c. **False.** Telomerase prevents the shortening of telomeres that would otherwise occur at each cell division, allowing a cell to divide indefinitely. Most cancer cells possess telomerase.

d. **True.** Asbestos fibres are inhaled and can produce lung fibrosis (asbestosis). They can also lead to the development of malignant mesothelioma (a pleural cancer). Most asbestos exposure is occupational and people who have mined asbestos, unloaded it at the docks or worked with it (e.g. lagging boilers) are at high risk of mesothelioma. There is often a long lag period between the time of exposure and onset of tumour. This may be many decades.

e. **True.** UV light is associated with the development of malignant melanoma, basal cell carcinoma and squamous cell carcinoma, as well as with many kinds of benign proliferative skin lesions. UV light causes damage to DNA, leading to mutations.

Case history answers

Case history 1

1. Dysplasia literally means abnormal growth, and has been used in different ways through the course of medical history. However, in the context of neoplasia it means the histological changes associated with intraepithelial neoplasia. Dysplasia encompasses a constellation of features, including: loss of polarity and tissue organisation, loss of cytoplasmic differentiation, nuclear abnormalities including enlargement, pleomorphism and hyperchromatism, increased mitoses (which may be of abnormal shape), and increased nuclear-cytoplasmic ratio.

2. *Comment*: Metaplasia is the adaptive change from one adult cell type to another adult cell type in a tissue. When you are asked for examples of metaplasia think of hollow viscera that may become inflamed or obstructed, since these are the commonest sites.

Chronically inflamed transitional epithelium of the urinary bladder will often show areas of squamous metaplasia. Gastro-oesophageal reflux causes glandular metaplasia of the lower oesophagus. The pseudo-stratified, ciliated columnar respiratory epithelium of the bronchus undergoes metaplasia to squamous cells in the presence of chronic irritation by cigarette smoke. When the noxious stimulus is removed (patient gives up smoking!) the epithelium can revert to normal.

3. *Comment*: There is much research into this area of cell biology. Metaplasia is mediated by gene expression in the stem cells replenishing an epithelium exposed to an adverse environment.

As certain genes are switched on or off, the new cells will have a different complement of intracellular and surface proteins. If the noxious stimulus continues or increases, the new cell type may begin to acquire mutations. This can occur because of increased cell proliferation (at each mitosis there is a risk of mutation), DNA damage caused directly by the noxious stimulus, or both. Ultimately a neoplastic clone may grow out of the epithelium.

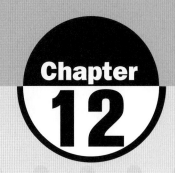

Neoplasia: classification, grading and staging

Chapter overview

Tumours exhibit a wide variety of behaviour and have a myriad of possible effects. Pathological analysis of neoplasms aims to allow sensible correlation with aetiological factors, to help select the best treatment, and to predict the prognosis. This is done by:

- classifying neoplasms according to the type of normal tissue they resemble
- grading them according to how closely they resemble normal tissue
- staging them by how far they have spread through the body.

12.1 Pathological characteristics of neoplasms

Learning objectives

You should:
- describe the pathological diagnostic process with respect to neoplasms
- discuss the role of tumour markers in managing neoplasia
- classify prognostic factors.

There are many characteristics of neoplasms that may be related to aetiology, response to treatment or prognosis. When examining neoplasms, pathologists may use a variety of diagnostic methods.

Macroscopic (naked eye) examination gives a preliminary idea of the nature of the tumour, since the growth pattern depends on the site of origin, speed of growth and cellular characteristics. Polypoid neoplasms stand above the adjacent tissue surface; exophytic neoplasms also do so but in an irregular way; fungating neoplasms are large, exophytic tumours with necrosis and surface ulceration; while the term ulcerating is used for ulcerated neoplasms that grow into the underlying tissue without a large exophytic component (Figure 30).

Some clues as to whether the tumour is benign or malignant may be obtained by macroscopic examination. Infiltration of surrounding tissues implies malignancy, while a well-circumscribed tumour surrounded by a capsule of reactive fibrous tissue is more likely to be benign. Neoplasms with extensive necrosis or a fungating appearance are probably malignant.

The mainstay of routine pathological classification is still light microscopy using sections stained with haematoxylin and eosin (H&E). Sometimes, special stains, immunohistochemistry or molecular techniques (see Ch. 2) may be needed for accurate classification. In some tumours, characteristics such as hormone receptor expression may give additional information about how the tumour is likely to respond to treatment.

Tumour markers

Some tumours secrete substances which can be detected in the blood or urine (Table 17). They may be:

- substances normally produced by the tissue but in excessive amounts, e.g. PSA produced by prostatic carcinoma
- substances not normally produced by the tissue (ectopic production), e.g. adrenocorticotrophic hormone from a lung cancer
- substances usually only seen in primitive or fetal tissues, such as CEA and AFP.

Tumour markers are used clinically in the initial diagnosis of a neoplasm and in monitoring its response to treatment. For example, detecting markedly raised PSA in the blood of a man with prostatic symptoms suggests prostatic carcinoma. After surgical resection of the cancer, the level of PSA should return to normal, but if it starts to rise again, it suggests recurrence of the cancer.

Prognostic factors in neoplasia

Many factors affect the prognosis of a patient with a neoplasm. It is useful conceptually to divide them into three groups:

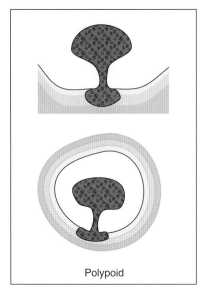
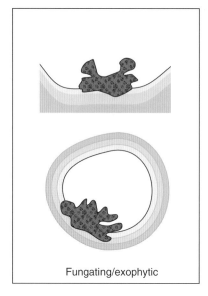
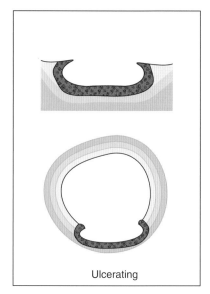

| Polypoid | Fungating/exophytic | Ulcerating |

Figure 30 Patterns of neoplastic growth.

Table 17 Tumour markers

Marker	Tumour
Carcinoembryonic antigen (CEA)	Colorectal disease, benign and malignant
Human chorionic gonadotrophin (hCG)	Malignant teratoma
Alpha-fetoprotein (AFP)	Malignant teratoma, hepatocellular carcinoma
Prostatic specific antigen (PSA)	Prostate cancer
Vanillyl mandelic acid (VMA)	Neuroblastoma
5-Hydroxy indole acetic acid (5HIAA)	Carcinoid tumour

- tumour-related factors
- host-related factors
- access to care.

Tumour-related factors

These are characteristics of the neoplasm itself: whether it is benign or malignant, its grade and stage (see later), whether it expresses certain hormone receptors, etc.

Host-related factors

These are characteristics of the patient. For example, other diseases, called co-morbidities in this context, may worsen the patient's overall condition, or prevent optimum therapy (e.g. respiratory disease may prevent an anaesthetic for surgical resection). The very old and very young sometimes have a worse prognosis than the rest of the population.

Access to care

The available treatment may be important in prognosis, i.e. whether optimum care is available and whether the

individual has access to that care. These are sometimes called 'environment-related factors'.

12.2 Classification of neoplasms

Learning objectives

You should:
- describe the principles of tumour nomenclature
- interpret the names of neoplasms.

Neoplasms are named according to whether they are benign or malignant (see Ch. 11) and by the type of tissue they resemble. In general, although there are important exceptions, benign neoplasms have the suffix -oma, malignant neoplasms arising from epithelial tissues are called carcinomas and malignant neoplasms arising from mesenchymal tissue are called sarcomas (Table 18, Figure 31). The rest of the name usually indicates the type of tissue the neoplasm resembles. Thus, adenoma means 'benign neoplasm of glandular epithelium', adenocarcinoma means 'malignant neoplasm of glandular epithelium', and chondrosarcoma means 'malignant neoplasm of cartilage'.

Unfortunately, there are exceptions to these rules. For example,

- melanoma and lymphoma are malignant despite the fact they end with -oma
- some neoplasms cannot be easily classified as benign or malignant; some are given names such as 'borderline tumour'.

Hamartomas (Box 16) are not generally considered to be neoplastic because they stop growing when the individual reaches adulthood. However, they may have genetic abnormalities similar to true neoplasms.

Table 18 Examples of the nomenclature of neoplasms

Tissue of origin	Benign	Malignant
Squamous epithelium	Squamous papilloma	Squamous cell carcinoma
Glandular epithelium	Adenoma	Adenocarcinoma
Smooth muscle	Leiomyoma	Leiomyosarcoma
Fat	Lipoma	Liposarcoma
Bone	Osteoma	Osteosarcoma
Skeletal muscle	Rhabdomyoma	Rhabdomyosarcoma

Box 16 Hamartomas and teratomas

Hamartomas are tumour-like masses of tissue but are not classified as neoplastic. They are composed of a mixture of tissues normally found at the site and grow slowly with the host. For example, hamartomatous polyps of the bowel consist of smooth muscle, glandular elements and blood vessels. Bronchial hamartomas contain cartilage, smooth muscle and bronchial epithelium.

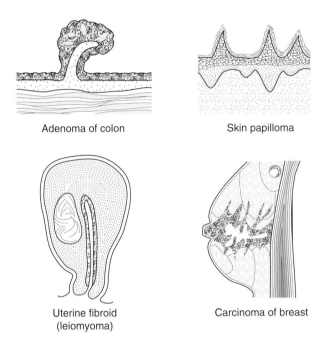

Adenoma of colon

Skin papilloma

Uterine fibroid (leiomyoma)

Carcinoma of breast

Figure 31 Examples of benign and malignant tumours.

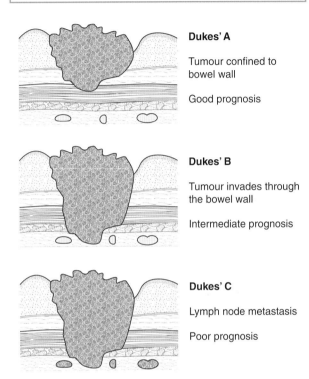

Dukes' A

Tumour confined to bowel wall

Good prognosis

Dukes' B

Tumour invades through the bowel wall

Intermediate prognosis

Dukes' C

Lymph node metastasis

Poor prognosis

Figure 32 Dukes' staging of colorectal cancer.

A teratoma is a neoplasm which is derived from tissues of more than one germ cell layer (and usually all three layers, namely endoderm, mesoderm and ectoderm). Some are benign but others are malignant.

Usually – though not always – tumours tend to resemble the tissue in which they arise. For example, squamous cell carcinomas are commonest in squamous epithelia (including metaplastic squamous epithelia).

12.3 Grading and staging

Learning objectives

You should:
- define and use the terms grade and stage
- describe the principles of grading and staging.

Grade and stage are two important features of a tumour that are commonly associated with prognosis and response to treatment.

Grade

The grade of a neoplasm describes how closely the tumour resembles normal tissue, i.e. the degree of cellular differentiation. A tumour that closely resembles its normal counterpart is called well differentiated or low grade, whereas a tumour that shows little resemblance to normal is called high grade or poorly differentiated. Moderately differentiated is a term for an intermediate degree of differentiation.

In some tumours, there are established numbered grading systems, usually of three of four groups, with grade 1 representing the most well differentiated neoplasms and grade 3 or 4 representing the least degree of differentiation. For example, breast carcinomas are divided into three grades based on the degree of tubular differentiation, nuclear pleomorphism and mitotic count. Renal cell carcinomas are divided into four grades based on nuclear characteristics such as size and shape.

The significance of grade is that it can be related to prognosis and response to treatment. High-grade neoplasms tend to grow faster and spread more rapidly than low-grade lesions. For example, in the case of large intestinal adenocarcinomas, well differentiated and moderately

Twelve

differentiated lesions have a better prognosis than poorly differentiated ones.

Stage

The stage of a neoplasm is determined by how far it has spread at the time of diagnosis. The concept only applies to malignant neoplasms, since benign tumours do not spread. In most cancers, it is the single most important tumour-related prognostic feature. Generally, the earlier a cancer is detected and treated, the better the outlook for the patient.

In the TNM system of tumour staging, a score is given for the extent of local spread (T category), local lymph node involvement (N category) and distant metastases (M category). These scores can then be used to calculate the stage group of the tumour. Each cancer has its own particular scoring system, but in general the higher the number the further the cancer has spread.

In the case of large intestinal carcinomas, another commonly used staging system is the Dukes' classification (Figure 32).

Self-assessment: questions

One best answer questions

1. A patient has a carcinoma of the colon. The tumour is resected and sent to the pathology laboratory, where its features are reported by the pathologist. Which of the following features, if present, is most likely to confer a poor prognosis?
   a. excision margins clear of neoplasm
   b. Dukes' A stage
   c. lymph node metastases
   d. moderate differentiation
   e. presence of a residual benign adenoma

2. Which one of the following is most likely to suggest a lymphoma?
   a. atypical lymphocytes in a lymph node aspirate
   b. papillary lesion of the oesophagus
   c. raised serum carcinoembryonic antigen
   d. reduced serum calcium
   e. reduced numbers of circulating lymphocytes

3. Which one of the following features is likely to suggest a neoplasm is benign?
   a. enlarged regional nodes
   b. extensive necrosis of the tumour
   c. growth of the tumour along nerves
   d. fungating appearance
   e. smooth external borders of the tumour

Extended matching items questions (EMIs)

EMI 1

Theme: Classification of neoplasms

A. adenocarcinoma
B. adenoma
C. chondroma
D. chondrosarcoma
E. hamartoma
F. leiomyoma
G. leiomyosarcoma
H. lymphoma
I. osteoma
J. osteosarcoma
K. teratoma

For each of the following questions, select the most appropriate response from the above list. Each response may be used once, more than once, or not at all.

1. A pathologist examines a tumour under the microscope and sees malignant glandular epithelium. What is the most appropriate classification?
2. Which name should be given to malignant tumour of smooth muscle?
3. tumour has arisen in the epithelium of the stomach and spread to regional lymph nodes. Which is the most likely tumour type?
4. Which lesion is not neoplastic?
5. A gynaecologist removes an ovarian tumour. He sees that it contains a mixture of tissues, including hair, teeth-like structures, bone and fat. What is the most likely diagnosis?

Case history questions

Case history 1

A 53-year-old woman presented to her doctor with a lump in her breast. On examination, the lump was in the upper outer quadrant of the right breast and was fixed to the skin which was puckered over the surface. The nipple was slightly inverted. The lump felt hard and craggy to palpation and was approximately 4 cm in diameter. The GP felt several enlarged lymph nodes in the axilla on the same side. The patient admitted that the lump had been present for at least a year, but she had been too scared to see her doctor before.

The GP referred her urgently to a breast surgeon. Fine needle aspiration with examination of the cells removed showed that the tumour was malignant and surgery was performed (lumpectomy with axillary node clearance). The pathologist reported that the tumour was a malignant carcinoma of ductal origin which had been completely excised. The lymph nodes contained metastatic tumour.

Several months later the patient presented with pain in the femur and a pathological fracture.

1. Why was the lump fixed to the skin?
2. How does breast cancer spread?
3. How might breast screening have altered the course of the disease in this patient?
4. What is the significance of the bone pain and fracture?

Self-assessment: answers

One best answer

1. c. The spread of neoplasm to the regional nodes is the most significant in this case, in keeping with the principle that high stage is the most important tumour-related adverse prognostic factor in most cancers. Such a lesion would be classified as Dukes' C. Complete excision would imply a better prognosis than if some tumour were left behind. The presence of a residual adenoma is irrelevant to the prognosis.

2. a. The presence of atypical (i.e. cytologically abnormal) lymphocytes is highly suggestive of a neoplastic proliferation. An oesophageal papillary lesion is most likely to be a squamous cell papilloma. CEA is typically raised in intestinal tumours. In lymphomas, the numbers of circulating lymphocytes are usually normal or increased.

3. e. Tumours with smooth external borders are described as well circumscribed. Benign tumours tend to have this appearance because they are confined to their site of origin. However, there are numerous exceptions! In contrast, enlarged regional nodes suggest that nodal metastases are likely, and extensive necrosis, perineural invasion and fungating growth are usually encountered in malignancies.

EMI answers

EMI 1

Theme: Classification of neoplasms

1. A. The nature of the lesion is reflected in the name: 'carcinoma' means malignant epithelial neoplasm, while 'adeno-' indicates glandular.

2. G. 'Leiomyo-' means smooth muscle; 'sarcoma' means malignant mesenchymal tumour.

3. A. The gastric epithelium is glandular, so glandular neoplasms are most common. This tumour must be malignant because it has spread to lymph nodes. Hence, it is an adenocarcinoma.

4. E. Hamartomas are not considered neoplastic because they behave as if they respond normally to constraints on cell growth. They are composed of tissues normally found at the site.

5. K. This lesion contains elements derived from at least two germ layers, ectoderm (teeth and hair) and mesoderm (fat and bone). Therefore, it is a teratoma. Most ovarian teratomas are benign and are called dermoid cysts. However, this lesion will require careful examination under the microscope to exclude any malignant elements.

Case history answers

Case history 1

1. Tumour fixation indicates that the tumour was invading the overlying skin. This gives it a puckered appearance. Sometimes tumour cells obstruct the lymphatics of the overlying skin, resulting in oedema and pitting of the surface rather like the skin of an orange. This clinical sign is called 'peau d'orange' and is a bad prognostic sign.

2. Breast cancer follows the general rules of spread of all cancers. It may invade locally into adjacent structures such as the skin, nipple and pectoralis muscles. Lymphatic spread to draining lymph nodes is common, in this case to axillary lymph nodes on the same side. Eventually, haematogenous spread may occur with metastases in the bones, lung, brain, liver or elsewhere.

3. If the patient had presented earlier, there may have been a chance that the tumour had not already spread either so extensively locally or to the lymph nodes. The earlier tumours are detected, usually, the better the prognosis. Breast screening programmes are designed to detect neoplasms before they become advanced, and should reduce the death rate from breast cancer.

4. The bone pain is caused by metastatic breast carcinoma (haematogenous spread) which has invaded the femur and caused it to become weak and fracture spontaneously (pathological fracture).

Pathological accumulations

Chapter 13

Chapter overview

This chapter covers several important pathological processes that used to be classified as 'tissue degenerations'. They are unified by the fact that they all involve abnormal accumulations of pigments or other substances that build up as a result of a variety of different pathological processes. These materials can be classified as endogenous if they are produced In the body, or exogenous if they are derived from outside.

13.1 Abnormal endogenous accumulations

Learning objectives

You should:

* state the main characteristics and pathological significance of fatty change, lipofuscin, haemosiderin and amyloid
* distinguish metastatic from dystrophic calcification
* recognise abnormal melanin accumulation
* understand the term hyaline
* discuss the principles of the inherited storage disorders.

Fatty change

Fatty change (steatosis) represents accumulation of triglyceride in cells and is usually an indicator of cell stress and reversible injury. Organs affected by fatty change appear enlarged, pale and have a greasy consistency. The liver is the most common site of fatty change, reflecting the central role of liver cells in fat metabolism. Common causes include excessive alcohol consumption, the metabolic syndrome, type 2 diabetes mellitus and drug reactions. The fat accumulates when cell damage compromises the ability of the hepatocyte to metabolise fatty acids or to bind lipid to protein and transport it out of the cell. Fatty change can also be seen in cardiac muscle cells as a result of severe anaemia or starvation (e.g. anorexia nervosa)

where protein deficiency results in a reduced capacity for the protein binding and transport of triglyceride out of cells.

Haemosiderin

Haemosiderin is a golden yellow to brown pigment found in lysosomes within the cell cytoplasm. It is composed of aggregates of partially degraded ferritin, which is protein-covered ferric oxide and phosphate. It can be visualised using the Prussian blue reaction, when haemosiderin appears dark blue.

Haemosiderin represents iron deposition and accumulates in tissues in two main circumstances. First, if there is haemorrhage into a tissue the haemoglobin is broken down and haemosiderin is deposited in macrophages locally. This process occurs in many chronic inflammatory conditions; the extravasated red blood cells are broken down and haemosiderin is produced from the iron they contain. The identification of haemosiderin in a tissue sample can be a clue to previous haemorrhage or inflammation.

Second, an excess of circulating iron can result in systemic haemosiderin accumulation. For example, primary haemochromatosis is an inherited disease in which there is excessive absorption and widespread deposition of haemosiderin in the tissues, especially the liver, pancreas, heart and skin. The iron is toxic to the tissues and leads to fibrosis of the liver (cirrhosis), fibrosis of the pancreas (leading to diabetes mellitus), and heart failure.

Other causes of systemic iron deposition include increased absorption of iron from the intestine, haemolytic anaemia and recurrent blood transfusions. The presence of iron in the tissues is termed haemosiderosis, which is not be confused with the disease haemochromatosis as described previously.

Melanin

Melanin is the brown/black pigment normally present in the cytoplasm of cells in the basal layer of the epidermis, called melanocytes. Melanin is derived from tyrosine, stored in melanosomes and distributed to the other epidermal cells. The function of melanin is to block harmful UV rays from reaching the epidermal nuclei. It may accumulate in excessive quantities in benign or malignant melanocytic neoplasms and its presence is a useful diagnostic feature for such lesions. In inflammatory skin lesions, where the epidermis is damaged, melanin may be released from injured basal cells and taken up by dermal macrophages. This gives rise to post-inflammatory pigmentation of the skin. Melanin can be identified in tissue sections by the use of the Masson–Fontana stain.

Excessive melanin pigmentation of the skin is a feature of certain diseases, e.g. Addison's disease and neurofibromatosis.

Lipofuscin

This is the yellow/brown 'wear-and-tear' pigment seen in atrophic tissues (see atrophy, Ch. 3). It also accumulates in ageing cells of the liver, myocardium and elsewhere. Lipofuscin does not seem to damage cells and does not cause clinical problems.

Calcification

Calcification is the deposition of calcium salts within tissues, often causing them to become chalky, hard or brittle. There are two main types of calcification:

- dystrophic
- metastatic.

Dystrophic calcification

This type of calcification occurs within diseased tissues. The plasma calcium and phosphate levels are normal. The exact mechanism by which dystrophic calcification occurs is not known. Examples include calcification within areas of necrosis, foci of old tuberculosis, atheromatous plaques, and in neoplasms. The calcification can often be identified on radiographs.

Metastatic calcification

Metastatic calcification occurs in normal tissues as a consequence of raised plasma calcium concentrations (hypercalcaemia). Common causes of hypercalcaemia include widespread metastatic cancer in the bones, hyperparathyroidism and multiple myeloma. Metastatic calcification does not often cause clinical problems, although occasionally renal failure can follow calcification of the kidneys.

Hyaline

Hyaline simply means 'glassy' and is used as a descriptive term by pathologists for a variety of materials that have a uniform pink (eosinophilic) appearance under the microscope. Deposits of protein in renal tubules and Mallory bodies in the liver can be described as exhibiting a hyaline appearance. In longstanding diabetes and hypertension, accumulation of proteins in the walls of arterioles causes them to become hyalinised.

Amyloidosis

The term amyloid means 'starch-like' and as such is misleading because amyloid is not a carbohydrate. Amyloid is a descriptive term used for a group of proteinaceous substances that may be deposited in tissues and organs to give characteristic naked eye, microscopic and ultrastructural appearances.

What is amyloid?

Amyloid is an abnormal protein characterised by a β-pleated sheet configuration deposited in the extracellular matrix. Many different proteins can produce amyloid, and the type of protein found in the amyloid deposits depends on the underlying disease. For example, in patients with multiple myeloma (a neoplastic proliferation of antibody-producing plasma cells), the amyloid is composed of antibody fragments. The β-pleated sheets form long, non-branching fibrils with a diameter of about 8 nm; they can be observed under the electron microscope. Once the β-pleated sheets have formed, the body's intra- and extracellular proteolytic enzyme systems find it almost impossible to digest; therefore, it accumulates inexorably.

Almost all types of amyloid also contain a second substance, a glycoprotein known as the P component (or P protein). The P component is a doughnut-shaped pentamer.

When amyloid is deposited in large amounts, the tissue becomes pale, smooth and waxy in texture. Histologically, amyloid stains pink with Congo red dye; the pink colour turns apple green under polarised light, a property unique to amyloid.

Where does amyloid accumulate?

Amyloid can accumulate within any tissue or organ. The disease may affect just one tissue or organ, i.e. localised amyloidosis, or several, i.e. systemic amyloidosis. It always accumulates outside cells and has a predilection for basement membranes and interstitial connective tissues.

Where there is abundant amyloid deposition, cells become 'strangled' and organ failure occurs. There is also evidence that some types of amyloid have a direct toxic effect on cells. For example, β-amyloid in the brain damages neurones, possibly by free radical production.

When does amyloid accumulation occur?

It is thought that defective proteolysis of the precursor protein results in amyloid production. The two most common examples of systemic amyloidosis are:

- **AL amyloid**: Patients with multiple myeloma typically have excessive amounts of circulating intact and fragmented immunoglobulin light chains. Defective proteolysis of these light chains gives an amyloid protein called AL amyloid.
- **AA amyloid**: This type of amyloid complicates long-term inflammatory conditions. These can be suppurative processes, such as bronchiectasis, or autoimmune diseases, such as rheumatoid disease. In these conditions, the liver produces a number of acute-phase proteins that have various functions in the inflammatory process. Among these is serum amyloid A protein (SAA). This normal protein can be converted into amyloid A (AA amyloid).

Examples of localised amyloid are:

- **β-amyloid**: Derived from amyloid precursor protein (APP) in the brain, this is a component of the plaques of Alzheimer's disease.

- **Amyloid deposits in endocrine neoplasms**: The hormones produced by neuroendocrine tumours can be converted into amyloid and deposited in the tumour stroma.

What are the effects of amyloid on tissues/organs?

The effects of amyloid deposition depend on the organs involved and the amount of amyloid deposited. The most serious complications of systemic amyloidosis are usually seen in the kidney and heart. Renal involvement can lead to the loss of large amounts of protein in the urine and even renal failure. Myocardial amyloid may stop the heart contracting properly and cause heart failure, or, if deposited in the conducting system, cause a lethal arrhythmia.

The storage disorders

These conditions are rare inborn errors of metabolism that cause accumulation of a macromolecule in cells. They are all due to a genetic disorder and generally show recessive inheritance. The genetic defect results in the massive accumulation of a substance within tissues, causing secondary cell injury. The majority of these conditions can be divided into two main groups: the glycogen storage diseases and lysosome storage diseases.

The glycogen storage diseases, or glycogenoses, are due to defects in an enzyme involved in glycogen metabolism. For example, deficiency of glucose 6-phosphatase causes glycogen to accumulate particularly in the liver and kidney. Other glycogen storage diseases may primarily affect muscle, or cause generalised systemic deposition of glycogen.

The lysosome storage diseases are due to a failure in lysosomal digestion. The defect is found in the activity of an enzyme that breaks down a macromolecule into its component subunits or in a transport protein that is required for moving the digested material out of the lysosome. Consequently, the macromolecule accumulates within lysosomes that become massively distended. For example, deficiency of glucocerebrosidase causes Gaucher's disease, in which gangliosides accumulate in macrophages in the bone marrow, spleen and liver, causing

reduction in blood cell production (pancytopenia) and hepatosplenomegaly.

13.2 Abnormal exogenous accumulations

> **Learning objectives**
>
> You should:
> - state the two main routes of entry for exogenous materials that accumulate in the body, and give examples of each
> - describe the general features of the pneumoconioses.

If insoluble substances that cannot be adequately eliminated enter the body, they will accumulate. A variety of pigments and other materials can do this. They may be toxic and produce inflammatory tissue reactions or they may be relatively inert. There are two main routes by which such materials enter the body: through the skin and the lungs.

Exogenous skin pigmentation is due to tattooing. The pigments are engulfed by dermal macrophages that become immobilised, retaining the pigments in the skin indefinitely.

Inhaled dusts entering the respiratory tract can accumulate in the lungs. They are taken up by pulmonary macrophages that remain in the walls of the airways. Carbon derived from soot is found in virtually everyone living where there is air pollution, and its accumulation is called anthracosis. Pure carbon is relatively inert, but other substances are toxic and can cause significant disease. The general term for a disease of the lungs caused by inhaled dust is pneumoconiosis. Coal dust, asbestos, silica and other dusts cause fibrosis of the lung that may compromise lung function and cause breathlessness and reduced exercise tolerance. By interfering with normal blood flow through the lungs, they can also cause cor pulmonale and right ventricular failure. In addition, some inhaled dusts are carcinogenic and can cause cancer.

Thirteen

Self-assessment: questions

One best answer questions

1. The following materials can form pathological accumulations. Which one of them is exogenous?
   a. amyloid
   b. calcium
   c. carbon
   d. lipofuscin
   e. melanin

2. A 25-year-old man has an appendicectomy for abdominal pain. The pathologist finds no evidence of acute inflammation in the appendix, but the deposition of a pigment suggests that the appendix has been inflamed in the past. Which one of the following is most likely to have led to this conclusion?
   a. carbon
   b. haematoxylin
   c. haemosiderin
   d. lipofuscin
   e. melanin

3. Which one of these materials shows apple-green birefringence when stained with Congo red?
   a. amyloid
   b. glycogen
   c. lipofuscin
   d. Mallory bodies
   e. melanin

True-false questions

1. The following are correctly paired:
   a. lipofuscin pigment – tattoos
   b. haemosiderin pigment – skin bruising
   c. asbestosis – pneumoconiosis
   d. AL amyloid protein – bronchiectasis
   e. parathyroid adenoma – metastatic calcification

2. The following statements are true:
   a. fatty change caused by alcoholic liver damage is reversible
   b. lipofuscin accumulation is associated with ageing
   c. calcification of atherosclerotic plaques is rare

   d. anthracosis is caused by silica
   e. Gaucher's disease is inherited as an autosomal dominant disorder

Extended matching items questions (EMIs)

EMI 1

Theme: Abnormal accumulations

A. AA amyloid
B. AL amyloid
C. β-amyloid
D. asbestos
E. calcium
F. glycogen
G. haemosiderin
H. intracellular lipid
I. lipofuscin
J. melanin

For each of the following scenarios, select the substance from the list that is most likely to be responsible for the clinical and pathological features.

1. A 95-year-old woman dies and an autopsy is performed. The pathologist finds the heart to be atrophic and to have a uniform brown appearance.

2. A 75-year-old woman with longstanding rheumatoid arthritis presents with proteinuria. A renal biopsy shows deposition of eosinophilic material in the glomeruli.

3. A 50-year-old man with type 2 diabetes mellitus has a routine blood test that shows abnormal levels of liver enzymes. Ultrasound of the liver shows diffuse increased echogenicity.

4. A 6-month-old baby boy dies of heart failure. Histological sections of the heart show the accumulation of large amounts of periodic acid-Schiff (PAS)-positive material in the cytoplasm of the myocytes. A section of liver shows similar material in the hepatocytes.

5. A 65-year-old retired docker has a history of poor lung function associated with extensive lung fibrosis. He presents with a lung mass, and squamous cell carcinoma is diagnosed by biopsy of the mass.

Case history questions

Case history 1

A 56-year-old woman presented with generalised symptoms of feeling unwell. She had noticed swelling of her ankles and face and was breathless. On examination, she had signs of heart failure and oedema. Her urine, collected over 24 hours, contained 11 g of protein (normal is less than 150 mg) and her serum albumin level was 20 g/L (normal is about 40 g/L).

A kidney biopsy was performed and showed amyloid deposition. Further examination of the urine and serum proteins showed increased amounts of λ light chain proteins. Electrophoresis of the blood revealed a monoclonal band of immunoglobulin. Bone marrow biopsy was performed.

1. What type of cell would you expect to see in excessive numbers in the bone marrow biopsy?

2. What type of amyloid would you expect to find in this case?

3. State two physical characteristics of the amyloid in this case.

4. Why might the loss of large amounts of protein in the urine lead to ankle swelling?

Case history 2

A 58-year-old accountant was noticed by his family and firm to have become unreliable, mentally slow, confused and have a poor memory. Over the next few years, he became progressively unable to walk and lead an independent existence. He died at the age of 67. Clinically, a diagnosis of Alzheimer's disease was made during his illness.

1. State the type of amyloid found in the plaques of Alzheimer's disease, and the normal protein from which it is derived.

2. Would you expect to find the amyloid inside or outside cells?

3. Why does the study of Down's syndrome help us in the understanding of Alzheimer's disease?

Self-assessment: answers

One best answer

1. c. Carbon is inhaled as coal dust or air pollution. The others are produced in the body.
2. c. Haemosiderin can be found in macrophages for some time after the inflammation has died down. Perl's stain is often used by pathologists to demonstrate it in tissue sections; this stain uses the Prussian blue reaction. Note that haematoxylin is a dye used in routine histological stains.
3. a. This staining reaction is a useful histological test for amyloid.

True-false answers

1. a. **False.** Lipofuscin is the brown intracellular pigment which accumulates in cells with age. It is present in autophagic vacuoles within cells and is often known as wear-and-tear pigment. Organs which are very atrophic may actually look brown to the naked eye from excessive amounts of this pigment. Tattoos gain their colour and permanence from the intradermal injection of inks and dyes, often based on carbon or mercury pigments. These are ingested by local macrophages which cannot digest them and become immobilised at the site of the tattoo, the colour remaining visible through the skin.
   b. **True.** Haemosiderin is the iron-based pigment resulting from the breakdown of haemoglobin. When haemorrhage occurs into tissues, red cell haemoglobin is degraded and ingested by macrophages. Haemosiderin is a brownish yellow pigment which gives the bruise its characteristic colour.
   c. **True.** Asbestosis is characterised by fibrosis of the lungs and reduced respiratory function. It is acquired by inhaling asbestos dust, and so it is a type of pneumoconiosis. Asbestos also causes other diseases, such as lung carcinoma and pleural malignant mesothelioma.
   d. **False.** AL amyloid is composed of κ or λ immunoglobulin light chains and is found in amyloid derived from immunoglobulin, most commonly in multiple myeloma. Multiple myeloma is a neoplastic monoclonal proliferation of plasma cells which produces abnormal amounts of a single immunoglobulin. Bronchiectasis leads to chronic infection of the lungs which can lead to AA protein amyloid formation.
   e. **True.** Parathyroid adenoma is a benign tumour of the parathyroid glands which can produce abnormal amounts of parathyroid hormone. This leads to increased levels of calcium in the bloodstream (hypercalcaemia), which causes fits, vomiting and excessive urine production (polyuria), and sometimes metastatic calcification.

2. a. **True.** Fatty change represents reversible tissue injury. In the liver, intracellular triglycerides must be complexed with protein in order to transport them through the cell. Alcohol interferes with this metabolic process and hence causes fatty change. The liver is the most common site for fatty change to be clinically apparent.
   b. **True.** Lipofuscin is associated with ageing and can be seen accumulating in many major organs in elderly people. Lipofuscin itself is not injurious to cells.
   c. **False.** Dystrophic calcification of atherosclerotic plaques is common.
   d. **False.** Anthracosis is caused by the accumulation of carbon pigment in lung macrophages. It is seen in coal miners and city dwellers.
   e. **False.** If only one allele is abnormal, the cell can produce enough normal enzyme. Only if both alleles are abnormal does the cell accumulate glucocerebroside. Gaucher's disease is inherited as an autosomal recessive condition; storage diseases in general show recessive rather than dominant inheritance.

EMI answers

EMI 1

Theme: Abnormal accumulations

1. I. The heart shows 'brown atrophy', i.e. the accumulation of 'wear and tear' lipofuscin pigment in the atrophic tissue has imparted a brown appearance.
2. A. AA amyloid complicates chronic inflammatory conditions such as systemic autoimmune diseases, tuberculosis and chronic inflammatory bowel disease. The nephrotic syndrome (see Ch. 23) can follow renal involvement. The eosinophilic material in the glomeruli is the amyloid; it will be positive with Congo red.
3. H. This patient has non-alcoholic fatty liver due to type 2 diabetes. The ultrasound findings are not specific but point to a diffuse abnormality of the liver, in this case accumulation of fat in hepatocytes.
4. F. This description is of Pompe's disease, a type of glycogen storage disease. Glycogen is positive with the PAS stain.

5. D. Asbestos causes asbestosis, which is a fibrotic disease of the lungs causing a restrictive lung defect. In addition, asbestos is carcinogenic and predisposes to malignant neoplasms of the lung (carcinoma, as in this case) and pleura (malignant mesothelioma). Individuals who worked in dockyards without adequate protection are likely to have been exposed to asbestos.

Case history answers

Case history 1

1. This patient has multiple myeloma, which is an uncontrolled proliferation of plasma cells. Therefore, the type of cell expected to be present in excess in the bone marrow is the plasma cell. Bone marrow biopsy is a useful diagnostic test in this condition. *Comment*: The specific clues to the diagnosis in the scenario are the light chain proteinuria and the monoclonal band in the plasma. They represent the excessive amounts of abnormal immunoglobulin being produced by the plasma cells.

2. AL amyloid (derived from the light chains).

3. *Comment*: A good response would be:
   - β-pleated sheet
   - fibrillary structure.

4. Protein loss in the urine leads to a reduced intravascular colloid osmotic pressure and hence hydrostatic pressure forces fluid out of the blood vessels into the interstitium. This is clinically seen as tissue oedema.

Case history 2

1. β-amyloid, derived from APP.

2. Outside: amyloid is an extracellular deposit.

3. Individuals with Down's syndrome (trisomy 21) who survive to middle age show similar neuritic plaques and neurofibrillary tangles in their cerebral cortex. Therefore, it has been postulated that genes on chromosome 21 have an important role in the development of these degenerative changes in Alzheimer's disease.

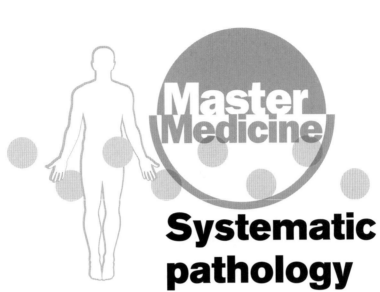

Systematic
pathology

Cardiovascular system

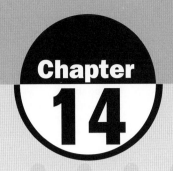

Chapter 14

Chapter overview

Pathology of the cardiovascular system, the heart and blood vessels, is responsible for a large proportion of deaths in the UK each year, and also causes considerable morbidity through heart failure, stroke and peripheral vascular disease. The major underlying disease processes responsible include atherosclerosis, hypertension and diabetes mellitus. Lifestyle modification can have a significant role in reducing disease risk, particularly in relation to smoking, exercise, body weight and fat consumption. This chapter covers atherosclerosis and its complications, ischaemic heart disease, hypertension, valvular heart disease, cardiomyopathies and congenital heart disease. Many cardiac pathologies result in heart failure, which may initially primarily involve either the left or right ventricle. The basic pathology of vasculitis and vascular tumours is also reviewed.

14.1 Atherosclerosis, aneurysms and ischaemic heart disease

Learning objectives

You should:

- understand the pathogenesis and clinical consequences of atherosclerosis
- be able to discuss pathology and complications of myocardial infarction
- know how lifestyle modifications can reduce the risk of ischaemic heart disease.

Atherosclerosis

Atherosclerosis (also called atheroma) is an inflammatory, degenerative disease of large and medium-sized arterial vessels. It is characterised by the development of fibrolipid plaques within the intima of the vessel wall. In smaller arteries, including the coronary vessels that supply the myocardium, these plaques can cause severe narrowing (stenosis) of the lumen, with significant impairment of blood flow. The clinical consequences depend on the speed of development of the stenosis, and on whether the affected tissue has any additional source of blood supply (known as collateral supply). In large arteries, such as the abdominal aorta, the inflammatory atherosclerotic process also damages the muscular wall causing weakness and dilatation. This is known as aneurysm formation (see Box 17). As the aneurysm enlarges there is an increasing risk of rupture, with resultant catastrophic haemorrhage.

Four major risk factors are recognised for atherosclerosis:

- smoking
- hypercholesterolaemia (raised low density lipoproteins)
- hypertension
- diabetes mellitus.

Minor risk factors include increasing age, male sex, obesity, family history and stress.

Pathogenesis of the fibrolipid atherosclerotic plaque

Atheromatous plaques are probably initiated by injury to the endothelial cells of the arterial intima. An inflammatory response is evoked to the damage, which results in an infiltrate of macrophages, and proliferation of smooth muscle cells from the media of the vessel wall. These smooth muscle cells migrate into the intima and begin to produce collagen. Both the macrophages and the smooth muscle cells may accumulate lipid within their cytoplasm, giving a vacuolated appearance on light microscopy ('foam cells'). Free cholesterol and necrotic inflammatory debris also become incorporated within the plaque lesion.

Figure 33 shows a normal muscular artery and a typical atheromatous plaque with a fibrous tissue cap and a lipid-rich, necrotic centre. It is important to realise that the actual composition of individual plaques varies, and can change over time. Plaques that are particularly rich in

---

Box 17 Aneurysms

Definition. Abnormal dilatation of a vessel wall, which communicates with the lumen – almost always arterial

Pathogenesis:

- Inflammation: atherosclerotic aneurysm (abdominal aorta, iliac arteries, popliteal arteries); polyarteritis nodosa; Kawasaki's disease (coronary arteries)

- Infection (mycotic aneurysm): syphilis; direct spread from adjacent infection

- Congenital defect: Berry aneurysm (circle of Willis, see Ch. 27)

- Metabolic: diabetes mellitus (retinal capillary microaneurysms)

- Hypertension: Charcot–Bouchard aneurysms (deep white matter of cerebral hemispheres)

- Trauma

Complications:

- Rupture with haemorrhage (often fatal if aorta or cerebral vessels involved)

- Compression of adjacent structures

- Thrombus formation (vessel occlusion and distal thromboembolism)

- Secondary infection

- Sclerosing periaortitis (dense fibrosis surrounding abdominal aortic aneurysm which can entrap ureters)

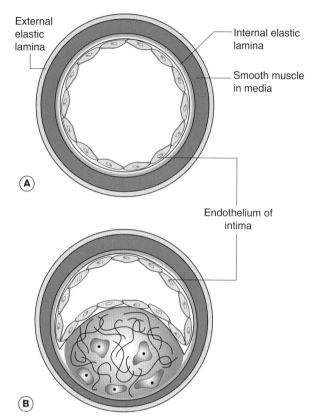

Figure 33 (A) Normal muscular artery structure within intima (endothelium), internal elastic lamina and media. (B) An atherosclerotic plaque composed of lipid and fibrous tissue is present in the intima causing internal narrowing (stenosis) of the vessel lumen and thinning of the underlying muscular media.

---

lipids may be more unstable and susceptible to rupture or haemorrhage. Older plaques can become heavily calcified. The plaque surface is prone to develop superimposed thrombosis, which can rapidly increase the severity of the obstruction to blood flow. At autopsy, it is common to find a recent thrombus complicating an atheromatous coronary artery plaque in patients who died after acute myocardial infarction.

Clinical complications of atherosclerosis

- **Coronary arteries**: angina, myocardial infarction, heart failure, sudden death (cardiac arrhythmia).
- **Cerebral arteries**: transient ischaemic attacks, stroke.
- **Aorta**: abdominal aneurysm formation (risk of rupture and death) (see Box 17).
- **Mesenteric arteries**: intestinal ischaemia and infarction.
- **Renal arteries**: renal artery stenosis (hypertension, ischaemic kidney).
- **Lower limbs**: intermittent claudication, gangrene.

Aortic dissection

Aortic dissection is also called dissecting aneurysm, although this is an inaccurate term as the aorta is not significantly dilated. In aortic dissection, blood tracks into the muscular wall of the blood vessel. The entry point of blood into the aortic media is through an intimal tear, usually within the proximal 10 cm of the ascending aorta. Occa-

sionally, there is a second distal luminal tear, through which blood re-enters the circulation, producing a 'double-barrelled' aorta. More commonly, however, the haemorrhage extends outwards with vessel rupture and catastrophic extramural haemorrhage into:

- the pericardium, causing cardiac tamponade
- the mediastinum, causing haemothorax
- the abdominal cavity (haematoperitoneum).

The dissection can also involve the great vessels of the neck, compromising cerebral blood flow. Dissection of the coronary arteries is a rare cause of acute myocardial ischaemia.

There is a strong association with systemic hypertension and with Marfan's syndrome.

Ischaemic heart disease

Ischaemia is due to lack of oxygen, and in the overwhelming majority of ischaemic heart disease (IHD) cases this is due to reduced blood flow through coronary arteries narrowed or occluded by atherosclerosis. However, the left ventricular myocardium is also at risk of ischaemia when there is pathological hypertrophy, for example in systemic hypertension or aortic valve stenosis. Under these conditions, cardiac perfusion may be insufficient to meet the metabolic needs of the increased muscle mass. Rarely, cardiac ischaemia can result from decreased oxygen-carrying capacity of the blood in severe anaemia (even though the coronary arteries may be normal).

Myocardial infarction

Cell death (necrosis) caused by ischaemia is known as infarction. Cardiac muscle cells cease to function within 30–60 seconds of loss of blood supply. Irreversible cell injury requires at least 20 minutes of anoxia (no oxygen). Cardiac muscle cells do not divide in post-natal life (i.e. they are 'permanent' cells) and infarcted myocardium is eventually replaced by fibrous scar tissue.

Regional (transmural) infarction

Regional (transmural) infarction is caused by occlusion of a single coronary artery. The arterial blockage results from atherosclerosis complicated by thrombosis or by intra-plaque haemorrhage, which rapidly expands the athero-matous plaque (see Figure 34). The commonest sites for clinically significant coronary atherosclerosis are:

- proximal left anterior descending artery (up to 50%)
- right coronary artery (30%)
- left circumflex artery (up to 20%)
- left main coronary artery.

Regional infarction most frequently affects part of the anterior wall of the left ventricle, or part of the interven-tricular septum, with extension into the right ventricle in a small proportion of cases. Isolated right ventricular infarction is very uncommon.

The subendocardial region of the myocardium is the muscle area most vulnerable to hypoxia.

Subendocardial infarction

Subendocardial infarction can occur when there is a global decrease in cardiac blood flow due to systemic hypoten-sion ('shock'). Myocardial necrosis is usually limited to the inner third of the muscle but can involve the territory of more than one coronary artery.

Unusual causes of myocardial infarction include coro-nary artery dissection, arteritis or spasm.

Macroscopic and microscopic changes in myocardial infarction

- Less than 24 hours – microscopic changes only (increased eosinophilic staining of cardiac muscle cells, loss of nuclei, muscle cells become buckled).
- From 24 to 72 hours – infarct becomes apparent macroscopically at autopsy as an area of pallor or yellow discoloration, with a peripheral rim of haemorrhage. Microscopically the dead muscle fibres provoke an inflammatory response, initially consisting of neutrophils followed by macrophages. The infarct becomes soft.

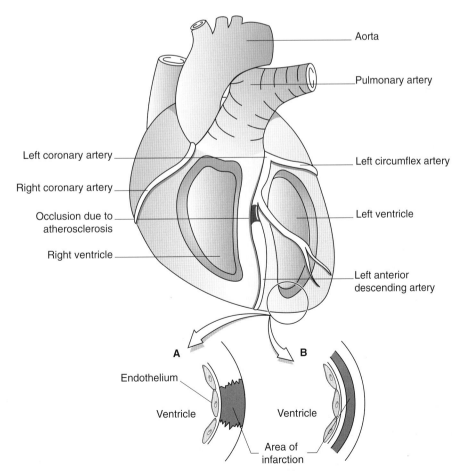

Figure 34 Major coronary arteries and types of myocardial infarction: (A) regional and (B) subendocardial.

- Up to 2–3 weeks – the dead tissue is removed and replaced by blood vessel proliferation and myofibroblasts (granulation tissue).
- Weeks to months – collagen is produced and the scar becomes progressively less cellular, less vascular and more fibrotic. See also brief summary on page 50 (Table 8).

Biochemical markers of myocardial infarction

Necrotic cardiac muscle releases enzymes, which can be measured in the serum and are helpful in confirming the diagnosis.

- **Heart-specific troponins** – released 2–4 hours after cell death, remaining raised for up to 1 week. Troponin T and I are highly specific for myocardial damage.
- **Creatine kinase (CK)** – starts to rise after a few hours of infarction, and falls again within 48 hours. CK is also released from injured skeletal muscle cells; measurement of the specific cardiac isoenzyme is therefore more diagnostically helpful.
- **Aspartate aminotransferase (AST)** – this is also non-specific as it is released by damaged liver cells.
- **Lactate dehydrogenase (LDH)** – peaks at 3–6 days and may remain elevated for 2 weeks. May be useful in patients presenting late after suspicious chest pain.

Complications of myocardial infarction

Immediate:

- arrhythmias
- acute cardiac failure
- cardiogenic shock
- sudden death.

Early:

- infarct rupture (3–7 days).

Late:

- mural thrombosis
- cardiac aneurysm.

Dressler's syndrome (pericarditis associated with circulating antibodies to heart muscle) occurs from 2 weeks to 2 years after infarction.

Reinfarction can occur at any time. Cardiac failure and arrhythmias may also be late complications. The presence of myocardial scarring increases the risk of sudden death from ventricular arrhythmia.

14.2 Hypertension, cardiomyopathies and myocarditis

Learning objectives

You should:

- know the aetiology, risk factors and complications of hypertension, so as to be able to identify patient risk factors amenable to treatment by lifestyle modification, and to investigate patients appropriately for causes of secondary hypertension
- understand the term cardiomyopathy, its classification, major causes and complications.

Hypertension

Chronically raised systemic blood pressure is a major cause of morbidity and mortality. Hypertension can cause, or significantly contribute to:

- atherosclerosis
- hypertensive heart disease (left ventricular hypertrophy)
- chronic renal failure
- cerebrovascular disease (intracerebral haemorrhage, ruptured Berry aneurysm)
- retinopathy.

'Normal' blood pressure varies within a population and with age, but evidence suggests that a sustained pressure of 140/90 mmHg or greater is associated with increased risk of disease. Persistent diastolic blood pressure in excess of 100 mmHg requires treatment. Very high blood pressure (e.g. 240/120 mmHg) can result in accelerated disease – 'malignant hypertension'.

In approximately 10% of cases, systemic hypertension is secondary to another disease (Box 18). The mechanism of primary hypertension is unclear but the following defects have been found in patients:

- abnormal renal excretion of sodium
- abnormal sodium and calcium metabolism in vascular smooth muscle
- abnormalities of renin-angiotensin mechanism, probably in part related to polymorphisms in key genes.

Family history, obesity and excessive alcohol intake are further associated factors. The aetiology of essential

---

Box 18 Secondary hypertension

Renal disease:

- Glomerulonephritis
- Polycystic kidney disease
- Renal artery stenosis
- Chronic pyelonephritis
- Renal cell carcinoma

Endocrine disease:

- Adrenal cortical tumours
- Cushing's disease
- Phaeochromocytoma
- Diabetes mellitus
- Acromegaly

Coarctation of the aorta

Iatrogenic:

- Steroid treatment

Note that hypertension can be either a cause or a consequence of chronic renal impairment.

hypertension is complex and clearly involves a combination of genetic and environmental factors. Modest, but clinically significant, reductions in blood pressure may be achieved by weight loss, regular physical exercise, moderation of alcohol intake and possibly by reduction of salt in the diet.

Blood vessel changes are similar in both primary and secondary hypertension, with homogeneous thickening of arteriolar walls and narrowing of the vascular lumen ('hyaline arteriosclerosis'). Marked cellular proliferation ('onion skinning') and necrosis of the blood vessel wall may occur in malignant hypertension. Hypertensive heart disease is characterised by concentric hypertrophy of the left ventricle.

Cardiomyopathy

Cardiomyopathy is defined as heart muscle disease not caused by ischaemic, hypertensive, valvular or congenital heart disease. Although uncommon, cardiomyopathies are an important cause of cardiac failure and sudden death in young adults. The aetiology of specific cardiomyopathies is shown in Box 19. Ninety per cent are of the dilated type.

Hypertrophic cardiomyopathy

Hypertrophic cardiomyopathy (HOCM) is characterised by asymmetrical left ventricular hypertrophy (as opposed to the concentric hypertrophy seen in hypertensive heart disease and aortic valve stenosis). The interventricular septum is particularly thickened. Microscopically, the cardiac muscle cells are enlarged and haphazardly organised (myocyte disarray). There is often fibrosis between muscle cells. Many cases show autosomal dominant inheritance. Genetic defects include cardiac myosin genes on chromosome 14. Complications of hypertrophic cardiomyopathy include:

- atrial fibrillation
- atrial thrombus and systemic embolism
- infective endocarditis of the mitral valve
- cardiac failure
- sudden death.

Dilated cardiomyopathy

Dilated cardiomyopathy is characterised by dilatation of all four cardiac chambers with progressive cardiac failure. The heart is typically enlarged (two to three times normal weight) and flabby at autopsy. Mural thrombi may be present. The microscopic findings are not specific, but there is often patchy ventricular fibrosis. Cardiomyopathy caused by alcohol, chemotherapy agents and haemochromatosis is of the dilated type.

Restrictive cardiomyopathy

Restrictive cardiomyopathy describes a condition of 'stiff' ventricles, which fail to relax, impeding diastolic filling. The ventricles are of normal size but the atria are dilated. Microscopically there is non-specific myocardial scarring. Causes include radiation fibrosis and cardiac involvement by amyloid.

Myocarditis

Myocarditis is inflammation of the heart muscle. It may be asymptomatic, or cause:

- acute cardiac failure
- sudden death
- chronic cardiac failure (usually due to dilated cardiomyopathy).

Acute myocarditis may be suggested at autopsy by a pale, flabby heart, but histological examination is necessary for diagnosis. Microscopically there is multifocal myocardial chronic inflammation associated with death of the cardiac muscle cells. The aetiology of myocarditis is shown in Box 20.

Fourteen

Box 19 Cardiomyopathy

Genetic:

- Hypertrophic cardiomyopathy (HOCM)
- Haemochromatosis

Post-infectious:

- Dilated cardiomyopathy (many cases are probably caused by viral infection)

Toxic:

- Alcoholic cardiomyopathy
- Drug induced (chemotherapy agents)

Metabolic:

- Amyloid heart disease

Idiopathic

Box 20 Causes of myocarditis

Infection:

- Viral (Coxsackie, ECHO)
- Bacterial (meningococcus)
- Fungal (*Candida*)
- Parasitic (Chagas' disease, toxoplasmosis)

Immune-mediated:

- Post-infective (including rheumatic fever)
- Systemic lupus erythematosus
- Transplant rejection

Idiopathic:

- Sarcoidosis

14.3 Congenital heart disease

Congenital heart disease describes abnormalities of the heart and major vessels that are present at birth. The incidence of congenital heart disease in liveborn infants is approximately 1:200. The common lesions include:

- isolated defects in cardiac chamber walls – atrial septal defect, ventricular septal defect
- persistence of embryonic structures – patent foramen ovale, patent ductus arteriosus
- stenosing lesions ('narrowings') – aortic valve stenosis, pulmonary stenosis, coarctation of the aorta
- transposition of the great arteries
- complex anomalies – Fallot's tetralogy.

The aetiology is unknown in many cases but there is evidence of genetic predisposition. A small percentage of cases are associated with chromosome abnormalities, particularly Turner's syndrome (45XO syndrome), with coarctation of the aorta, and Down's syndrome (trisomy 21), with atrial and ventricular septal defects. Intrauterine infection with rubella may cause multiple congenital cardiac defects. Atrial septal defects are a feature of fetal alcohol syndrome.

Some congenital heart defects, such as small atrial septal defects, may be clinically inconsequential or present only in later adult life.

Abnormal connections between the cardiac chambers permit shunting of blood from one side of the circulation to the other. In post-natal life, atrial and ventricular septal defects usually cause shunting of blood from the left side of the heart (high pressure) to the right side (low pressure). This increases the work of the right ventricle (pressure and volume overload) and can lead to right ventricular hypertrophy and pulmonary hypertension. Structural narrowing of pulmonary arteries occurs in response to chronically raised pulmonary vascular pressure, and the flow of blood through the shunt may be reversed (i.e. it becomes a right-to-left shunt, known as Eisenmenger syndrome).

Some congenital cardiac defects cause right-to-left blood shunts from their onset. Deoxygenated blood bypasses the lungs and passes directly from the right heart into the systemic circulation. If the shunt is large enough, cyanosis will be clinically apparent as blue discoloration of the skin and nail beds. Cyanotic congenital heart defects include the following.

Fallot's tetralogy

- Ventricular septal defect
- Outflow obstruction to the right ventricle
- Aorta overriding the ventricular septal defect
- Right ventricular hypertrophy

Transposition of the great vessels

The aorta emerges from the right ventricle and the pulmonary artery arises from the left ventricle. To be compatible with post-natal life, there must also be either an atrial or ventricular septal defect.

14.4 Valvular heart disease

Valvular stenosis and incompetence

Damage to the cardiac valves can result in stenosis (narrowing of the valve orifice with obstruction to blood flow) or incompetence (regurgitation of blood back through a leaking valve). Valve disease can be congenital (see Section 14.3) or acquired. In non-congenital cases the clinically important lesions almost always affect the mitral or aortic valves.

Abnormal movement of deformed valves and abnormal blood flow causes characteristic murmurs and added sounds on cardiac auscultation.

Rheumatic heart disease

Rheumatic heart disease (RHD) is a major cause of acquired mitral valve disease. The incidence has dramatically decreased in the UK over recent decades but is still relatively common in the developing countries. The initiating event is usually a pharyngeal infection by group A β-haemolytic streptococci, followed several weeks later by rheumatic fever, an immunologically mediated multisystem disorder. Rheumatic fever (RF) results from the cross-reaction of antistreptococcal antibodies with normal host tissues – direct bacterial infection does not occur. During acute RF there is often a pancarditis with inflammation of pericardium, myocardium and endocardium. Myocarditis can occasionally cause acute heart failure, arrhythmias and death. However, it is recurrent attacks of rheumatic fever that produce the most significant cardiac lesions. Repeated acute inflammation of the endocardium covering heart valves leads to fibrosis and deformity. Valve leaflets become thickened and fused, resulting in 'fish-mouth' or 'buttonhole' mitral valve stenosis. The aortic valve may also be affected. Complications include:

- atrial fibrillation
- valvular and atrial thrombus formation with systemic embolism

- cardiac failure
- infective endocarditis.

Mitral valve prolapse

Mitral valve prolapse, also known as 'floppy mitral valve', is a common condition involving approximately 5% of adults. Young females and individuals with Marfan's syndrome are particularly affected. One or both mitral valve leaflets are enlarged and prolapse into the left atrium during systole. The condition is usually incidental but occasionally can cause mitral regurgitation, infective endocarditis, valvular thrombosis or arrhythmias.

Infective endocarditis

Infection of the endocardium or vascular endothelium can occur in:

- previously damaged heart valves (e.g. rheumatic heart disease, calcific aortic stenosis)
- congenital heart disease
- prosthetic heart valves or vascular tissue
- normal heart valves (uncommon causes, acute severe endocarditis).

Infective endocarditis (see also Box 21) is usually a chronic/subacute illness caused by low-virulence organisms colo-nising abnormal tissue. Normal heart valves can be infected by high-virulence bacteria or fungi, especially in intravenous drug users or immunosuppressed individuals (those with acquired immune deficiency syndrome (AIDS) or diabetics, alcoholics, transplant recipients).

The causes and consequences of valvular heart disease are summarised in Table 19.

14.5 Heart failure

Learning objectives

You should:
- understand the pathological causes of heart failure in order to appropriately investigate patients with this condition
- be able to describe the typical changes seen at autopsy in the organs of a patient who has died from cardiac failure
- understand the clinical features of left and right heart failure and be able to relate these to the underlying pathological changes.

Box 21 Infective endocarditis: clinical notes

Acute endocarditis

Acute endocarditis typically presents with fever and acute valvular incompetence. In intravenous drug users the tricuspid valve is often affected (organisms are injected directly into arm or leg veins). Blood cultures will often be positive for the causative virulent organism. Early antibiotic treatment is necessary and emergency valve replacement may be indicated if valve destruction has caused cardiac failure.

Subacute endocarditis

Subacute endocarditis may give rise to non-specific chronic symptoms of malaise, fatigue, weight loss and anorexia. There is often a fluctuating pyrexia and a heart murmur (particularly a regurgitant or changing murmur). Extracardiac clinical features frequently reflect embolisation of cardiac vegetations, immune complex deposition or sepsis, and include:

- splinter haemorrhages in the nails
- petechial haemorrhages in the skin and conjunctivae
- glomerulonephritis
- cerebral infarction (or history of transient ischaemic attacks)
- finger clubbing
- splenomegaly
- disseminated abscesses or infarcts.

Common pathogenetic bacteria in infective endocarditis include:

- *Streptococcus viridans* – normal flora of upper respiratory tract; low virulence.
- *Streptococcus faecalis* – normal flora of perineum and gut; low virulence.

- *Staphylococcus aureus* – can be member of normal mucocutaneous flora; high virulence.
- *Staphylococcus epidermidis* – normal skin flora; low virulence.

Other organisms include *Coxiella*, *Escherichia coli*, *Chlamydia* and *Candida*.

Colonisation occurs following transient bacteraemia (bacteria floating in the bloodstream, distinct from septicaemia, which is clinical illness caused by bacteria multiplying in the blood). Such bacteraemia may result from dental work, endoscopy, surgery or established infection elsewhere in the body. Organisms may be introduced in prosthetic material or by intravascular catheters such as central venous pressure lines. Patients known to have damaged or prosthetic heart valves are at risk of developing infective endocarditis after episodes of transient bacteraemia with low virulence organisms, and so require prophylactic antibiotic therapy prior to undergoing any procedure that might seed organisms into the bloodstream.

Layers of microorganisms and fibrinous inflammatory debris build up at the site of colonisation, forming 'vegetations', which can be seen on an echocardiogram. Complications include:

- valve perforation with acute incompetence
- valve thrombosis
- perivalvular abscess
- dehiscence of prosthetic valves
- septic embolisation of the vegetations with distant infarction and abscess formation in the brain, kidney, spleen, bone, and elsewhere.

Table 19 Causes and consequences of valvular heart disease

Valve lesion	Causes	Consequences
Mitral stenosis	Rheumatic heart disease	Increased left atrial pressure; left atrial dilatation, atrial fibrillation Increased pulmonary venous pressure, leading to pulmonary hypertension and right ventricular hypertrophy
Mitral incompetence	Rheumatic heart disease Infective endocarditis Left ventricular dilatation Papillary muscle ischaemia, fibrosis or rupture Mitral valve prolapse Leaking prosthetic valve	Left atrial dilatation Left ventricular hypertrophy, due to volume overload (acute mitral incompetence caused by rupture of necrotic papillary muscle in myocardial infarction can result in acute cardiac failure)
Aortic stenosis	Senile calcification of normal tricuspid valve Calcification of congenitally bicuspid valve Rheumatic heart disease	Left ventricular hypertrophy, due to pressure overload (increased gradient across stenotic valve); ischaemia of hypertrophic ventricular myocardium (angina, arrhythmias, cardiac failure, sudden death)
Aortic incompetence	Rheumatic heart disease Infective endocarditis Leaking prosthetic valve Aortic root dilatation (aortic dissection, arthritis, Marfan's syndrome, syphilis)	Left ventricular hypertrophy, due to volume overload; left ventricular failure

Heart failure

Heart failure occurs when one or both cardiac ventricles cannot maintain an output sufficient for the body's metabolic needs. Although at first the left or the right ventricle may fail (depending on the underlying pathology), eventually both ventricles will fail, producing congestive cardiac failure and generalised enlargement of the heart (cardiomegaly). However, it is helpful to consider the aetiology and clinical effects of left and right heart failure separately.

Left ventricular failure

Left ventricular failure results from a loss of myocardial contractility, due to the sudden or gradual dysfunction, or death, of cardiac muscle cells. Less frequently, there may be marked impairment of ventricular filling during diastole. The latter situation occurs when the left ventricular wall is abnormally 'stiff' and unable to distend adequately.

Loss of myocardial contractility

- Ischaemic heart disease
- Hypertensive heart disease
- Valvular heart disease
- Dilated cardiomyopathy

Inability to fill ventricle adequately

- Massive ventricular hypertrophy (hypertension, hypertrophic cardiomyopathy, aortic stenosis)
- Amyloidosis (restrictive cardiomyopathy)

Other causes

- Pericardial disease that impedes cardiac filling (pericardial effusion or constrictive pericarditis)
- High-output cardiac failure (anaemia or thyrotoxicosis)

Markedly increased blood volume due to iatrogenic fluid overload or renal failure can precipitate or exacerbate cardiac failure.

Right ventricular failure

Right ventricular failure is most often encountered as a consequence of left ventricular dysfunction. Myocardial infarction only infrequently involves the right side of the heart, and then this is usually as an extension of a predominantly left ventricular infarct. Primary right ventricular failure can occur as a result of chronic lung disease. The right ventricle is spared the effects of systemic hypertension. However, raised pressure in the pulmonary circulation will affect the right ventricle, causing hypertrophy. This is recognised by the pathologist at post mortem by an increase in the thickness of the right ventricular wall, which is normally less than 5 mm, and an increase in isolated right ventricular weight (normally less than 50–60 g; total heart weight depends on sex and body weight, but is usually 250–350 g in the absence of any cardiac disease). Lung diseases causing pulmonary hypertension include:

- pulmonary embolism
- obstructive lung diseases
- interstitial lung diseases.

Clinical features of heart failure

Ventricular failure causes back-damming of blood in the supplying veins, venules and capillaries. This raises the hydrostatic pressure, in capillaries and venules, to the point where the hydrostatic pressure exceeds the plasma oncotic pressure throughout the course of the vessel. The result is that tissue fluid is not reabsorbed into the circulation and accumulates extravascularly, causing oedema. Dilated congested capillaries and venules may also rupture, causing microscopic tissue haemorrhages.

In left ventricular failure, these changes first appear in the pulmonary circulation. Back-pressure is transmitted through pulmonary veins into the alveolar capillaries of the lungs. Thus, oedema develops first in the pulmonary air spaces, causing shortness of breath. Patients dying with pulmonary oedema have dark-red, 'wet' lungs at post mortem, due to the accumulation of blood and oedema. Lung weights (normally 250–300 g) are often doubled or trebled by the fluid, which is easily demonstrated when the lung surfaces are cut with a knife and the fluid squeezed out, like water from a sponge. Microscopically, 'heart failure cells' are often prominent – these are alveolar macrophages containing haemosiderin pigment, a marker of previous capillary haemorrhage. Fluid accumulation within the pleural cavities may produce bilateral serous effusions.

In right ventricular failure, the inferior and superior vena cavae and their feeding veins become congested. Clinically this is evident as raised jugular venous pressure in the neck. Congestion may extend into many organs, especially the liver, which becomes enlarged and shows a characteristic patchy, pale and reddish cut surface at post mortem (which pathologists like to describe as 'nutmeg liver'). Splenomegaly is also common. Oedema develops in the dependent areas of the body, affecting the legs of seated and ambulant patients, and the sacral area in patients confined to bed. Ascites (straw-coloured fluid) may develop in the peritoneal cavity.

In severe left ventricular failure, symptoms and signs will also result from failure to adequately perfuse the systemic organs. The systemic blood pressure is decreased, the skin appears pale and cold as circulation is diverted to conserve vital organs, especially the brain. Intestinal ischaemia can result in haemorrhage or infarction. Renal ischaemia stimulates the renin-angiotensin system, causing fluid retention that may exacerbate oedema. Severe kidney ischaemia causes acute tubular necrosis and acute renal failure. In advanced heart failure, even the cerebral circulation may be compromised sufficiently to cause symptoms of confusion and diminished consciousness. The effects of low cardiac output are confounded as many patients with cardiac failure also have significant atherosclerotic disease in their major visceral arteries, which further limits blood flow to the organs.

14.6 Thrombosis, embolism and vasculitis

Learning objectives

You should:
- understand the basic pathology of thrombogenesis, and the risk factors for development of deep vein thrombosis
- know the types of embolus that can occur, and the pathology of pulmonary embolism
- know the common causes of vasculitis.

Thrombosis and embolism

See Chapter 6 and Figure 35.

Vasculitis

Inflammation of blood vessels can affect arteries, veins and capillaries. The aetiology most frequently appears to be immunological, with deposition of immune complexes in vessel walls. Some vasculitides are associated with antineutrophil cytoplasmic antibodies (ANCA). These antibodies show two distinct patterns on direct immunofluorescence examination – perinuclear (p-ANCA) and cytoplasmic (c-ANCA). Over 80% of patients with Wegener's

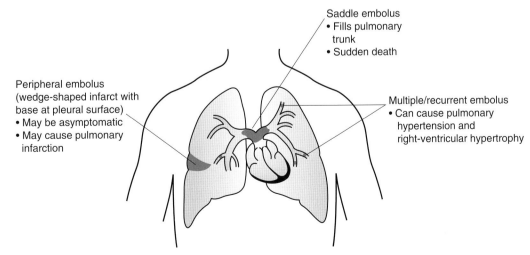

Peripheral embolus (wedge-shaped infarct with base at pleural surface)
- May be asymptomatic
- May cause pulmonary infarction

Saddle embolus
- Fills pulmonary trunk
- Sudden death

Multiple/recurrent embolus
- Can cause pulmonary hypertension and right-ventricular hypertrophy

Figure 35 Pulmonary embolism.

Fourteen

Table 20 Vasculitis

Disease	Vessel type	Clinico-pathological features	Mechanism of disease
Giant cell arteritis	Temporal arteries, also aorta	Segmental granulomatous inflammation, headache, visual impairment	Unknown
Polyarteritis nodosa	Medium-sized (muscular) arteries	Focal vessel wall necrosis, aneurysm formation, multiple organ involvement with ulceration, infarcts and haemorrhage	Unknown (possibly immune complex related)
Wegener's granulomatosis	Arteries, arterioles, capillaries, venules	Necrotising vasculitis, granulomatous inflammation of the respiratory tract, glomerulonephritis (often severe)	Immunologically mediated, c-ANCA raised in active disease
Kawasaki's disease	Coronary arteries	Acute illness – necrotising vasculitis, cervical lymphadenopathy, skin rash and erythema; coronary artery aneurysm is a late complication	Unknown (possibly infection, possibly immune system dysfunction)
Henoch–Schönlein purpura	Arterioles, capillaries, venules	Haemorrhagic rash on buttocks and legs due to acute necrotising vasculitis, 30% have glomerulonephritis	Immunological (IgA immune complexes)
Cutaneous hypersensitivity vasculitis	Arterioles, capillaries, venules	Skin rash, vessel necrosis with acute inflammation (neutrophil polymorphs)	Immunological reaction to drugs, microorganisms or other antigens

granulomatosis have circulating c-ANCA at some stage of their disease. The pathogenetic role of ANCA is uncertain, but the antibodies are useful in diagnosis and in monitoring disease activity and the effects of treatment.

The more commonly encountered and important vasculitides are shown in Table 20. Vasculitis can also occur in connective tissue disease such as rheumatoid arthritis. Infectious vasculitis occurs when microorganisms invade blood vessels from an adjacent source of sepsis, or via haematogenous spread from distant sites of infection.

14.7 Pericardial disease

Learning objective

You should:
- know the causes of pericardial fluid accumulation and pericarditis.

Pericardial serous effusions occur in congestive cardiac failure. Haemopericardium (blood in the pericardium) is seen in ruptured myocardial infarction, aortic dissection and trauma. Rapid accumulation of greater than about 200 ml of blood into the pericardium prevents ventricular filling and causes cardiac arrest.

Pericardial inflammation (pericarditis) has various causes:

Infections:

- bacterial
- viral
- tuberculosis
- fungal.

Immunological:

- rheumatic fever
- systemic lupus erythematosus
- post-myocardial infarction (Dressler's syndrome).

Other causes:

- uraemia
- post-surgery
- neoplasia
- trauma.

14.8 Vascular and cardiac neoplasms

Learning objective

You should:
- know the common benign and malignant tumours that arise in blood vessels.

Haemangiomas

Haemangiomas are common benign neoplasms of blood vessels, usually of capillary type. Haemangiomas occur in the skin and in many solid organs.

Kaposi's sarcoma

Kaposi's sarcoma is a low-grade vascular proliferation usually classified as a neoplasm, but recently linked to human herpes virus 8 infection. Kaposi's sarcoma occurs in elderly eastern European men as an indolent disease, and also arises in African children (more aggressive). Kaposi's sarcoma often develops in patients with AIDS.

Angiosarcoma

Angiosarcoma is an uncommon malignant tumour of endothelial cells, usually arising on the head and neck of elderly patients. It can also arise in solid organs. Hepatic angiosarcoma is associated with industrial exposure to polyvinyl chloride.

Cardiac myxoma

Cardiac myxoma is the commonest tumour of the heart, arising in the atria. Although benign, cardiac myxomas can cause valvular obstruction.

The heart and pericardium can become secondarily involved by malignant tumours, particularly by direct spread of bronchial carcinoma or malignant pleural mesothelioma.

Fourteen

Self-assessment: questions

One best answer questions

1. Systemic hypertension is not associated with:
   a. left ventricular hypertrophy
   b. renal artery stenosis
   c. retinopathy
   d. obesity
   e. mitral valve prolapse

2. A 28-year-old man is admitted to hospital with fever and acute left ventricular failure. He admits to regular intravenous drug misuse. He has no previous significant medical history. The likely diagnosis is:
   a. viral myocarditis
   b. hypertrophic cardiomyopathy
   c. congenital heart disease
   d. acute endocarditis
   e. subacute endocarditis

True-false questions

1. The following investigations may be indicated in a young adult with hypertension:
   a. urinary tract ultrasound
   b. urinary catecholamine measurement
   c. urinary oestrogen measurement
   d. renal artery angiography
   e. plasma glucose measurement.

2. The following are correctly paired:
   a. patent ductus arteriosus – infective endocarditis
   b. Fallot's tetralogy – tricuspid stenosis
   c. atrial septal defect – early cyanotic heart disease
   d. Turner's syndrome – coarctation of the aorta
   e. ventricular septal defect – pulmonary hypertension

3. Early complications of myocardial infarction include:
   a. papillary muscle rupture
   b. complete heart block
   c. cardiogenic shock
   d. ventricular aneurysm
   e. Dressler's syndrome

4. The following conditions can cause a dilated cardiomyopathy:
   a. haemochromatosis
   b. amyloidosis
   c. viral myocarditis
   d. alcohol misuse
   e. chemotherapeutic agents

5. The following are normal constituents of atherosclerotic plaques:
   a. cholesterol
   b. smooth muscle cells
   c. collagen
   d. neutrophil polymorphs
   e. foamy macrophages

6. Isolated left ventricular failure causes:
   a. pulmonary oedema
   b. haemosiderin-laden alveolar macrophages
   c. ascites
   d. 'nutmeg' liver
   e. raised jugular venous pressure

7. The following are risk factors for coronary heart disease:
   a. alcohol consumption of 1 unit per day
   b. raised high density lipoprotein (HDL) cholesterol
   c. post-menopausal state
   d. modest hypertension
   e. diabetes mellitus

8. The following are correctly paired:
   a. giant cell arteritis – temporal artery involvement
   b. atherosclerosis – granulomatous inflammation
   c. Wegener's granulomatosis – respiratory-tract disease
   d. polyarteritis nodosa – c-ANCA
   e. Henoch–Schönlein purpura – IgA nephropathy

9. Aortic dissection:
   a. is a complication of atherosclerosis
   b. often commences distal to the aortic arch
   c. is associated with systemic hypertension
   d. can occur in patients with inherited connective tissue disorders
   e. is inevitably fatal

10. Regarding myocardial infarction:
    a. macroscopic changes will be evident in the myocardium after 10 hours
    b. the right ventricle alone is affected in 10% of cases
    c. the underlying pathology always involves coronary artery atherosclerosis
    d. irreversible myocardial cell injury requires at least 20 minutes of anoxia
    e. the subepicardial region of the heart muscle is the most susceptible to hypoxia

11. Regarding vascular tumours:
    a. Kaposi's sarcoma occurs only in HIV-positive patients
    b. Kaposi's sarcoma is associated with cytomegalovirus infection
    c. angiosarcoma often arises in the skin
    d. angiosarcoma can be an industrial disease
    e. capillary haemangiomas have potential for malignant behaviour

12. The following are correctly paired:
    a. mitral stenosis – left ventricular hypertrophy
    b. rheumatic fever – *Staphylococcus aureus*
    c. mitral incompetence – myocardial infarction
    d. aortic stenosis – sudden cardiac death
    e. mitral valve disease – cerebrovascular accident

13. The following are risk factors for infective endocarditis:
    a. rheumatic heart disease
    b. prosthetic heart valves
    c. immunosuppression
    d. endoscopy
    e. myocardial infarction

Case history questions

Case history 1

A 67-year-old woman presents with angina. An electrocardiogram (ECG) shows changes of left ventricular hypertrophy. An echocardiogram shows left ventricular thickening and an abnormal bicuspid aortic valve.

1. What are the pathological causes of left ventricular hypertrophy?
2. What is the significance of a bicuspid aortic valve?
3. What other cardiovascular complications might occur in this patient?

Case history 2

A 58-year-old man presents with chest pain. He has a history of hypertension. The blood pressure in his left arm is 180/100 mmHg, whereas that in his right arm is 140/90 mmHg. A chest X-ray shows minor widening of the mediastinal structures, which may be related to the aorta. Electrocardiogram (ECG) shows no evidence of acute ischaemia. He collapses and dies suddenly and a coroner's autopsy is performed to ascertain the cause of death. On opening the chest, a haemopericardium is apparent.

1. What are the possible causes of haemopericardium?
2. What is the clinical significance of hypertension and of the blood pressure difference between the arms?
3. What inflammatory conditions can affect the aorta?

Case history 3

A 27-year-old drug misuser is seen in Accident and Emergency after taking an overdose of heroin. Clinical examination and investigations during admission show swinging pyrexia, splinter haemorrhages and a cardiac murmur.

1. Which other investigations are indicated?
2. Of what further cardiovascular complications is the patient at risk?

Case history 4

A 48-year-old woman consults her general practitioner for advice on coronary heart disease prevention. Her mother and paternal grandfather both died of 'heart attack' before their seventieth birthday. She has no history of cardiac symptoms herself, and is reluctant to take any regular medications.

1. What lifestyle advice would you give to this patient?
2. In view of her family history, what investigations might be considered?

Viva questions

1. What changes would you expect to see in the organs at the post-mortem examination of a patient with congestive cardiac failure?
2. Discuss the risk factors for pulmonary embolism.

Self-assessment: answers

One best answer

1. e. Hypertension is a common cause of concentric left ventricular hypertrophy. Renal artery stenosis is a cause of secondary hypertension. Retinopathy is a late complication of prolonged or severe hypertension. Weight loss in obese patients can significantly reduce blood pressure.

2. d. Whilst all of these conditions can cause left ventricular failure, the history of fever and intravenous drug use is most suggestive of acute infective endocarditis, with high-virulence organisms damaging previously normal heart valves.

True-false answers

1. a. **True.** If there are indications from urinalysis (proteinuria, haematuria) or from serum urea, creatinine and electrolyte measurements, that renal disease is present. Renal ultrasound can demonstrate kidney size, scarring and the presence of tumour masses or polycystic renal disease.
   b. **True.** If phaeochromocytoma is suspected (see Ch. 19).
   c. **False.**
   d. **True.** If renal artery stenosis is suspected.
   e. **True.** Fasting hyperglycaemia would suggest an underlying endocrine pathology – diabetes, acromegaly or Cushing's disease – with secondary hypertension.

2. a. **True.**
   b. **False.** There is pulmonary outflow tract stenosis; the tricuspid valve is unaffected.
   c. **False.**
   d. **True.**
   e. **True.** With larger defects, there is a significant left-to-right shunt, increasing pressure in the pulmonary circulation.

3. a. **True.** Infarct rupture is most common in the first 3–7 days.
   b. **True.**
   c. **True.**
   d. **False.** Ventricular aneurysm develops within the scar that forms as the infarcted muscle is replaced by fibrous tissue; it is a late complication, arising weeks or months after the infarct.
   e. **False.** This is an immunological reaction that develops at least 2 weeks after infarction.

4. a. **True.**
   b. **False.** Amyloid produces a restrictive cardiomyopathy.
   c. **True.**
   d. **True.**
   e. **True.**

5. a. **True.**
   b. **True.**
   c. **True.**
   d. **False.**
   e. **True.**

6. a. **True.**
   b. **True.**
   c. **False.**
   d. **False.**
   e. **False.**

7. a. **False.** This level of alcohol consumption is probably associated with a lower risk of coronary heart disease than abstinence. However, high alcohol intake is associated with greater cardiovascular morbidity.
   b. **False.**
   c. **True.** Women are relatively protected against ischaemic heart disease during reproductive years.
   d. **True.**
   e. **True.** Diabetes is associated with a twofold increase in ischaemic heart disease.

8. a. **True.**
   b. **False.**
   c. **True.**
   d. **False.**
   e. **True.**

9. a. **False.**
   b. **False.** The dissection usually commences in the proximal 10 cm of the aorta.
   c. **True.**
   d. **True.** There is an increased incidence in patients with Marfan's syndrome.
   e. **False.**

10. a. **False.** Naked-eye changes are unlikely to be evident until at least 24 hours after infarction.
    b. **False.** Isolated right ventricular infarction accounts for only 3% of all infarcts, but the frequency of partial right ventricular involvement in inferior left ventricular infarcts is approximately 40%.

c. **False.** The rare causes of myocardial infarction (with little or no coronary artery atheroma) include coronary artery aneurysm, dissection, arteritis and embolism. Beware the 'always' and 'never' questions!

d. **True.**

e. **False.** The most sensitive region to hypoxia is the subendocardium.

11. a. **False.**

b. **False.** Herpes virus 8.

c. **True.** Especially the head and neck of elderly patients.

d. **True.** Vinyl chloride exposure has been associated with angiosarcoma in the liver.

e. **False.** They are entirely benign neoplasms.

12. a. **False.** The left atrium is usually hypertrophic.

b. **False.** Rheumatic fever follows Group A β-haemolytic streptococcal infection.

c. **True.** If the infarct involves the papillary muscle.

d. **True.**

e. **True.** Both mitral stenosis and regurgitation can cause atrial enlargement and fibrillation, with a high risk of atrial thrombo-embolism to the brain.

13. a. **True.**

b. **True.**

c. **True.**

d. **True.** In patients with previously damaged or prosthetic valves, or certain types of congenital heart disease (e.g. patent ductus arteriosus).

e. **False.**

Case history answers

Case history 1

1. Pathological causes of left ventricular hypertrophy include:

- hypertension
- aortic stenosis
- mitral valve incompetence
- hypertrophic cardiomyopathy.

The first two are the commonest.

2. Congenitally bicuspid aortic valves occur in 1–2% of the UK population, and are more susceptible to becoming pathologically narrowed due to valve calcification. This occurs at an earlier age than calcific stenosis developing on a previously normal three-cusped aortic valve.

3. A congenitally abnormal valve is a risk factor for infective endocarditis, with its multiple complications. Bicuspid aortic valves can become incompetent as well as stenotic. Left ventricular hypertrophy can cause angina, sudden cardiac death (through a fatal cardiac arrhythmia), or gradual left ventricular failure.

Case history 2

1. Causes of haemopericardium include:

- ruptured myocardial infarction (commonest)
- aortic dissection
- trauma.

2. Hypertension and differing arm blood pressures may be features of aortic dissection. If the dissection involves the aortic arch, blood tracking in the aortic media can partly obstruct the major arterial vessels (carotid and left subclavian arteries), and therefore reduce blood flow and pressure in the upper limbs. Of course hypertension is very common in the UK population, and very few patients presenting with raised blood pressure and chest pain will have aortic dissection. Remember that hypertension is a major risk factor for ischaemic heart disease.

3. Aortic inflammation (vasculitis/aortitis) can occur in giant cell arteritis and in Takayasu disease (a histologically similar but clinically distinct granulomatous vasculitis). In previous decades, tertiary syphilis was a common cause of aortitis with thoracic aortic aneurysm, but this condition is now extremely rare in the UK. Atherosclerosis is, of course, an inflammatory condition that commonly results in distal abdominal aneurysms. Rarely, infective aortitis results in mycotic aneurysm formation.

Case history 3

1. The features are highly suggestive of infective endocarditis. Blood cultures are required for identification of the organism(s) responsible – these are more likely to be positive in acute endocarditis than in subacute cases, where multiple culture specimens can be negative, especially if antibiotics have been started. An echocardiogram will demonstrate valvular vegetations.

2. *Comment*: Complications are discussed in Box 21, page 125, but include:

- valve incompetence, with or without acute cardiac failure
- septic embolisation and infarction
- glomerulonephritis
- distant organ abscess formation.

Case history 4

Comment: Remember that the four main risk factors for atherosclerosis, and therefore for coronary heart disease, are: smoking, hypertension, diabetes and hypercholesterolaemia. Giving up cigarettes, maintaining a normal body weight, taking regular physical exercise, moderating excess alcohol intake and reducing cholesterol and saturated fats in the diet can all help reduce the risk of ischaemic heart disease.

Heart disease is very common, so it may be mere coincidence that this patient reports a family history. However, hypercholesterolaemia and type 2 diabetes certainly can show familial clustering, so fasting cholesterol and dipstick urine testing or fasting blood glucose might be appropriate. A strong history of multiple young cardiac deaths in the family raises the possibility of a more unusual inherited cause, such as an uncommon form of hyperlipidaemia, hypertrophic cardiomyopathy or an unusual conduction defect.

Viva answers

1. Changes in the heart will reflect the underlying cause of the cardiac failure – there may be fibrosis of the left ventricle in ischaemic heart disease, with hypertrophy in hypertension, aortic stenosis or mitral incompetence. There is often generalised cardiac chamber enlargement (cardiomegaly) in biventricular failure. Other features can include valvular heart disease (vegetations, valve thickening, distortion or calcification), and right ventricular hypertrophy in patients with pulmonary hypertension. Ventricular hypertrophy is confirmed by measuring the isolated ventricular weight but is suggested by increased muscle thickness. The lungs frequently show marked vascular congestion and pulmonary oedema. The pleural cavities may contain straw-coloured effusions (transudates). The liver has a 'nutmeg' appearance on its cut surface, due to venous congestion, which is most severe in the perivenular (centrilobular) part of the liver lobules. The liver may show mild enlargement. Vascular congestion is also seen in the spleen and kidneys. Pitting subcutaneous oedema can be demonstrated in the dependent areas (usually lower legs).

2. *Comment*: You need to know what pulmonary embolism is, its clinical consequences, and the risk factors for deep vein thrombosis. Be prepared to discuss the basic pathophysiology of thrombogenesis. This is all covered in Chapters 6 and 15.

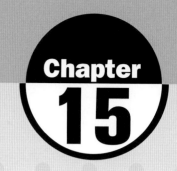

Respiratory system

Chapter overview

The respiratory system extends from the nasal orifices to the periphery of the lungs and the pleura, and includes the nasal passages, paranasal sinuses, larynx and lungs. The pathology of these structures will be discussed in this chapter. Respiratory diseases are so common that you will inevitably encounter them in whichever branch of medicine you decide to follow. Many bed-ridden patients develop some degree of bronchopneumonia. Pneumonia is also a frequent cause of hospital admission, and is often fatal in the elderly and infirm. Obstructive and restrictive (interstitial) lung diseases are common, causing significant morbidity among the general population. Last but not least, lung cancer is not only the most common malignancy in men, with increasing frequency in women, but it is also the most frequently fatal malignancy. Lung disease in general is a major cause of morbidity and mortality across the globe, and its importance in clinical practice cannot be overemphasised.

15.1 Nasal passages and paranasal sinuses

Learning objective

You should:
- know the major inflammatory conditions and tumours that can affect the nasal passages and paranasal sinuses.

Structure and function

The nasal passages and sinuses lie in continuity and are lined by respiratory-type epithelium. The function of the nasal sinuses is to warm, humidify and clean inspired air.

Inflammatory disorders

Inflammatory diseases are the commonest disorders to affect the nasal passages and paranasal sinuses.

Rhinitis

Inflammation of the nasal passages has two main causes:

- **The common cold** (infective rhinitis). This is almost invariably initiated by a virus.
- **Hay fever** (allergic rhinitis). This is initiated by allergens, the inflammatory reaction being mediated via type I and type III hypersensitivity reactions (see Ch. 8).

Nasal polyps

These inflammatory swellings are common and result from recurrent inflammation of the nasal passages. They are often bilateral (in contrast with nasal tumours which are usually unilateral).

Sinusitis

Inflammation of the sinuses is frequently a complication of acute rhinitis. Swelling of the nasal mucosa obstructs the drainage orifices of the sinuses. This leads to stasis of the secretions within the sinuses, with consequent infection and inflammation.

Tumours

Tumours of the nasal passages and sinuses are uncommon.

Benign

The most frequent benign tumours are:

- squamous papilloma
- inverted papilloma (transitional cell papilloma)
- haemangioma
- angiofibroma.

Malignant

Malignant tumours of the nasal passages and paranasal sinuses include:

- squamous cell carcinoma
- transitional cell carcinoma
- adenocarcinoma
- plasmacytoma
- olfactory neuroblastoma.

15.2 The larynx

Structure and function

The larynx connects the trachea to the pharynx. It is a complex organ with numerous connective tissue elements. The lining epithelium varies from non-keratinising stratified squamous to respiratory-type epithelium. The function of the larynx is to allow air into the trachea and to produce sound for speaking. The epiglottis prevents food from entering the trachea.

Inflammatory disorders

Laryngitis

Inflammation of the larynx can be the result of infection, overuse of the voice, mechanical irritation or exposure to tobacco, other chemical agents, or allergens. Infective laryngitis can be caused by a number of viruses and bacteria. The laryngeal inflammation is usually mild, but if it is severe, such as in diphtheria, the resultant oedema and exudate can cause laryngeal obstruction, particularly in children.

Epiglottitis

The most commonly implicated organism in epiglottitis is the bacteria *Haemophilus influenzae.* Infection results in marked oedema and enlargement of the epiglottis, which can cause life-threatening airway obstruction in children.

Tumours

Benign

The commonest benign tumours are:

- laryngeal polyps ('singers' nodes'). These are most often found in smokers or people who overuse their larynx
- squamous papilloma.

Malignant

The most frequent malignant tumour of the larynx is squamous cell carcinoma, which typically affects males over 40. This tumour is associated with cigarette smoking, and there may be an increased risk in those exposed to asbestos. Arising most often on the vocal cords, the carcinoma invades locally and can later cause widespread distant metastases.

15.3 The lungs

Structure and function of the lungs

The function of the lungs is to exchange gases between the inspired air and the blood. Inspired air passes from the trachea into the main left and right bronchi. Each bronchus then branches dichotomously giving rise to progressively smaller airways, hence the term 'respiratory tree' (Figure 36). Progressive branching of the bronchi forms bronchioles. Bronchioles branch until they form terminal bronchioles. The part of the lung distal to each terminal bronchiole is called the acinus, or terminal respiratory unit. Branching of the terminal bronchioles gives rise to respiratory bronchioles, which in turn branch into alveolar ducts. Each alveolar duct branches and empties into blind-ended alveolar sacs, where gas exchange occurs. A group of 3–5 acini is referred to as a lobule.

The trachea, bronchi and bronchioles are lined by respiratory-type epithelium. The alveoli are lined by type I and type II pneumocytes, beneath which lies a thin connective tissue membrane. This membrane separates the alveoli from the pulmonary capillaries but allows rapid and efficient diffusion of gases.

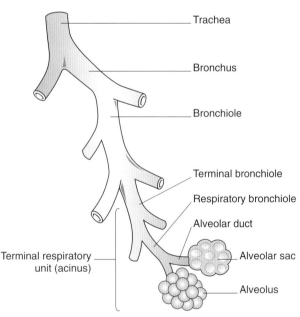

Figure 36 Structure of the lower respiratory tract.

Trachea

Bronchus

Bronchiole

Terminal bronchiole

Respiratory bronchiole

Alveolar duct

Alveolar sac

Alveolus

Terminal respiratory unit (acinus)

Disorders of the lungs can be divided into five major groups:

- Inflammatory
- Obstructive
- Restrictive (interstitial)
- Vascular
- Neoplastic.

Inflammatory disorders

Bronchitis

Acute bronchitis can be caused by infection or exposure to irritant chemical agents such as tobacco smoke, sulphur dioxide and chlorine. Infective inflammation of the bronchi is usually accompanied by inflammation of the trachea and larynx (acute laryngotracheobronchitis), which is clinically more severe in children ('croup'). Acute infective bronchitis is most commonly initiated by viruses such as respiratory syncytial virus (RSV), although bacteria can also be a cause. Episodes of acute bronchitis are often seen in people with chronic bronchitis, causing an exacerbation of the established disease.

Bronchiolitis

There are three main types of bronchiolitis:

- **Primary bronchiolitis**: This is most commonly seen in infants, in whom it can cause symptoms of acute respiratory distress. The inflammation is usually caused by viruses, especially RSV. Resolution is usual, but a minority of patients develop bronchopneumonia.
- **Follicular bronchiolitis**: This is seen in patients with rheumatoid arthritis. Lymphoid aggregates with germinal centres compress the airways.
- **Bronchiolitis obliterans**: This can occur from a number of diseases and disease states, and is characterised by the obliteration of bronchiolar lumina by masses of organising inflammatory exudate.

Bacterial pneumonia

Pneumonia is defined as an inflammatory condition of the lung characterised by consolidation (solidification) of the pulmonary tissue. In infective pneumonia, the causative organism infects the lung parenchyma, causing the formation of an inflammatory exudate within the alveolar spaces with consequent consolidation.

Pathogenesis

The respiratory system uses a number of defence mechanisms to clear or destroy any inhaled microorganisms. These include:

- nasal secretions
- the mucociliary apparatus
- alveolar clearance by macrophages
- coughing and sneezing.

Pneumonia can result whenever these defence mechanisms are impaired (see Table 21).

Table 21 Defects in lung defence mechanisms predisposing to infection

Defect in defence mechanism	Causes
Loss or suppression of the cough reflex	Coma, sedation, neuromuscular disorders, drugs
Impairment of ciliary function	Immotile cilia syndrome (Kartagener syndrome)
Injury to the mucociliary apparatus	Cigarette smoking
Accumulation of secretions	Cystic fibrosis, bronchiectasis
Interference with alveolar macrophage function	Cigarette smoking, hypoxia
Flooding of the alveoli	Pulmonary congestion and oedema
Reduction in immune response	Immunosuppression

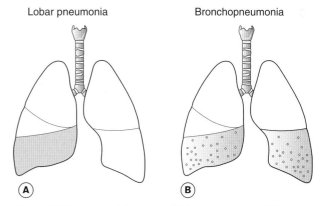

Figure 37 Distribution of disease in (A) lobar pneumonia and (B) bronchopneumonia.

Classification

Classically, pneumonia is classified according to the main anatomical pattern of consolidation into bronchopneumonia and lobar pneumonia (Figure 37).

Bronchopneumonia Bronchopneumonia is characterised by patchy consolidation of the lung. Those individuals most at risk are elderly people, infants, and people with debilitating illnesses. Typical aetiological organisms include streptococci, staphylococci, pneumococci, *H. influenzae*, *Pseudomonas aeruginosa* and coliform bacteria. The consolidation is multilobular and frequently bilateral and basal. Histologically, a neutrophil-rich exudate fills the bronchi, bronchioles and adjacent alveolar spaces.

Lobar pneumonia Lobar pneumonia is characterised by consolidation of a large portion of a lobe or an entire lobe, and it typically affects otherwise healthy adults aged between 20 and 50 years. The most common pathogenic organism is *Streptococcus pneumoniae*. Less common causal organisms are *Klebsiella pneumoniae*, staphylococci, strep-tococci and *H. influenzae*.

The four stages in the pathological progress of untreated lobar pneumonia are:

1. **Congestion** – This stage lasts for about 24 hours. It is characterised by vascular engorgement and the passage of exudate (protein-rich fluid) into the alveolar spaces. The affected lung is heavy and red.
2. **Red hepatisation** – This stage lasts for a few days. The exudate in the alveolar spaces now contains inflammatory cells, red blood cells and fibrin. A pleural fibrinous exudate forms (pleuritis/pleurisy). The lung is airless, red and solid.
3. **Grey hepatisation** – This stage also lasts for a few days. The inflammatory cells and red cells are destroyed while the fibrin continues to accumulate. The lung is firm and has a grey-brown, dry surface.
4. **Resolution** – This occurs on about the eighth day. The exudate undergoes enzymic digestion and is then resorbed or coughed up. The lung parenchyma returns to normal. The pleural exudate is either resorbed or undergoes organisation.

Atypical pneumonia

The term 'atypical' in the context of pneumonia is used when the inflammatory changes in the lungs are confined to the alveolar septa and interstitium, without a significant alveolar exudate. Characteristically, patients have few localising symptoms even with severe atypical pneumonia. As such, atypical pneumonia should be suspected when the chest X-ray findings are much worse than the symptoms.

Immunocompromised patients are particularly at risk.

Aetiology

In immunocompetent individuals, the causes of atypical pneumonia are:

- Viruses, e.g. influenza, RSV, adenovirus
- Bacteria, e.g. *Legionella pneumophila* (Legionnaire disease)
- Mycoplasma
- *Coxiella burnetii* (Q fever).

In immunocompromised individuals the causes of atypical pneumonia are:

- Viruses, e.g. CMV, measles, varicella
- Bacteria, e.g. *Pneumocystis carinii*, *Chlamydia*
- Fungi, e.g. *Candida*, *Aspergillus*.

Aspiration pneumonia

When food or liquid is aspirated into the lung, there is irritation of the pulmonary tissue by the acidic gastric contents and introduction of organisms from the oropharynx. Inflammation and consolidation of the affected part of the lung may ensue. At-risk clinical situations include sedation, coma, anaesthesia and acute alcoholism.

Lung abscess

A lung abscess is a local suppurative process within the lungs (often walled off), accompanied by necrosis of the lung tissue.

Aetiology and pathogenesis

Under the right conditions, almost any pathogen can cause a lung abscess. An abscess may form as a result of:

- Aspiration or bacterial pneumonia
- Entrapment of septic emboli in the lungs (e.g. embolisation of vegetations in infective endocarditis)
- Infection of a pulmonary infarct
- Airway obstruction. An abscess may form beyond the obstruction, which may be a tumour or a foreign body
- Miscellaneous situations, such as following penetrating trauma to the lung or the spread of infection from neighbouring organs.

Complications

With antibiotic therapy, many resolve and heal completely leaving a fibrous scar. A persistent abscess may require surgical treatment. Possible complications of a lung abscess include an empyema (pus in the pleural space), pyo-pneumothorax, haemorrhage and spread of infection to distant sites to cause, for example, brain abscesses or meningitis.

Tuberculosis

The term 'tuberculosis' refers to the disease caused by *Mycobacterium tuberculosis* (found within infected respiratory secretions and air droplets) and less commonly *Mycobacterium bovis* (found in the milk of diseased cows). Tuberculosis is the single most important infectious cause of death in the world. Up until the mid-1980s, Western countries had seen a decline in the number of clinical cases because of:

- improved hygiene and social conditions
- the introduction of effective antibiotics against the bacilli
- the introduction of immunisation with bacille Calmette–Guérin (BCG).

At present the incidence of tuberculosis is rising in the USA, Europe and Africa, most probably due to the increasing incidence of human immunodeficiency virus (HIV) infection. Furthermore, antibiotic-resistant strains are now being isolated. The lung is the commonest site for infection. Tuberculosis is classically divided into two phases, primary and post-primary (secondary) tuberculosis (Figure 38).

Primary tuberculosis

Inhaled *M. tuberculosis* passes into the lungs and initiates a non-specific inflammatory response. Alveolar macrophages phagocytose the organism and transport it to the hilar lymph nodes. These naive macrophages are unable to kill the organism, and so more macrophages are recruited. Meanwhile, the bacilli multiply, lyse the host cell and then infect more macrophages. At this point, the organisms can potentially disseminate via the bloodstream

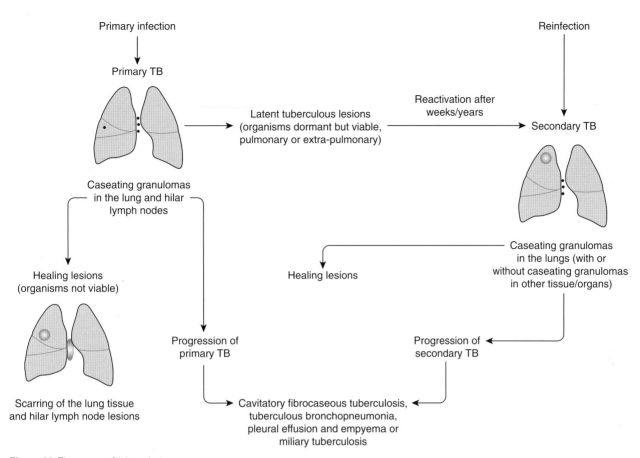

Figure 38 The course of tuberculosis.

to other parts of the lung and more distant sites. In immunocompetent hosts, the mycobacteria activate the T cells, which can cause lysis of infected macrophages and stimulate macrophages to mature into epithelioid cells, which are effective killers of *M. tuberculosis*. Some epithelioid cells fuse to become multinucleated giant cells. Consequently, a granuloma forms consisting of epithelioid cells, giant cells and a central area of caseous necrosis corresponding to lysed infected macrophages (see Ch. 4). The bacilli are unable to survive in such acidic and oxygen-poor conditions, and so infection is controlled. A calcified scar forms in both the affected lung parenchyma (Ghon focus) and the hilar lymph nodes, which together are called the primary Ghon complex. Importantly, bacilli may still survive in these scarred foci for many years. Primary tuberculosis is asymptomatic in most cases. Rarely, particularly with infants, children or immunocompromised adults, the primary lesion may progress, resulting in cavitation, tuberculous bronchopneumonia, pleural effusion and empyema, or miliary tuberculosis (tuberculosis spreading around the body).

Post-primary (secondary) tuberculosis

Most post-primary tuberculosis represents reactivation of previous primary tuberculosis. During primary infection, the bacilli may attempt to disseminate and establish themselves at sites of high oxygen tension and low blood flow, such as the lung apices. Development of post-primary tuberculosis may occur if the host is susceptible, with the formation of typical caseating granulomas. These lesions either heal spontaneously, or with treatment, resulting in a fibrocalcific scar. Alternatively, post-primary tuberculosis may progress, resulting in cavitatory fibrocaseous tuberculosis, tuberculous pneumonia, pleural effusion and empyema, or miliary tuberculosis.

Miliary tuberculosis

If the tuberculous bacteraemia becomes heavy during primary or post-primary tuberculosis, miliary tuberculosis may result. Miliary tuberculosis is characterised by numerous granulomas in many organs, and may be fatal if left untreated.

Obstructive airways disease

This group of disorders is characterised by an increase in resistance to airflow, owing to partial or complete obstruction at any level of the respiratory tree. The major obstructive disorders are chronic bronchitis, emphysema, asthma and bronchiectasis. The symptom common to all these disorders is 'dyspnoea' (difficulty breathing), but each have their own clinical and anatomical characteristics.

Chronic bronchitis and emphysema almost always coexist, and the term chronic obstructive pulmonary disease (COPD) is often used to refer to them.

Chronic bronchitis

Chronic bronchitis is defined clinically as cough with sputum production for at least 3 months in at least 2 consecutive years. The condition tends to affect middle-aged men who are smokers. Typically, patients with severe disease are cyanotic (blue) and are then referred to as 'blue bloaters'.

Aetiology

Undoubtedly, the single most important cause is cigarette smoking.

Pathogenesis

Irritants, such as tobacco smoke, cause two main abnormalities, which lead to airway obstruction.

- Increase in size (hypertrophy) of submucosal glands and a marked increase in the number (hyperplasia) of goblet cells. There is consequent hypersecretion of mucus, mainly in the large airways, which results in mucous plugging and overproduction of sputum.
- A respiratory bronchiolitis affecting the smaller airways of less than 2 mm in diameter.

Infection does not seem to play a role in the initiation of chronic bronchitis, but is an important cause of exacerbations.

Emphysema

Emphysema is characterised by abnormal permanent dilatation of the air spaces distal to the terminal bronchioles, accompanied by destruction of their walls without obvious fibrosis. The clinical symptoms of emphysema do not appear until at least a third of the lung parenchyma is destroyed. Typically, patients overventilate to remain well oxygenated, and are then referred to as 'pink puffers'.

Classification

Emphysema is classified into four main types according to the anatomical distribution of the lesions and based on the appearance of the lungs with the naked eye or hand lens (Figure 39).

Centrilobular (centriacinar) emphysema In this type there is involvement of the central or proximal parts of the acinus with sparing of the distal alveoli. The lesions are closely associated with cigarette smoking and are more common in the upper lobes.

Panlobular (panacinar) emphysema In this type all airways distal to the terminal bronchioles (i.e. the entire acinus) are involved. The lower lobes are more commonly affected, particularly the bases. Panacinar emphysema is associated with α_1-antitrypsin deficiency.

Paraseptal emphysema In this type the distal (peripheral) part of the acinus is involved, with sparing of the proximal part. It is usually more severe in the upper lobes. The affected airways can become very dilated, forming cyst-like structures which are termed 'bullae' if they reach over 10 mm in diameter. These bullae may rupture, resulting in a spontaneous pneumothorax.

Irregular emphysema In this type the acinus is irregularly involved. Irregular emphysema is almost invariably associated with scarring.

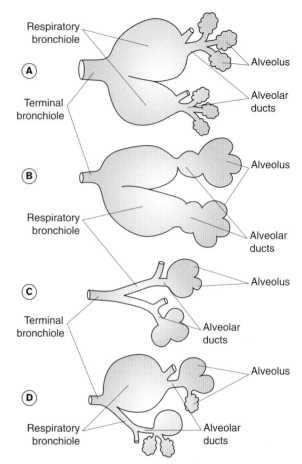

Figure 39 Classification of emphysema. (A) Centrilobular, (B) panacinar, (C) paraseptal and (D) irregular emphysema.

Pathogenesis

Current evidence indicates that emphysema is due to an imbalance between protease and antiprotease activity in the lung. Support for this theory is based on the association between α_1-antitrypsin deficiency and the development of emphysema. α_1-Antitrypsin inhibits the actions of proteases, particularly elastase, which is secreted by neutrophils. α_1-Antitrypsin deficiency is a genetic disorder showing an autosomal recessive pattern of inheritance. Homozygous patients have reduced levels of the enzyme and have a tendency to develop emphysema because they are unable to inhibit elastase secreted by inflammatory cells. Destruction of the airway wall ensues. The process is further compounded by smoking, mainly because smokers have more inflammatory cells in their lungs.

Irregular emphysema is thought to be due to air trapping because of fibrotic scarring. The scars are the result of a previous inflammatory process.

Pathology

In the advanced stages of the disease, the lungs may appear voluminous and bullae may be seen. Microscopically, there are abnormal fenestrations in the walls of the alveoli with complete destruction of the septal walls.

Asthma

Asthma is a chronic relapsing disorder characterised by hyper-reactive airways leading to episodic, reversible bronchoconstriction, owing to increased responsiveness to various stimuli. These sudden episodes of bronchoconstriction are manifested by sudden attacks of dyspnoea, coughing and wheezing. Between attacks, patients are often asymptomatic. Rarely, symptoms may be severe and prolonged (status asthmaticus). Severe asthma and status asthmaticus are both medical emergencies and can prove fatal.

Asthma is divided into two basic types:

* extrinsic asthma
* intrinsic asthma

Extrinsic asthma

This type of asthma is induced by exposure to an extrinsic allergen, and is mediated by a type I hypersensitivity reaction.

Atopic allergic asthma This is the most common type of asthma. It usually begins in childhood and patients may also have other atopic disorders such as hay fever or eczema. There is often a family history of asthma, hay fever or eczema. The asthma is triggered by environmental allergens such as dust, pollen, food and animal dander. Inhalation of such allergens triggers a type I, IgE-mediated hypersensitivity reaction characterised by an immediate response and a late phase reaction caused by the local release of inflammatory mediators from a variety of cell types (Figure 40). The precise pathogenesis of asthma involves interactions between many cell types and mediators, and these interactions are not fully understood. A number of chemical mediators are implicated in the asthma response. Histamine, prostaglandin D_2, leukotrienes, platelet-activating factor, tumour necrosis factor (TNF), chemokines and various interleukins are among those substances thought to be important.

The following morphological changes are seen in the lungs in cases of severe asthma:

* mucous plugging of bronchi. These plugs may contain whorls of shed epithelium (Curschmann's spirals)
* oedema and inflammation of the bronchial walls. Histologically, there is prominence of eosinophils. Eosinophil membrane protein can be seen as crystals called Charcot–Leyden crystals
* over-inflation of the lungs distal to the obstruction
* mucous gland hypertrophy
* bronchial wall smooth muscle hypertrophy
* thickening of the bronchial basement membrane.

Occupational asthma This form of asthma is triggered by agents inhaled at work, e.g. fumes, dusts, gases and other chemicals. The airway reaction is thought to be mediated by type I and type III hypersensitivity.

Allergic bronchopulmonary aspergillosis This type of asthma is induced by the inhalation of spores of the fungus *Aspergillus fumigatus*. The inhaled spores induce type I and type III hypersensitivity reactions.

Intrinsic asthma

Intrinsic asthma can be induced by pulmonary infection (usually viral), ingestion of aspirin, cold, exercise and stress. The mechanism leading to the bronchoconstriction seems to be non-immunological. The pathogenesis remains uncertain.

Bronchiectasis

Bronchiectasis is characterised by permanent dilatation of bronchi and bronchioles. Patients suffer from cough with the production of copious amounts of foul-smelling sputum.

Pathogenesis

Both obstruction and infection are usually necessary for development of bronchiectasis. Obstruction of the bronchial lumen results in secondary inflammation and fibrosis. The damaged bronchial walls weaken and eventually become irreversibly dilated. The obstruction can be due to a foreign body, tumour, inspissated mucus or external compression. Persistent infection results in inflammation and leads to extensive weakening and destruction of the airway walls. Either infection or obstruction may be the initiating factors in the development of bronchiectasis. Persistent infection may lead to obstruction of airways, and obstruction may lead to secondary infection.

It therefore follows that bronchiectasis may be associated with congenital or hereditary disorders such as cystic fibrosis, Kartagener syndrome or immunodeficiency states.

Complications

Complications such as empyema formation, brain abscess and amyloidosis are now rare.

Interstitial (restrictive) lung diseases

The interstitium of the lung consists of the basement membrane of the endothelial and epithelial cells, collagen fibres, elastic tissue, fibroblasts and occasional inflammatory cells. In interstitial (restrictive) lung diseases, there is diffuse infiltration of the interstitium, leading to increased amounts of tissue in the lung and causing reduced lung compliance and lung volume, and reduced oxygen diffusing capacity. The functional changes are restrictive rather than obstructive, and affected patients develop symptoms of progressive breathlessness and cough.

Many conditions belong to this group of disorders. Although each begins as a distinct entity, they all ultimately cause scarring and destruction of the lung, referred to as 'honeycomb lung'.

Pathogenesis

Regardless of the type of interstitial lung disease, the earliest change seen in the lungs is the influx of inflammatory cells into the alveoli and alveolar walls. This distorts the normal structure of the alveoli and results in the release of chemical mediators, which injure parenchymal cells and promote fibrosis. Ultimately, with remodelling, the alveoli are replaced by cystic spaces separated by fibrous connective tissue (honeycomb lung).

Fifteen

141

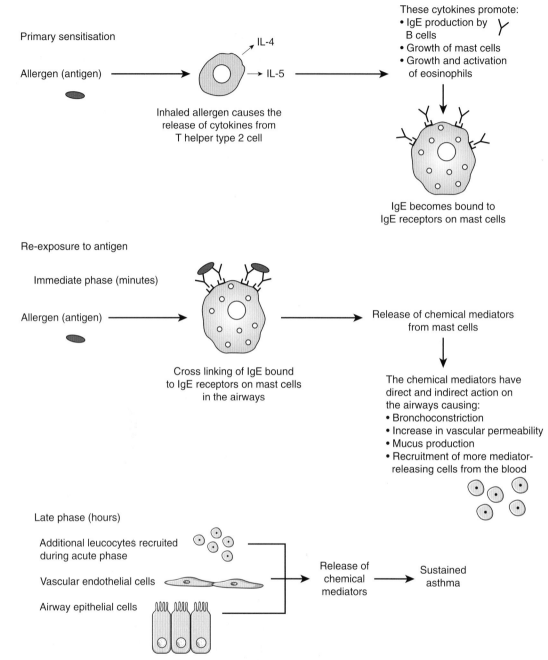

Figure 40 A model of mechanisms in the pathogenesis of asthma.

Classification

There are different ways in which the interstitial lung diseases can be classified (Table 22).

Pneumoconiosis

This term is used to refer to a group of lung diseases resulting from the inhalation of dusts, fumes and vapours.

Coalworker pneumoconiosis

Coalworker pneumoconiosis (CWP) is caused by inhalation of coal dust. Because coal dust particles are less than 2–3 μm in size, they travel all the way to the alveoli. The coal dust is ingested by alveolar macrophages, which then aggregate around the airways and lymphatics. During their attempts to degrade the particles, macrophages release inflammatory chemical mediators, which cause parenchymal injury and induce fibrosis. The effect of coal dust on the lungs progresses through three stages. Progression through the stages, with continued exposure to coal dust, varies significantly from person to person.

1. **Anthracosis** refers to the presence of coal-dust pigment within the lung and is asymptomatic.
2. **Simple CWP** refers to focal accumulations of dust-laden macrophages within the lung. This stage can be further subdivided into macular and nodular CWP. Coal macules are lesions measuring 1–2 mm

Table 22 Classification of interstitial lung diseases

Classification according to aetiology		Classification according to speed of onset of damage	
Known aetiology	Unknown aetiology	Acute interstitial diseases	Chronic interstitial diseases
Environmental agents	Idiopathic pulmonary fibrosis	ARDS	Idiopathic pulmonary fibrosis
Radiation		Drugs and toxins	Pneumoconiosis
Hypersensitivity pneumonitis	Sarcoid	Acute radiation pneumonitis	Sarcoid
Following adult respiratory distress syndrome (ARDS)	Goodpasture's syndrome Idiopathic pulmonary haemosiderosis	Diffuse pulmonary haemorrhage syndromes	Collagen vascular diseases
Drugs and toxins	Collagen vascular diseases		

in diameter, while coal nodules are larger and contain collagen fibres. The effect of simple CWP on lung function is minimal.

3. **Complicated CWP/progressive massive fibrosis** refers to the presence of large, blackened nodules (>10 mm) within the lung with extensive scarring. The condition generally takes several years to develop, but ultimately the progressive fibrosis results in severely compromised lung function.

Silicosis

Silicates are inorganic minerals found in stone and sand. Silica particles are particularly fibrogenic and, after inhalation, enter the terminal respiratory units, where they stimulate the release of chemical mediators from macrophages. They also have toxic effects on macrophages and epithelial cells, denaturing their cell membranes. Grossly, affected lungs contain multiple fibrous nodules, which may coalesce to form large scars. Fibrotic lesions may also occur in the hilar lymph nodes and their characteristic appearance on radiography is referred to as 'eggshell calcification'. With progression of the disease there is severe impairment of lung function.

Asbestosis

Asbestos is a family of silicates that form fibres. There are two distinct geometric forms of asbestos:

- serpentine: curly flexible fibres; includes the chrysotile form
- amphibole: straight stiff fibres; includes the crocidolite and amosite forms.

Amphiboles are more pathogenic than serpentines. The long, thin fibres have a small enough diameter (0.25–0.5 μm) to reach all the way to the alveoli and become impacted there. Alveolar macrophages attempt to ingest and degrade the fibres but, in so doing, release chemical mediators that cause tissue injury and fibrosis resulting in asbestosis. The fibrosis tends to be diffuse rather than nodular. During the attempts at engulfment and digestion, asbestos fibres become coated by mucopolysaccharides and haemosiderin, producing a beaded appearance under microscopy (asbestos bodies). As well as asbestosis,

exposure to asbestos can cause other pathological changes in the lungs:

- pleural plaques – the commonest manifestation of asbestos exposure (they are asymptomatic)
- pleural effusion
- diffuse pleural fibrosis
- bronchogenic carcinoma
- mesothelioma
- other extrapulmonary neoplasms, e.g. laryngeal, gastrointestinal.

Berylliosis

Berylliosis results from prolonged exposure to beryllium. Workers in the nuclear and aerospace industries are at risk, but new cases of chronic berylliosis are now rare. Beryllium induces the formation of pulmonary and systemic granulomatous lesions. The pulmonary granulomas eventually become fibrotic.

Caplan's syndrome

This refers to the coexistence of rheumatoid nodules with pneumoconiosis.

Idiopathic pulmonary fibrosis

In this condition there is diffuse pulmonary fibrosis of unknown aetiology. The disorder typically affects individuals between 45 and 65. With progression of the disease, respiratory failure with or without cor pulmonale ensues. Although some patients benefit from treatment with corticosteroids, median survival is less than 5 years.

Hypersensitivity pneumonitis (extrinsic allergic alveolitis)

This is caused by intense prolonged exposure to antigens which evoke type III and type IV hypersensitivity responses. Conditions such as farmer's lung, pigeon breeder's lung, and humidifier lung are included in this type of interstitial lung disease.

Drugs and toxins

After they are absorbed into the body, some drugs (e.g. bleomycin, nitrofurantoin, gold, penicillamine and amiodarone) and some other toxic substances (e.g. paraquat) can cause fibrosis within the lungs.

Ionising radiation

The toxic effects of radiation on the lungs is dose dependent, with increased exposure to radiation increasing the risk of diffuse alveolar damage (acute radiation pneumonitis). The condition is most commonly seen in those undergoing radiotherapy for pulmonary or other thoracic tumours. Some cases of acute radiation pneumonitis respond to corticosteroid treatment, but others progress, leading to interstitial fibrosis in the affected area (chronic radiation pneumonitis).

Sarcoidosis

This condition is characterised by non-caseating granulomas within many tissues and organs. There is lung and lymph node involvement in the vast majority of cases. The chest X-ray of affected individuals typically shows bilateral hilar lymphadenopathy.

Pulmonary involvement in collagen vascular disorders

- Systemic sclerosis (scleroderma)
- Systemic lupus erythematosus (SLE)
- Rheumatoid arthritis, pulmonary involvement occurs in one of four forms:
  - *chronic pleuritis*
  - *diffuse interstitial fibrosis*
  - *intrapulmonary rheumatoid nodules*
  - *rheumatoid nodules with pneumoconiosis (Caplan's syndrome).*

Diffuse pulmonary haemorrhage syndromes

Goodpasture's syndrome

In this condition, circulating anti-glomerular basement membrane (anti-GBM) antibodies cross-react with pulmonary alveolar basement membrane, resulting in intrapulmonary haemorrhage.

Idiopathic pulmonary haemosiderosis

Typically affects children and is manifest by recurrent episodes of intra-alveolar haemorrhage.

Vasculitides causing intra-pulmonary haemorrhage

Involvement of the lung by vasculitides such as hypersensitivity angiitis, Wegener's granulomatosis and SLE can cause intrapulmonary haemorrhage.

Adult respiratory distress syndrome

Adult respiratory distress syndrome (ARDS) is characterised by rapid onset of respiratory distress, initiated by the delivery of a massive insult to the alveolar capillary walls. Endothelial damage allows leakage of proteins and fibrin into the alveoli with the formation of hyaline membranes, which act as barriers to gas exchange. The insult can occur in a number of clinical settings, but infection and physical injuries such as burns and head injuries are the most common causes. The condition is fatal within a few days in 50% of cases despite intensive therapy. For the majority

of survivors, there is permanent lung damage with fibrosis. Resolution of the inflammation and complete recovery is unusual.

Bronchiolitis obliterans organising pneumonia

The major pathological finding in bronchiolitis obliterans organising pneumonia (BOOP) is polypoid plugs of loose fibrous tissue (Masson bodies) filling the bronchioles. Aetiologies include infections, inhaled toxins, drugs, collagen vascular diseases and bronchial obstruction.

Miscellaneous

Other less common causes of interstitial lung disease include conditions such as Langerhans' cell histiocytosis X, pulmonary eosinophilia and pulmonary alveolar proteinosis.

Vascular diseases of the lungs

Pulmonary oedema and congestion

Pulmonary oedema signifies increased fluid in the lung interstitium, causing breathlessness and cough productive of frothy, pink sputum. There are several causes of pulmonary oedema.

- Common cause:
  - *increased venous hydrostatic pressure.*
- Uncommon causes:
  - *injury to the alveolar capillary bed, e.g. acute respiratory distress syndrome (ARDS)*
  - *blockage of lymphatic drainage*
  - *lowered plasma oncotic pressure.*

The commonest cause of pulmonary oedema is increased venous hydrostatic pressure, most often resulting from left ventricular failure. When the increasing hydrostatic pressure exceeds the oncotic pressure within the pulmonary capillaries, fluid is forced out of the vessels and into the lung interstitium, with resultant pulmonary oedema. Oedematous lungs are heavy, congested and wet. Histologically, the alveolar capillaries are engorged, and frothy, pink precipitate can be seen within the alveoli. Alveolar microhaemorrhages may be seen with associated haemosiderin-laden macrophages ('heart failure cells').

Pulmonary embolism

An embolus is a detached intravascular solid, liquid or gaseous mass, which is carried by the blood to a site distant from its point of origin. Pulmonary embolism refers to the occlusion of some part of the pulmonary arterial tree by an embolus.

Pulmonary thrombo-embolism

This is by far the commonest type of embolus. In most cases, the thrombotic mass originates in the deep veins of the legs above the level of the knee. After detachment, the embolic mass travels via the bloodstream to the right side of the heart and into the main pulmonary artery. Thereafter, the calibre of the blood vessels decreases progressively and the embolus eventually becomes lodged. The consequences of this depend on the volume of lung tissue subsequently deprived of blood. Emboli that occlude the main pulmonary artery or impact across the bifurcation (saddle embolus, see Ch. 14, Figure 35) or occlude the right or left pulmonary artery, often cause sudden death. Death is usually due to acute right heart failure.

Smaller emboli can pass into and occlude smaller arteries supplying a lobe or a segment of the lung, causing severe chest pain with dyspnoea. Small emboli occluding the smaller arterioles may be clinically silent, but entrapment of multiple small emboli over the course of time eventually causes occlusion of the vascular pulmonary bed, resulting in pulmonary hypertension and cor pulmonale. Rarely, an embolus may pass through an interatrial or interventricular septal defect to gain access to the systemic circulation (paradoxical embolism).

Because of the dual blood supply to most parts of the lungs, pulmonary embolism causes infarction only when the circulation is already inadequate, e.g. patients with cardiac or respiratory disease. Infarcts are typically wedge shaped. Most emboli eventually resolve by fibrinolysis. However, since patients who have had one pulmonary embolus are at high risk of having more, therapy with fibrinolytic agents is usually initiated. Prevention of deep vein thrombosis is of major clinical importance.

Fat embolism

Fat emboli result from fracture of bones containing fatty marrow (usually the long bones, e.g. femur), or by massive injury to subcutaneous fat. The globules of fat enter torn veins and become emboli.

Gas embolism

Air emboli can occur after chest trauma. Nitrogen can come out of solution in divers during decompression ('decompression sickness').

Amniotic fluid embolism

This type of embolus can occur during delivery or abortion. During labour, amniotic fluid may enter torn uterine veins. Flakes of keratin and epithelial cells shed from the fetal skin embolise to the lungs, where they become lodged. If the patient survives the initial crisis, thrombogenic substances contained within the amniotic fluid trigger disseminated intravascular coagulation.

Tumour embolism

Clusters of tumour cells may enter the venous circulation and, if large enough, occlude the pulmonary veins.

Pulmonary hypertension

Pulmonary hypertension is defined as the point when the mean pulmonary blood pressure reaches a quarter of the systemic level. Patients present with dyspnoea and fatigue, or anginal-type chest pain. Over time, symptoms worsen and right ventricular hypertrophy develops with ensuing cor pulmonale.

Pulmonary hypertension can be primary, but it is most often secondary to other cardiopulmonary conditions such as:

- pulmonary embolism
- obstructive lung diseases
- interstitial lung diseases
- left ventricular failure
- mitral stenosis.

Pathology

Changes seen within the arteries include the deposition of atheroma, an increase in the thickness of the muscular media (medial hypertrophy) and intimal fibrosis. Changes relating to the underlying cause are also seen.

Lung tumours

Bronchogenic carcinoma

Bronchogenic carcinoma is the commonest malignancy in the UK, and has the worst prognosis. It accounts for around a third of all cancer deaths in men, and the incidence is rising in women. Typically, patients are aged between 40 and 70 years.

Aetiology

Cigarette smoking There is overwhelming evidence implicating cigarette smoking as a major risk factor for the development of lung cancer.

Occupational hazards There is a high correlation between asbestos exposure and the risk of lung cancer, especially adenocarcinoma. The risk is heightened dramatically if the individual also smokes. All types of radiation may be carcinogenic. There is also an increased risk of lung cancer among people who work with nickel, chromates, coal, mustard gas, arsenic, beryllium and iron.

Scarring Some lung cancers, especially adenocarcinomas, appear to arise in areas of previous scarring, e.g. old tuberculous foci. It has been proposed that scarring induces dysplasia of pneumocytes, predisposing to lung cancer in that area.

Classification

Bronchogenic carcinoma is classified according to the appearance under light microscopy:

- squamous cell carcinoma (25–40%)
- adenocarcinoma (25–40%)
- small cell carcinoma (20–25%)
- large cell carcinoma (10–15%).

Occasionally, lung carcinomas are simply classified as either small cell carcinoma or non-small cell carcinoma. The relevance of this type of classification is that small cell carcinomas are more responsive to chemotherapy than any of the other types of lung cancer.

Squamous cell carcinoma This type of lung cancer is closely associated with smoking. The tumour commonly arises in the central bronchi and spreads locally, usually at a rapid rate. Metastases usually occur later than with the other types of lung cancer. The tumours are thought to arise from areas of squamous metaplasia through grades of dysplasia.

Adenocarcinoma This type of cancer is usually peripheral and is sometimes associated with scarring. It is the most common type of lung cancer in women and non-smokers. Adenocarcinomas grow more slowly than the squamous cell carcinomas.

Small cell carcinoma Small cell carcinoma is a neuroendocrine tumour and is strongly related to cigarette smoking. The tumours often arise centrally in the lungs and metastasise widely but, unlike other types of lung cancer, they are sensitive to radiotherapy and chemotherapy. Small cell carcinoma is also referred to as 'oat-cell' carcinoma, because the cells are thought to resemble oat grains; they are small, round to oval, and have little cytoplasm. The nuclei often appear smudged under microscopy. As these tumours originate from neuroendocrine (Kulchitsky's) cells present in the bronchial epithelium, they show the following additional features:

- the cytoplasm contains neurosecretory granules similar to those seen in Kulchitsky's cells
- some of these tumours secrete polypeptide hormones
- the cells stain positively for neuroendocrine markers on immunohistochemistry.

Large cell carcinoma These are usually central, highly aggressive tumours. Histologically, the cells are highly pleomorphic with numerous bizarre mitoses. Large cell carcinoma may represent squamous cell carcinomas and adenocarcinomas that are so poorly differentiated that they can no longer be recognised.

Gross pathology

The tumour starts as an irregular thickening, which grows either exophytically (outwards into the lumen), to produce an intraluminal mass, or endophytically (into the bronchial wall), causing erosion of the bronchial wall. Spread is by local extension to neighbouring tissues, spread to lymph nodes and distant metastases.

Clinical features

The clinical features of lung cancer are the result of local spread within the lung, direct spread to neighbouring structures, distant spread or paraneoplastic syndromes.

Effects of local intrapulmonary spread:

- cough – due to irritation of the airways
- haemoptysis – due to erosion of small blood vessels
- wheezing, stridor, atelectasis, pneumonia, bronchiectasis, lung abscess – due to airway obstruction.

Effects of direct spread to neighbouring structures:

- pain – with involvement of nerves, or the pleura (pleuritis)
- shortness of breath – extension to the pleura causes pleural effusions
- hoarse voice – with involvement of the recurrent laryngeal nerve
- paralysis of the diaphragm – with involvement of the phrenic nerve
- symptoms caused by a tumour in the lung apex (Pancoast's tumour):
  - *Horner's syndrome (sunken eye, small pupil, eyelid drooping and loss of sweating on the same side of the lesion) due to involvement of the sympathetic ganglia*
  - *pain and weakness in the shoulder and arm due to involvement of the branchial plexus*

- vena caval syndrome – characterised by facial congestion, oedema of the face, neck and upper arms, and distension of the veins in the neck and over the chest.

Effects of distant spread: depend on the sites of the secondary deposits.

Paraneoplastic syndromes These are signs or symptoms in cancer patients that are not explicable in terms of local or metastatic spread of the tumour. General paraneoplastic syndromes include weight loss, fever and loss of appetite.

Paraneoplastic syndromes may be associated with the secretion of hormones (endocrinopathies). All types of bronchogenic carcinoma can secrete hormones, including antidiuretic hormone (ADH), adrenocorticotrophic hormone (ACTH), parathormone, parathyroid hormone-related peptide, some cytokines, calcitonin, gonadotrophin and serotonin, and the syndromes associated with secretion of these hormones may become clinically apparent (e.g. development of Cushing's syndrome with the secretion of ACTH).

Other paraneoplastic syndromes that can occur are:

- Lambert–Eaton myasthenic syndrome
- peripheral neuropathy
- hypertrophic pulmonary osteoarthropathy.

Treatment and prognosis

The stage of the tumour at presentation is of prognostic significance (the tumour node metastasis (TNM) staging system is usually adopted), but the prognosis is generally poor. The only hope of cure is total resection of the tumour, which is only possible with peripheral tumours without metastases. Some patients with small cell carcinoma benefit from radiotherapy and chemotherapy, which can induce remission (occasionally sustained).

Neuroendocrine tumours

Three types of malignant neuroendocrine tumours are found in the lung:

- small cell carcinoma (discussed above)
- bronchial carcinoid
- large-cell neuroendocrine carcinoma.

Bronchial carcinoids are considered to be tumours of low-grade malignancy and resemble carcinoid tumours found elsewhere, e.g. intestine. They are capable of producing the classic carcinoid syndrome. Growth of these tumours is slow and they may be amenable to resection. Consequently, the survival figures for bronchial carcinoids are much better than those for bronchogenic carcinoma.

Large-cell neuroendocrine tumours are more aggressive than bronchial carcinoids.

Miscellaneous primary lung tumours

Included in this category of lung tumour are:

- benign and malignant tumours of salivary gland-type
- benign and malignant mesenchymal tumours
- benign and malignant lymphoreticular tumours

- lung hamartomas
- adenomas.

Metastatic lung tumours

The lung is a frequent site for metastatic neoplasms. Just about any carcinoma, sarcoma or lymphoma can spread to the lung, but those most commonly implicated are carcinomas from the breast, kidney and gastrointestinal tract. Multiple discrete tumour nodules may be scattered throughout the lungs, or if the spread is via the lymphatics, the metastatic growth may be confined to peribronchial and perivascular tissue, leading to the characteristic appearance of grey-white streaking of tumour in the lungs (lymphangitis carcinomatosis).

15.4 The pleura

Learning objectives

You should:
- understand what is meant by the term 'pleural effusion' and know the various clinical settings in which it may arise
- understand what is meant by the term 'pneumothorax' and know the various types
- know about malignant mesothelioma.

Structure of the pleura

The pleura are composed of two opposing layers of connective tissue lined by mesothelial cells. The visceral pleura covers the lungs and the parietal pleura lines the internal thoracic wall and covers the thoracic surface of the diaphragm, the heart and the mediastinum. The potential space between these two layers is called the pleural cavity or pleural space.

Pleural effusion

This term denotes an increased accumulation of fluid between the two layers of the pleura, causing shortness of breath. Pleural effusions can occur in the following settings:

- increased hydrostatic pressure, e.g. congestive cardiac failure

- increased capillary permeability, e.g. pneumonia, bronchogenic carcinoma, mesothelioma
- decreased intrapleural negative pressure, e.g. atelectasis
- decreased lymphatic drainage, e.g. mediastinal carcinomatosis
- decreased oncotic pressure (hypoalbuminaemia), e.g. nephrotic syndrome, liver cirrhosis.

Pleural effusions can be either inflammatory, when they are associated with a pleuritis, or non-inflammatory (see Table 23). To try to establish the cause of the effusion, a diagnostic aspiration of the pleural fluid is useful. If the fluid is a transudate (protein <20 g/L), then heart failure or hypoalbuminaemia is the cause; if the fluid is an exudate (protein >30 g/L), then all other causes should be considered.

Pneumothorax

Pneumothorax refers to air/gas in the pleural cavity. When severe, a pneumothorax can cause symptoms of respiratory distress and may be fatal. Resorption of the air in the pleural space occurs slowly, and if deemed necessary, interventional procedures may be used to remove the air from the pleural cavity, e.g. chest drain.

Spontaneous pneumothorax

This type of pneumothorax occurs in people with pre-existing disease that causes rupture of an alveolus. It is most often seen in association with emphysema, asthma and tuberculosis.

Traumatic pneumothorax

This can occur following penetrating injuries to the chest.

Therapeutic pneumothorax

Intentional deflation of the lung was a method once used to enhance healing of tuberculous lesions.

Spontaneous idiopathic pneumothorax

This condition occurs in young healthy people, and seems to be due to rupture of small peripheral usually apical subpleural blebs. Recurrent attacks are common.

Table 23 Types of pleural effusion and their causes

	Type of pleural effusion	Common associations
Inflammatory	Serofibrinous effusion	Inflammation of the adjacent lung, e.g. pneumonia, lung abscess, tuberculosis, collagen vascular diseases
	Suppurative effusion (empyema, pyothorax)	Suppuration in the adjacent lung
	Haemorrhagic effusion	Neoplastic infiltration, pulmonary infarction
Non-inflammatory	Serous effusion (hydrothorax)	Cardiac failure, renal failure, liver failure
	Haemothorax	Trauma to chest wall, ruptured aortic aneurysm
	Chylothorax (lymph in the pleural space)	Obstruction of the lymphatics by tumour

Fifteen

Tension pneumothorax

This term refers to when the defect responsible for the pneumothorax acts as a valve, allowing air into the pleural cavity during inspiration, but not permitting its escape during expiration. Consequently, the pressure in the pleural cavity rises swiftly and progressively. The condition is a medical emergency, and is fatal if the pressure is not relieved.

Tumours

Tumours of the pleura may be benign or malignant.

Benign

The solitary fibrous tumour of the pleura is a tumour that is often attached to the pleura by a peduncle. These benign tumours can become enormous.

Malignant

Malignant tumours of the pleura may be primary or secondary. Secondary (metastatic) tumours (e.g. from lung carcinomas or breast carcinomas) are much more common than primary tumours of the pleura.

Malignant mesothelioma

This term refers to a malignant tumour of mesothelial cells, and when applied to the pleura, means a primary malignant tumour of the pleura.

Aetiology Malignant mesothelioma is associated with exposure to asbestos, particularly crocidolite ('blue' asbestos) and amosite ('brown' asbestos). It should be noted, however, that for any individual asbestos worker, the risk of developing malignant mesothelioma is much lower than the risk of developing lung carcinoma.

Pathology The tumour begins as pleural nodules that enlarge and extend over the surface of the lung, gradually encasing it. Infiltration of the chest wall and intercostal muscles by the tumour causes severe pain. Histologically, mesotheliomas may be composed of epithelial cells (epithelioid type) or spindle cells (sarcomatoid type) or a mixture of both.

Self-assessment: questions

One best answer questions

1. An 83-year-old woman undergoes emergency surgery for fracture of the femur following a fall at her nursing home. On the sixth postoperative day she suddenly collapses and dies. The case is reported to the coroner and an autopsy is performed. The most likely cause of death identified at post-mortem examination is:

   a. bronchopneumonia
   b. ruptured myocardial infarction
   c. pulmonary thrombo-embolism
   d. fat embolism
   e. tension pneumothorax

2. A 79-year-old retired shipyard worker complains of marked progressive weight loss over the last 4 months and increasing breathlessness. On chest imaging he is found to have a large unilateral pleural effusion and diffuse pleural thickening encasing the lung. The most likely diagnosis is:

   a. bronchial carcinoma
   b. asbestosis
   c. silicosis
   d. mesothelioma
   e. empyema

True-false questions

1. The following statements are correct:

   a. epiglottitis is usually caused by the bacterium *Haemophilus influenzae*
   b. squamous cell carcinoma of the larynx is strongly associated with cigarette smoking
   c. epithelial dysplasia precedes squamous cell carcinoma of the larynx
   d. laryngeal cancer often presents with persistent hoarseness of voice
   e. laryngeal cancer may present with haemoptysis

2. The following statements are correct:

   a. smokers are at an increased risk of developing pneumonia
   b. bronchopneumonia is characterised by consolidation of a large portion of a lobe or of an entire lobe
   c. *Pneumocystis carinii* is the organism frequently implicated in the development of bronchopneumonia
   d. lobar pneumonia is most frequently caused by the bacterium *Streptococcus pneumoniae*
   e. pneumonia can be treated with antibiotics and is now never fatal

3. The following statements regarding tuberculosis are correct:

   a. since the 1980s, Western countries have seen a decline in the incidence of tuberculosis
   b. primary pulmonary tuberculosis is always symptomatic
   c. histologically, tuberculosis is characterised by the presence of caseating granulomas
   d. tuberculosis may affect the gastrointestinal tract
   e. miliary tuberculosis represents lymphohaematogenous dissemination of the infection

4. The following statements regarding obstructive airways disease are correct:

   a. in the pathogenesis of chronic bronchitis, smoking induces hypersecretion of mucus in airways
   b. in emphysema there is abnormal permanent dilatation of the bronchi
   c. emphysema may be associated with α_1-antitrypsin deficiency
   d. asthma is characterised by irreversible bronchoconstriction
   e. obstruction and infection are important influences in the pathogenesis of bronchiectasis

5. Interstitial lung disease:

   a. is associated with reduced vital capacity of the lung
   b. is associated with reduced peak expiratory flow rate (PEFR)
   c. may be caused by inhalation of mineral dusts
   d. may lead to cardiac failure
   e. in its advanced form results in a macroscopic appearance referred to as 'honeycomb lung'

6. The following statements are correct:

   a. the most common cause of pulmonary oedema is left ventricular failure
   b. an embolus may be a solid, liquid or gas
   c. pulmonary thrombo-embolism may cause pleuritic chest pain
   d. pulmonary thrombo-emboli most commonly originate from the arteries of the lower limbs
   e. pulmonary hypertension is almost always idiopathic

7. The following statements regarding lung cancer are correct:

   a. smoking is associated with an increased risk of developing small cell carcinoma of the lung

   b. non-small cell carcinomas are particularly sensitive to chemotherapy

   c. bronchogenic carcinoma may cause development of a hoarse voice

   d. there is an association between bronchogenic carcinoma and Cushing's syndrome

   e. lung cancer may be associated with a pleural effusion

8. The following statements are correct:

   a. a tension pneumothorax is a medical emergency that requires immediate management

   b. pneumonia is the likely cause of a pleural effusion that has a protein content of <20 g/L

   c. involvement of the pleural cavity by tumour induces a haemorrhagic pleural effusion

   d. mesothelioma is a benign tumour of the pleura

   e. asbestos exposure is a risk factor for the development of mesothelioma

9. The following statements are true:

   a. pleural effusions are always bilateral

   b. idiopathic pulmonary fibrosis is one of the diseases associated with finger clubbing

   c. cystic fibrosis is a recessively inherited disorder

   d. exposure to asbestos is called 'asbestosis'

   e. there may be a significant time lag between exposure to asbestos and development of an asbestos-related disease

10. The following statements are true:

   a. malignant tumours can cause pulmonary embolism

   b. status asthmaticus is a medical emergency

   c. patients with chronic bronchitis have an increased risk of developing pneumonia

   d. small cell carcinomas of the lung are the only lung tumours that can secrete hormones

   e. Goodpasture's syndrome is an example of a type II hypersensitivity reaction

Case history questions

Case history 1

A 58-year-old man was admitted to hospital for repair of an inguinal hernia under a general anaesthetic. He smoked 10 cigarettes a day for 40 years (20 pack years). On the third postoperative day, he became pyrexial and developed a cough productive for green sputum. A blood count showed a raised white cell count with increased neutrophil polymorphs. A chest X-ray showed patchy opacities.

1. From these symptoms, signs and investigations, what is the most likely diagnosis?

2. What predisposing factors are present in this case?

3. Describe the pathological changes in the lungs.

Case history 2

A 72-year-old woman presents to her general practitioner with a persistent cough, haemoptysis, shortness of breath, weight loss and a hoarse voice. She is an ex-smoker. On clinical examination, she has finger clubbing, wasting of the small muscles of the left hand and left-sided Horner's syndrome.

1. What is the most likely diagnosis?

2. What is the pathological basis for these signs and symptoms?

3. What further investigations should be performed?

Short note questions

Write brief notes on the following:

1. The classification and pathogenesis of emphysema.

2. Respiratory tract pathology caused by asbestos exposure.

3. The differential diagnosis of a pleural effusion.

Viva questions

1. What diseases of the respiratory tract are related to smoking?

2. What defence mechanisms are employed by the respiratory tract to reduce the risk of infection by microorganisms?

Self-assessment: answers

One best answer

1. c. This is the commonest cause of sudden death in hospitalised patients; risk factors include immobility, trauma, surgery, acute infection and severe cardiac or respiratory disease. This patient has multiple risk factors for venous thrombo-embolism. Ruptured myocardial infarction is the next most likely explanation – myocardial infarction is another common cause of sudden death, and infarcts are most likely to rupture at 3–7 days' duration, so a ruptured perioperative myocardial infarction would be a distinct possibility in this case. Fat embolism can occur following bone fracture and bone surgery, but clinical manifestations would become apparent more immediately following the initiating event.

2. d. The clinical symptoms and signs suggest a malignant disease process; the pleural thickening encasing the lung is characteristic of malignant mesothelioma (it is not usually seen with bronchial carcinoma). Occupational history of asbestos exposure is aetiologically important in mesothelioma; workers in a wide range of construction industries may have been exposed to carcinogenic asbestos fibres. Pneumoconioses (including silicosis and asbestosis) cause fibrosis within the lung, as opposed to pleural thickening.

True-false answers

1. a. **True.**
   b. **True.**
   c. **True.**
   d. **True.**
   e. **True.**

2. a. **True.** Cigarette smoke interferes with alveolar macrophage function and causes injury to the mucociliary apparatus.
   b. **False.**
   c. **False.**
   d. **True.**
   e. **False.** Despite antibiotic treatment pneumonia may still be fatal, especially in the debilitated.

3. a. **False.** Since the 1980s, Western countries have seen a *rise* in the incidence of tuberculosis.
   b. **False.** Primary tuberculosis is frequently asymptomatic.
   c. **True.**
   d. **True.** Either during lymphohaematogenous dissemination or during primary infection due to ingestion of *Mycobacterium bovis* (unpasteurised milk).
   e. **True.**

4. a. **True.**
   b. **False.** There is permanent dilatation of the airways distal to the terminal bronchioles.
   c. **True.**
   d. **False.** The bronchoconstriction is characteristically *reversible*.
   e. **True.**

5. a. **True.**
   b. **False.** The PEFR is usually normal.
   c. **True.**
   d. **True.** Interstitial lung disease can lead to cor pulmonale.
   e. **True.**

6. a. **True.**
   b. **True.**
   c. **True.**
   d. **False.** They most frequently originate from the *veins* of the lower limbs.
   e. **False.** Most cases of pulmonary hypertension are secondary to other pathology.

7. a. **True.**
   b. **False.** *Small cell* carcinomas are particularly sensitive to chemotherapy.
   c. **True.** If a lung tumour spreads into the mediastinum, there may be involvement of the recurrent laryngeal nerve as it passes close to the aortic arch.
   d. **True.** Some bronchogenic tumours secrete hormones. Secretion of ACTH may induce Cushing's syndrome.
   e. **True.**

8. a. **True.**
   b. **False.** A protein content of <20 g/L indicates that the effusion is a transudate. Pneumonia would cause an exudative effusion.
   c. **True.**
   d. **False.** Although the name of this tumour suggests that it is benign, mesotheliomas are in fact malignant.
   e. **True.**

9. a. **False.**
   b. **True.**
   c. **True.**
   d. **False.** Asbestosis refers to *interstitial fibrosis* due to asbestos.
   e. **True.**

10. a. **True.**
    b. **True.**
    c. **True.**
    d. **False.**
    e. **True.**

Case history answers

Case history 1

1. A cough productive of green sputum associated with pyrexia is highly suspicious for pneumonia. A raised white cell count with increased neutrophil polymorphs suggests bacterial infection. Patchy opacities on the chest X-ray would support a diagnosis of bronchopneumonia in which the consolidation is patchy throughout the lung. In view of the history of recent surgery, the most likely diagnosis is postoperative pneumonia.

2. *Comment*: You need to know the defence mechanisms that are in operation in the respiratory tract to prevent infection, and ways in which they may be impaired predisposing individuals to pneumonia. There are several predisposing factors in this case. First, general anaesthesia would cause suppression of the cough reflex. Second, coughing increases intra-abdominal pressure and so any pain associated with the abdominal surgical wound would be increased when the patient coughs. Hence he may try to avoid coughing. Third, the patient is a smoker, and cigarette smoke interferes with alveolar macrophage function and injures the mucociliary apparatus.

3. In bronchopneumonia there is often widespread but patchy consolidation. The primary infection is centred on the bronchi, with spread to involve the adjacent bronchioles and alveolar spaces. In this case, the changes may be seen mostly in the dependent parts of the lung, where the retained secretions would accumulate. Macroscopically, the lungs would show firm red/grey airless areas and pus may be present in the airways. Microscopically, there is acute inflammation in the airways.

Case history 2

1. This combination of symptoms in an elderly person who is an ex-smoker is highly suggestive of a malignant process. The findings on clinical examination support a diagnosis of a lung cancer. The Horner's syndrome, together with the muscle wasting seen in the hands, is particularly suggestive of an apical (Pancoast's) tumour.

2. The cough may be due to distal infection, airway irritation, or airway obstruction by a tumour or lymph node mass. Haemoptysis results from ulceration of the tumour and consequent bleeding into the airway. Shortness of breath may be due to pleural effusions or obstruction of a main airway by tumour. The hoarse voice is caused by recurrent laryngeal nerve palsy secondary to mediastinal spread. Wasting of the small muscles of the hand is due to infiltration of the branchial plexus. Horner's syndrome results when there is involvement of the cervical sympathetic plexus.

3. A tissue diagnosis should be sought so that an appropriate management plan can be formulated. Small cell carcinomas may be more sensitive to chemotherapy and radiotherapy than non-small cell carcinomas. Several methods may be used. Cells in sputum, bronchoscopy-obtained bronchial brushings and washings, or pleural fluid can be examined under the microscope for any cytological features of malignancy. In the vast majority of cases small cell and non-small cell carcinomas can be distinguished. For central tumours, tissue may be obtained during bronchoscopy (bronchial biopsy). Biopsy of peripheral tumours may be done percutaneously (needle biopsy). After tissue diagnosis, further investigations are directed towards tumour staging, e.g. CT scan.

Short note answers

1. *Comment*: Start your answer with the definition of emphysema. Then go on to explain how emphysema is classified into four main types according to the anatomical distribution of the lesions, and the appearance of the lungs with the naked eye or hand lens. The four main types are centrilobular, panlobular, paraseptal and irregular, and you should be able to describe each of them. The pathogenesis of emphysema is not fully understood, but evidence suggests that emphysema is due to an imbalance between protease and anti-protease activity in the lung. Hence its association with smoking (which causes increased recruitment of neutrophil polymorphs to the lung where they release elastase) and α_1-antitrypsin deficiency.

2. Exposure to asbestos is linked to the development of a number of disorders of the respiratory tract, namely pleural plaques (asymptomatic), pleural effusions, asbestosis, bronchogenic carcinoma, mesothelioma and laryngeal carcinoma. These conditions usually develop in the setting of occupational exposure to asbestos, where the fibres can be inhaled.

3. Pleural effusion denotes the presence of fluid within the pleural space. There are several causes of a pleural effusion, but they can be divided into 'inflammatory' and 'non-inflammatory'. *Comment*: you should know the various causes of each. Pleural effusions can be detected either during physical examination of the chest or on imaging (e.g. chest X-ray), and to determine the cause of an effusion you must extract as much information as possible from these, as well as taking a thorough history. A diagnostic tap can also be performed. The appearance of the fluid may provide clues. Note if the fluid is clear, cloudy or bloodstained, or composed entirely of blood, pus or lymph. If the

protein content is measured, you can determine whether the fluid is a transudate or an exudate – inflammatory effusions are exudates and therefore have a higher protein content. If neoplastic infiltration is suspected, the fluid can be examined under the microscope for the presence of malignant cells.

Viva answers

1. Several diseases of the respiratory tract are related to smoking, including chronic bronchitis, emphysema, laryngeal carcinoma and bronchogenic carcinoma. Remember that smokers are also predisposed to pneumonia because cigarette smoke interferes with alveolar macrophage function and injures the mucociliary apparatus. These conditions together cause significant morbidity and mortality in the general population.

2. The respiratory tract employs several defence mechanisms to clear or destroy inhaled microorganisms. These include: nasal mucus (in which particles are trapped); coughing and sneezing; the mucociliary apparatus (which traps particles in the lung and moves them within the mucous layer towards the nasopharynx where they are swallowed or expectorated); and alveolar clearance (particles that reach the alveoli are phagocytosed by alveolar macrophages). Pneumonia results whenever these defence mechanisms are impaired.

Upper gastrointestinal tract

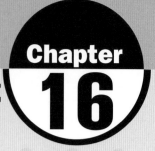

Chapter overview

This chapter covers the common pathology of the mouth, salivary glands, oesophagus, stomach and proximal duodenum. Inflammatory conditions of this region are frequent, and include oral ulcers, oesophagitis, gastritis and gastroduodenal (peptic) ulceration. Carcinoma of the oesophagus and stomach has a particularly poor prognosis. While the incidence of gastric cancer is decreasing in the UK, oesophageal carcinoma is rising in frequency. The role of *Helicobacter pylori* infection in gastric pathology, and the significance of lower oesophageal epithelial metaplasia (Barrett's oesophagus) will be discussed. Oral squamous cell cancer is relatively uncommon in the Western world but is a major health problem in India and other parts of Asia.

Part 1: Mouth and salivary glands

16.1 Inflammation and infection

Learning objectives

You should:
- know the common benign pathologies affecting the oral cavity
- understand the terms leucoplakia and erythroplakia and their clinical significance.

The following conditions are common in the mouth:

- non-specific ulceration ('aphthous ulcers')
- herpes simplex type 1 infection ('cold sore')

- candidiasis, especially in diabetic and immunosuppressed patients
- benign fibroepithelial polyp (reactive fibrous proliferation secondary to chronic irritation)
- cysts associated with teeth (developmental or inflammatory).

The oral mucosa can manifest several inflammatory conditions seen in the skin, such as lichen planus, bullous pemphigoid and erythema multiforme. Xerostomia (dry mouth) can be a feature of autoimmune disease in Sjögren's syndrome (see below).

Salivary gland inflammation can be due to:

- viral infection, e.g. mumps
- bacterial infection – staphylococcal and streptococcal, associated with salivary duct calculi (stones) and dehydration
- autoimmune disease.

Sjögren's syndrome results from autoimmune inflammatory damage to the salivary glands, lacrimal glands and small mucous glands of the nasal mucosa. Clinically this can present with dry mouth and dry eyes. There is a close association between Sjögren's syndrome and rheumatoid arthritis.

Leucoplakia is a clinical term describing a 'white patch' of oral mucosa. Leucoplakia does not reflect a specific pathological diagnosis and is often caused by inflammation or reactive hyperkeratosis (thickened keratin layer), but on occasion it can represent epithelial dysplasia or malignancy (Box 22). A more sinister lesion is erythroplakia, a velvety red patch of oral mucosa, which typically shows high-grade epithelial dysplasia on biopsy.

16.2 Oral and salivary gland neoplasia

Learning objectives

You should:
- know the pathology of oral squamous cell carcinoma
- know the common benign and malignant tumours of the salivary glands.

Box 22 Causes of leucoplakia

- *Candida* infection
- Smoking-related keratosis
- Traumatic keratosis from rubbing denture plate
- Lichen planus
- Squamous epithelial dysplasia

Table 24 Cancer checklist: oral squamous cell carcinoma

Incidence	Age 50–70 years. Less than 5% of non-skin cancers in Western world; up to 40% of all cancers in India
Risk factors	Smoking, alcohol, betel nut chewing (India/Asia), chronic inflammation
	UV light and pipe smoking in lip carcinoma
Protective factors	Fruit and vegetable consumption
Associated lesions	Epithelial dysplasia, may be erythroplakia (over 50% progress to invasive cancer) or less frequently leucoplakia
Clinical presentation	Mass noted by patient or dentist
Location	Floor of mouth, tongue and hard palate most frequent
Macroscopic appearance	Raised firm mass ± ulceration
Histological features	Vary from well-differentiated tumours with orderly keratinisation to anaplastic (undifferentiated) tumours
Pattern of spread	Local infiltration of oral structures, regional lymph nodes, lung, liver, bone
Prognosis (per cent 5-year survival)	Dependent on site: lip 90%; anterior tongue 60%; other sites 20–30%

Table 25 Cancer checklist: salivary gland carcinoma

Incidence	Uncommon; adults; slight female predominance
Risk factors	Irradiation (muco-epidermoid carcinoma)
Associated lesions	Small percentage of pleomorphic adenomas undergo malignant transformation
Common clinical presentation	Mass, pain, facial nerve involvement (parotid tumours)
Location	Parotid, 15% of tumours are malignant
	Submandibular, 40% malignant
	Minor salivary glands, majority malignant
Macroscopic appearance	Variable, usually infiltrative margin
Histological features	Variable
Pattern of spread	Adenoid cystic, local perineural invasion, late dissemination to lung, liver, bone, brain (50%)
	Muco-epidermoid, low-grade lesions recur locally, high-grade lesions may disseminate widely
Prognosis (per cent 5-year survival)	Adenoid cystic, 60% at 5 years, but 15% at 15 years
	Muco-epidermoid, 50–90%, depending on grade

Benign tumours of the oral cavity include squamous cell papilloma (analogous to skin lesions) and haemangiomas. Squamous cell carcinoma accounts for over 95% of oral malignancies (Table 24).

Salivary gland tumour pathology is complex, as both epithelial cells and associated myoepithelial cells may give rise to neoplasms. Most tumours arise in the parotid gland, and over 80% of these are benign. Neoplasms arising in the submandibular and sublingual glands and the minor salivary glands scattered throughout the oral mucosa have a much higher likelihood of being malignant (approximately 50%).

Pleomorphic adenoma

Pleomorphic adenoma is the commonest salivary tumour, arising most frequently in the parotid gland. The histological appearance is very variable, with epithelial glands or cell sheets, embedded in a connective tissue stroma showing myxoid changes, fibrosis, cartilaginous areas or even bone formation. Pleomorphic adenomas are benign tumours that appear well circumscribed macroscopically and do not infiltrate local structures (the facial nerve is, therefore, usually spared by pleomorphic adenomas arising in the parotid). However, there are often microscopic projections of tumour into the adjacent tissues, and attempted removal by enucleation carries a significant risk of multifocal recurrence, which can be difficult to treat. Up to 5% of pleomorphic adenomas may undergo malignant transformation to a high-grade carcinoma. The risk of malignant change is increased in longstanding adenomas.

Warthin's tumour

This tumour accounts for approximately 10% of salivary neoplasms, and arises almost exclusively in the parotid. There is a strong male preponderance. Ten per cent of tumours are bilateral, and a similar number are multifocal. The microscopic appearance is distinctive, with a double layer of eosinophilic epithelial cells covering reactive lymphoid tissue. The eosinophilic cells (oncocytes) are the neoplastic population. Warthin's tumour is benign and malignant change does not occur.

Salivary gland carcinoma

Many different histological variants of salivary gland carcinoma (Table 25) are now recognised. The two commonest are:

- **Muco-epidermoid carcinoma** – as the name implies, this carcinoma is composed of both glandular and squamous epithelium. Low-grade tumours are often partly cystic with well-differentiated glandular epithelium. High-grade carcinomas have a more solid growth pattern and are composed largely of squamous cells.
- **Adenoid cystic carcinoma** – this malignancy appears low grade on histological grounds, but is locally invasive and 50% will metastasise. The long-term survival is poor. Adenoid cystic carcinoma is composed of regular small epithelioid cells in a cribriform ('sieve-like') architectural pattern, associated with basement-membrane-like material. Perineural invasion by the tumour is a characteristic feature.

Part 2: Oesophagus, stomach and proximal duodenum

16.3 Inflammation, infection and benign conditions

Learning objectives

You should:
- understand gastro-oesophageal reflux disease and Barrett's oesophagus
- know the causes and complications of acute and chronic gastritis, and of peptic ulcer disease.

Oesophagitis

This disease may be due to infection, particularly by *Candida* in debilitated and immunosuppressed patients. Gastro-oesophageal reflux disease (GORD) is the commonest cause of oesophagitis in the UK, and its prevalence appears to be increasing. It is associated with sliding hiatus hernia, smoking, obesity, pregnancy and ingestion of certain foods. GORD classically presents with burning epigastric pain, which may be accentuated by bending or lying down, but is often asymptomatic. Histology shows hyperplasia of squamous oesophageal epithelium with inflammation (eosinophils, neutrophils and lymphocytes) and ulceration in more severe cases. Complications include:

- haematemesis
- anaemia
- inflammatory stricture
- Barrett's oesophagus (see below).

Other causes of oesophagitis include alcohol, corrosive chemical ingestion, chemotherapy, radiotherapy and graft-versus-host disease.

Barrett's oesophagus

This syndrome describes a metaplastic change of the squamous epithelium of the lower oesophagus into glandular epithelium. The metaplastic glandular epithelium may resemble gastric or small intestinal mucosa. Barrett's usually occurs in patients with more severe longstanding GORD. Endoscopically the metaplastic focus has a red, velvety appearance. Barrett's may progress to glandular dysplasia and eventually to invasive adenocarcinoma. Both Barrett's oesophagus and oesophageal adenocarcinoma have increased in incidence in recent years. For this reason, regular surveillance endoscopies are usually performed in patients with known Barrett's change, to identify high-grade dysplasia and early stage malignancy. However, the degree of increased cancer risk associated with Barrett's remains unclear, and less than half of all patients with oesophageal adenocarcinoma will describe any clinical history of reflux disease.

Achalasia

This is a motility disorder in which reduced oesophageal peristalsis and failure of relaxation of the lower oesophageal sphincter cause lower oesophagus dilatation. Resulting symptoms include dysphagia and food regurgitation. In most cases the pathogenesis is unknown. Achalasia can be secondary to Chagas' disease, caused by the protozoon *Trypanosoma cruzi* (frequent in Central America, Chagas' disease also causes acute myocarditis and chronic dilated cardiomyopathy).

Hiatus hernia

This is a common condition in which part of the stomach herniates up through the oesophageal opening of the diaphragm and into the mediastinum (Figure 41). The great

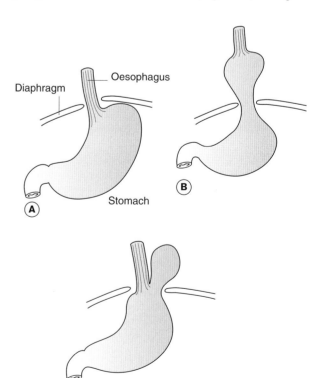

Figure 41 Hernias of the stomach. (A) Normal. (B) Sliding hernia. (C) Rolling hernia.

majority are sliding, and are often associated with reflux oesophagitis. Rolling hernias are less common.

Oesophageal varices

These are an important cause of serious haemorrhage and death in patients with portal hypertension. They are discussed further in Chapter 18.

Gastritis and benign ulcer disease

- **Gastritis**: inflammation of gastric mucosa, which may be acute or chronic.
- **Gastric erosion**: superficial loss of gastric mucosal tissue, not extending beyond muscularis mucosa. Erosions are associated with acute inflammation and are transient.
- **Gastric ulcer**: ulceration that extends through, and often well beyond, the mucosa, and may be acute or chronic.

Acute gastritis

Acute gastritis is most commonly due to:

- non-steroidal anti-inflammatory drugs (NSAIDs)
- excess alcohol
- heavy smoking
- 'stress' (burns, trauma, shock) causing mucosal ischaemia
- chemotherapy and radiotherapy.

Clinical consequences include haematemesis (vomiting blood), melaena (dark, altered blood in faeces), epigastric pain, nausea and vomiting.

Acute gastric ulceration

Acute gastric ulceration can also be caused by severe stress. Sepsis, shock, trauma, burns and raised intracranial pressure are the commonest predisposing factors and up to 10% of patients admitted to intensive care units will develop acute gastric erosions or ulcers. The ulcers are small (less than 10 mm diameter), frequently multiple and occur anywhere in the stomach. The adjacent mucosa rarely shows chronic gastritis. Acute ulcers are transient lesions that heal with complete restoration of normal structure and without scarring.

Chronic gastritis

Chronic gastritis can be classified into three major groups:

- Autoimmune – in pernicious anaemia, with autoantibodies to gastric acid producing parietal cells in the body of the stomach.
- Bacterial – *H. pylori* infection (most common cause of chronic gastritis, preferentially affecting the antrum)
- Chemical – due to biliary reflux or NSAIDs.

Other causes include alcohol, smoking, Crohn's disease and graft-versus-host disease.

Chronic mucosal inflammation can lead to intestinal metaplasia and gastric atrophy, and predisposes to development of gastric carcinoma. However, chronic gastritis and *Helicobacter* infection are very common, and clearly only a small percentage of those afflicted will eventually develop malignancy. Chronic gastritis itself is often asymptomatic.

Chronic peptic ulceration

Chronic peptic ulceration occurs in the gastric antrum, but is most frequent in the proximal duodenum. Lesions are usually solitary (if multiple, think of Zollinger–Ellison syndrome, see below). Peptic ulcer disease is common in adulthood and more frequent in men than women. The pathogenesis of peptic ulceration involves breakdown of mucosal defence mechanisms and increased injurious stimuli. The majority of cases (especially duodenal ulcers) are associated with *H. pylori* chronic gastritis. Other risk factors include smoking, chronic NSAID use, liver cirrhosis, chronic lung disease, hyperparathyroidism and chronic renal failure. Significant complications of peptic ulcer include:

- haemorrhage (clinically serious in up to 33%)
- perforation with peritonitis (5%)
- gastric outlet obstruction secondary to scarring.

Malignant change does not occur in duodenal peptic ulcers and is very unusual in gastric peptic ulcers.

Recurrent peptic ulcers occur in the Zollinger–Ellison syndrome. Hypersecretion of gastric acid is provoked by a gastrin-secreting tumour (usually located within the pancreas). The peptic ulcers can be multiple and arise in the stomach, proximal and distal duodenum and jejunum.

16.4 Oesophageal and gastric neoplasia

> ### Learning objectives
>
> You should:
> - understand the pathology of gastric and oesophageal carcinoma
> - be aware of the role of *H. pylori* infection in gastric inflammation and neoplasia.

Oesophagus

Benign tumours in the oesophagus are very uncommon, but can be of epithelial (squamous cell papilloma) or of connective tissue origin (lipoma, haemangioma). The vast majority of malignant oesophageal tumours are squamous cell carcinomas or adenocarcinomas (Table 26).

Stomach

Benign epithelial neoplastic polyps (adenomas) are rare in the stomach, in contrast to the colon. Up to a third are associated with invasive carcinoma at the time of diagnosis, either within the polyp itself or in the adjacent mucosa. Gastric adenocarcinoma (Table 27) has classically been divided into two based on the histological growth patterns (Figure 42): intestinal type (with gland formation) and diffuse type (also known as 'signet-ring' carcinoma).

Sixteen

Table 26 Cancer checklist: oesophageal tumours

	Oesophageal squamous cell carcinoma	Oesophageal adenocarcinoma
Incidence	Over 50s; decreasing in incidence in Western world More common in men; high incidence in parts of China, Iran, former USSR	Increasing incidence; over 40s, more common in men
Risk factors	Smoking, alcohol (particularly spirits), ?vitamin deficiencies, ?food contamination – fungal organisms, nitrosamines	GORD, Barrett's oesophagus, smoking; obesity
Associated lesions	Chronic oesophagitis; squamous dysplasia/carcinoma-in-situ	Barrett's oesophagus
Common clinical presentation	Gradual development of dysphagia, first to solids then to liquids	As for squamous cell carcinoma
Location	Upper third 25% Middle third 50% Lower third 25%	Lower third of oesophagus
Macroscopic appearance	Polypoid usually, but can be flat or ulcerated	Variable
Histological features	Squamous differentiation, with or without keratinisation	Glandular differentiation; may be histologically indistinguishable from gastric cancer
Pattern of spread	Local submucosal spread beyond area of grossly visible tumour, can erode locally into trachea (fistula formation, aspiration pneumonia) or aorta (haemorrhage) Regional lymph nodes, liver and lung	Local invasion into stomach and through oesophageal wall into adjacent structures Regional lymph nodes, liver and lung
Prognosis (per cent 5-year survival)	5%; often advanced stage tumour at presentation	As for squamous cell carcinoma

Table 27 Cancer checklist: gastric adenocarcinoma

Incidence	Geographical variation – highest in Far East, Central America, Scandinavia. Incidence of intestinal type variant has declined in UK over last 50 years
Risk factors	Chronic gastritis; dietary factors (nitrosamines, smoked/salted foods)
Protective factors	Fresh fruit and vegetable consumption
Associated lesions	*Helicobacter* gastritis, intestinal metaplasia
Common clinical presentation	Non-specific symptoms; weight loss, pain, nausea and vomiting
Location	Most frequent in antrum, but can occur anywhere
Macroscopic appearance	Polypoid, flat or ulcerated Diffuse thickening of stomach wall, 'linitis plastica', especially with signet-ring type
Histological features	Gland forming (intestinal type) or diffuse infiltration of single adenocarcinoma cells (signet-ring type)
Pattern of spread	Through serosal surface; local invasion of duodenum and pancreas Regional lymph nodes (also supraclavicular node) Peritoneal spread (especially to ovaries, resulting in Krukenberg's tumour)
Prognosis (per cent 5-year survival)	Less than 5% Early gastric cancer (confined to mucosa or submucosa, with or without lymph node spread) has a better prognosis

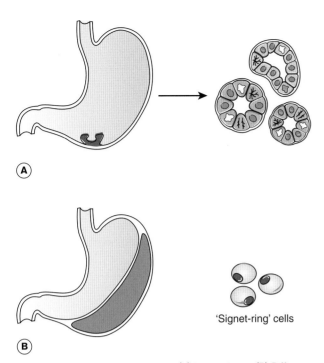

(A)

(B)

'Signet-ring' cells

Figure 42 Types of gastric carcinoma. (A) Intestinal type. (B) Diffuse type.

Lymphoma

Lymphoma can arise as a primary tumour in the stomach. There is a strong association with *Helicobacter* infection. It seems that hyperplasia of mucosal-associated lymphoid tissue (MALT) induced by chronic bacterial infection provides fertile soil for development of a monoclonal neoplastic lymphoid proliferation. In contrast with lymphomas arising in lymph nodes, MALT lymphomas tend to remain localised to their site of origin and may be amenable to surgical resection. Indeed, some apparent gastric lymphomas may regress following treatment of *Helicobacter* infection, blurring the distinction between hyperplasia and neoplasia (recall that the latter is an uncontrolled proliferation, which does not regress when the precipitating stimulus is removed).

Sixteen

Self-assessment: questions

One best answer question

1. A 58-year-old man presents with an ulcerated, hard, irregular 20 mm mass on his tongue. He smokes 30 cigarettes a day and drinks a tumbler of whisky every night. The likely diagnosis is:

   a. lichen planus

   b. benign fibroepithelial polyp

   c. oral carcinoma-in-situ

   d. invasive adenocarcinoma

   e. invasive squamous cell carcinoma

True-false questions

1. *Helicobacter* infection in the stomach is associated with:

   a. gastric carcinoma

   b. acute gastric ulceration

   c. chronic duodenal ulceration

   d. intestinal metaplasia

   e. gastric lymphoma

2. Regarding salivary gland tumours:

   a. malignant tumours arise most commonly in the parotid gland

   b. pleomorphic adenomas have a 20% risk of malignant transformation

   c. facial nerve impairment is an ominous sign

   d. adenoid cystic carcinoma has a good long-term prognosis

   e. enucleation of pleomorphic adenoma is appropriate treatment

3. Barrett's oesophagus:

   a. is a dysplastic change

   b. confers an increased risk of oesophageal squamous carcinoma

   c. can contain small intestinal-type epithelium

   d. can be complicated by benign oesophageal stricture

   e. increases in frequency with increased duration of gastro-oesophageal reflux symptoms

4. Oral leucoplakia (white mucosal patches) can be caused by:

   a. *Candida* infection

   b. smoking

   c. epithelial dysplasia

   d. ill-fitting dentures

   e. invasive carcinoma

5. Concerning gastric cancer:

   a. it is commoner in the UK than in Japan

   b. diffuse type (signet-ring) adenocarcinoma is decreasing in incidence

   c. many cancers arise from pre-existing benign peptic ulcers

   d. overall 5-year survival is 25%

   e. histological type is the most important prognostic factor

6. Acute gastric ulcers:

   a. are often multiple

   b. are common in severely ill patients

   c. are usually >25 mm in diameter

   d. are confined to the antrum

   e. usually heal without scarring

7. Concerning chronic gastritis:

   a. autoantibodies to gastrin-producing cells are present in autoimmune gastritis

   b. squamous metaplasia is often seen on biopsy

   c. chemical gastritis can be secondary to bile reflux

   d. it confers a high risk of development of gastric cancer

   e. it is frequently seen in patients taking long-term steroids

8. Concerning squamous cell carcinoma of the mouth:

   a. the incidence is higher in the Far East than the UK

   b. prognosis is best for anterior tumours

   c. there is an association with sun exposure

   d. the tumour rarely spreads beyond the oral cavity

   e. erythroplakia is a risk factor

Case history questions

Case history 1

A 63-year-old man presents to his general practitioner with swallowing problems. He describes gradually increasing difficulty with swallowing solid food, but no problems with liquids. He has recently lost half a stone in weight, and has a several years' history of 'heartburn'.

1. What is your differential diagnosis based on this history?

2. What changes might be present within oesophageal biopsies taken at endoscopy?

Case history 2

A 78-year-old woman is admitted to hospital as an emergency with abdominal pain and haematemesis. Urgent endoscopy is performed and a 15 mm ulcer is identified in the proximal duodenum as the source of the bleeding.

1. What specific questions would you ask the patient to help establish the cause of the ulcer?
2. Why might the endoscopist take a biopsy from the stomach (rather than the duodenal lesion)?

Viva questions

1. What are the causes and complications of acute gastritis?
2. Discuss the epidemiology of upper gastrointestinal tract cancer.

Self-assessment: answers

One best answer

1. e. Over 95% of oral malignancies are squamous cell carcinomas. Oral squamous cell carcinoma-in-situ is most likely to present as a velvety red patchy (erythroplakia), or as a white hyperkeratotic area (leucoplakia), and not as a tumour mass. Adenocarcinomas are much less common in the mouth but can arise from salivary gland tissue.

True-false answers

1. a. **True.**
   b. **False.**
   c. **True.**
   d. **True.**
   e. **True.**

2. a. **True.** Although only 10–15% of parotid tumours are malignant, neoplasms develop more frequently at this site than in the other salivary tissues, so that salivary gland cancers are still most common in the parotid.
   b. **False.** Less than 5%.
   c. **True.** As it indicates tumour infiltration of the nerve.
   d. **False.**
   e. **False.** Microscopic residual deposits cause subsequent clinical recurrence.

3. a. **False.** Barrett's is a metaplastic change; replacement of one adult differentiated epithelium by another. Although Barrett's itself is a benign process, there is a greater risk of developing glandular epithelial dysplasia and adenocarcinoma within the area of Barrett's change.
   b. **False.** It is the risk of adenocarcinoma that is increased.
   c. **True.**
   d. **True.**
   e. **True.**

4. a. **True.**
   b. **True.**
   c. **True.**
   d. **True.**
   e. **True.** Early stage invasive carcinoma may develop within a leucoplakic patch of dysplasia or carcinoma-in-situ.

5. a. **False.**
   b. **False.** It is the intestinal type of adenocarcinoma that is declining in frequency.
   c. **False.**

d. **False.** It is 5%.
e. **False.** Surgical resectability, which is related to tumour stage, is the most important prognostic factor.

6. a. **True.**
   b. **True.**
   c. **False.**
   d. **False.**
   e. **True.** Acute gastric ulcers are usually superficial.

7. a. **False.** The antibodies present are against acid-producing parietal cells.
   b. **False.** Intestinal metaplasia may be present.
   c. **True.**
   d. **False.** Chronic gastritis is very common, and the percentage of patients developing malignancy is low.
   e. **False.** Steroids can cause acute ulceration if given in high doses. Chemical gastritis can be caused by NSAIDs.

8. a. **True.**
   b. **True.**
   c. **True.** For carcinoma of the lip, which shares the same risk factors as skin cancer at other sites (see Ch. 26).
   d. **False.**
   e. **True.**

Case history answers

Case history 1

1. The symptoms suggest oesophageal obstruction and are most likely to be due to a benign inflammatory stricture or a malignancy. The history of heartburn points to GORD. Another much less common possibility is achalasia. Dysphagia due to cerebrovascular accident is of sudden onset. Benign strictures can complicate severe oesophagitis from any cause, including physical and chemical injury (such as caustic substance ingestion, irradiation and cancer chemotherapy). Oesophageal stricture also occurs in systemic sclerosis (scleroderma).

2. In benign strictures, oesophageal mucosal biopsies may show inflammatory changes with squamous epithelial hyperplasia. Ulceration may be present. The fibrosis causing a benign stricture may not be seen histologically as the scar tissue lies deeper within the wall of the oesophagus and may not be sampled in a superficial biopsy. Inflammation and squamous hyperplasia would be seen in GORD. Identification of glandular epithelium within the anatomical oesophagus would signify Barrett's

metaplasia. If a malignant tumour is present, biopsy will confirm whether this is squamous cell carcinoma, adenocarcinoma, or a more unusual tumour type (such as sarcoma or melanoma). Even if no mass is seen, in the presence of Barrett's oesophagus there is an increased risk of malignancy and of premalignant (dysplastic) changes in the glandular epithelium. For this reason, patients known to have Barrett's change may undergo regular endoscopies, although the effectiveness of this surveillance in identifying early stage, potentially curable, oesophageal tumours is not yet clearly established.

Case history 2

1. A careful drug history to exclude non-steroidal anti-inflammatory medication is essential. Many elderly patients may have osteoarthritis and buy medications over the counter. Smoking and alcoholic liver disease are associated with peptic ulceration and the relevant history of these habits should be obtained. Other relevant medical history would include chronic lung disease, chronic renal disease and hyperparathyroidism.

2. *Helicobacter pylori* gastritis is frequently present in association with peptic duodenal ulceration. A rapid urease detection test for *Helicobacter* can be performed with the tissue sample in the endoscopy suite, or the biopsy material can be submitted for histopathological examination. A patient breath test can also be used to make the diagnosis. Duodenal peptic ulcers do not undergo malignant transformation and can be safely assumed to be benign in nature without histological confirmation.

Viva answers

1. *Comment*: See text, Section 16.3.

2. *Comment*: Important points to include in your answer are:

   - the worldwide geographical variation in oral, gastric and oesophageal cancers

   - the changing incidence of certain cancers (increasing oesophageal adenocarcinoma, decreasing intestinal-type gastric carcinoma in the UK) and possible reasons for this (increasing incidence of GORD and Barrett's metaplasia in oesophageal adenocarcinoma; ?decreasing frequency of *Helicobacter* gastritis with improved general health and sanitation corresponding to reduced gastric cancer incidence)

   - the role of environmental factors including smoking, alcohol and dietary habits.

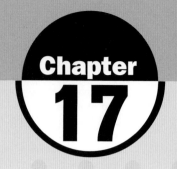

Chapter overview

This chapter covers pathological processes affecting the distal duodenum, jejunum, ileum, colorectum and anus. Worldwide, infective disease of the small and large intestines is one of the most important causes of mortality; approximately half of all deaths below the age of 5 years are due to infectious enterocolitis. In developed countries, bowel infections are still a common cause of morbidity but are rarely fatal. Modern standards of sanitation, healthcare and nutrition have eradicated the epidemics of cholera and typhoid prevalent in the UK before the mid-twentieth century. However, civilisation comes at a price. The average diet of the developed world appears to be a contributory factor to several common large bowel diseases – in particular diverticular disease and colorectal cancer.

17.1 Inflammation and infection

Learning objectives

You should:
- be aware of the types of pathogens that can cause enterocolitis
- be able to describe the differences between ulcerative colitis and Crohn's disease
- understand the pathogenesis and complications of acute appendicitis and diverticular disease.

Infectious enterocolitis

Infectious diseases of the bowel most commonly present with diarrhoea, which is an increase in stool mass, stool frequency or stool fluidity. Diarrhoea can result from a number of mechanisms (see Table 28). The pathogen responsible – which may be bacterial, viral, parasitic, pro-tozoal or fungal – varies with patient age, nutrition, immune status and environment, and is identifiable in only approximately half of all cases.

Viruses

Rotavirus affects primarily children aged 6 months to 2 years, and is responsible for an estimated 140 million cases of infective enterocolitis and 1 million deaths per year. Viral infection damages mature surface epithelial cells in the small intestine mucosa, which are replaced by immature secretory cells. This results in a loss of absorptive ability and increased gut secretions, producing a mixed osmotic and secretory diarrhoea (see Table 28). In older children and young adults, the majority of non-bacterial gastroenteritis is due to Norwalk-like viruses. Viral infection typically provokes cellular immunity involving cytotoxic T lymphocytes. Biopsies of intestinal mucosa are rarely undertaken in suspected viral infection, as symptoms of vomiting and diarrhoea are often self-limiting and of short duration. However, in an immunocompetent individual, the microscopic appearance of established viral infection would characteristically include epithelial cell damage and lymphocytic infiltration of the mucosa indicative of host immune response.

Bacteria

Bacteria cause disease in the gut by a number of mechanisms:

- effects of preformed bacterial toxins present in contaminated food
- toxin production by organisms within the gut
- enteroinvasive infection, in which organisms proliferate, invade and destroy the intestinal mucosal epithelium.

Enterotoxins Enterotoxins are polypeptides which cause diarrhoea. Some, such as cholera toxin, cause massive secretion of fluid in the absence of tissue damage (secretory and osmotic diarrhoea). Cholera toxin exerts its effects by persistently activating the cytoplasmic enzyme adenylate cyclase, causing profound secretion of chloride, sodium and water.

Secretory toxins Secretory toxins produced by *Escherichia coli* are the major cause of traveller's diarrhoea.

Cytotoxins Cytotoxins produced, for example, by *Shigella* and cytotoxic strains of *E. coli*, cause tissue damage

Table 28 Mechanisms and causes of diarrhoea

Type of diarrhoea	Mechanism	Major causes
Secretory diarrhoea	Stimulation of gut secretion	Viral infection Bacterial infection Neoplasms producing secretagogues
Osmotic diarrhoea	Excessive osmotic forces exerted by increased concentration of luminal solutes	Laxative therapy Malabsorption (many causes) Lactase deficiency
Exudative diarrhoea	Stools containing blood and inflammatory debris secondary to tissue damage	Crohn's disease Ulcerative colitis Bacterial infections Protozoal infections
Abnormal gut motility	Various causes of altered gut transit time and motility	Irritable bowel syndrome Diabetic neuropathy Post-bowel surgery

with epithelial cell necrosis and an acute inflammatory reaction. Cytotoxins usually induce 'dysentery' – low volume, painful, bloody diarrhoea.

Although bacterial infection is frequently confined to the gut, systemic disease may occasionally occur. Organisms may enter the bloodstream (causing a bacteraemia), multiply (septicaemia) and spread to other organs (dissemination). Inflammatory mediators activated by bacterial toxins or by products of damaged host cells may result in fever, lowered blood pressure and ultimately septic shock (see Ch. 5), which is often fatal. Typhoid fever is the name given to the generalised illness caused by infection by *Salmonella typhimurium*, which can include chronic inflammation of the biliary tree, joints, bones and meninges in addition to intestinal involvement.

Pseudomembranous colitis

Pseudomembranous colitis is an acute infectious disease of the colorectum, which is a common cause of diarrhoea in hospitalised patients receiving broad spectrum antibiotic therapy. The organism responsible (*Clostridium difficile*) is a normal toxin-producing commensal of the gut. Antibiotic therapy appears to alter the balance of the gut flora, allowing *C. difficile* to flourish. The toxin damages the colonic mucosa, causing an acute inflammatory reaction with the formation of a typical 'pseudomembrane'. The pseudomembrane is visible endoscopically as an irregular dark yellow coating over the bowel surface; microscopically it contains mucus and acute inflammatory debris including fibrin and degenerate neutrophils. The toxin of *C. difficile* can be identified in the stool of symptomatic patients.

Acute appendicitis

Acute inflammation of the appendix is the most common acute abdominal condition requiring surgery. It can occur at any age, although it is relatively rare in the very young and very old. Most cases are thought to arise secondary to obstruction of the appendiceal lumen by faeces. The exact

sequence of events is unknown, but may involve a combination of bacterial proliferation and increased intraluminal pressure causing vascular obstruction and ischaemia. The affected appendix shows the hallmarks of acute inflammation – intense neutrophil polymorph infiltration and oedema, with tissue necrosis and peritonitis in advanced cases. The serosal surface of the organ becomes covered with an acute inflammatory exudate composed of fibrin and neutrophils. If surgery is delayed there is a risk of appendiceal rupture, with localised abscess formation or generalised peritonitis with septicaemia. Chronic inflammation is very unusual in the appendix. Small scarred appendices, presumably representing the fibrotic end stage of repeated acute inflammation, are sometimes seen in older adults.

Peritonitis

Generalised acute inflammation of the peritoneum can arise secondary to bacterial invasion or chemical irritation. Bacterial peritonitis may complicate many inflammatory processes, including acute appendicitis, cholecystitis, perforated peptic ulcer, diverticulitis, bowel ischaemia and salpingitis. Infective peritonitis may also follow abdominal trauma or medical intervention (e.g. peritoneal dialysis). Chemical inflammation of the peritoneum may occur when bile, pancreatic enzymes, foreign material or blood (endometriosis, trauma, surgery) are released into the peritoneal cavity. Healing of peritonitis can result in the formation of fibrous adhesions between bowel loops. These adhesions can subsequently cause abdominal pain and bowel obstruction.

Crohn's disease and ulcerative colitis

Crohn's disease and ulcerative colitis are often grouped together under the term chronic idiopathic inflammatory bowel disease. As this term suggests, Crohn's disease and ulcerative colitis are of unknown aetiology, and it has been suggested that they may represent different parts of the spectrum of a single disease process. However, there are important clinical and pathological differences between these two conditions.

Crohn's disease

Crohn's disease is a granulomatous inflammatory condition, which can affect any part of the gastrointestinal tract from mouth to anus, but most frequently involves the small intestine and colon. Annual incidence in the developed world is 1–3 per 100 000, with equal sex incidence; white people are affected more frequently than non-Caucasians. Crohn's disease often presents in the second and third decades, but can manifest at any age. In the gut, approximately 40% of cases are restricted to the small bowel, 30% involve both small and large intestines and the remaining 30% show isolated colonic disease. About a quarter of patients have extra-intestinal involvement, which can include skin lesions, arthritis and eye disorders.

Crohn's disease is characterised by discontinuous, sharply demarcated areas ('skip lesions') of transmural chronic inflammation. Microscopically, aggregates of lymphocytes are seen in all layers of affected bowel wall. Non-necrotising granulomas, composed of epithelioid macrophages with multinucleated giant cells, are seen in approximately 60% of cases. Fissuring ulcers are another characteristic histological feature of Crohn's disease; these linear ulcers can also be seen with the naked eye, and often impart a 'cobblestone' appearance to the bowel mucosa when viewed endoscopically or in a surgical resection specimen. The intestinal wall becomes thickened by oedema in acute stages and flare-ups of Crohn's disease, and by fibrosis in chronic disease, leading to stricture formation. Extension of fissuring ulceration through to the serosal surface of the bowel can result in perforation, abscess formation, adhesions, fistulas and sinus tracts. A **fistula** is an abnormal communication between two epithelial surfaces (e.g. a colovesical fistula joins colonic mucosa to bladder mucosa). The fistulous tract itself is lined by epithelium or by granulation tissue. A **sinus** is a blind-ending tract, which connects with the skin or another epithelial surface at one end.

Crohn's disease manifests clinically with intermittent diarrhoea, fever and abdominal pain. Symptoms of the initial attack may mimic acute appendicitis. The terminal ileum is the commonest single site of disease and involvement of this region by Crohn's disease can cause symptoms relating to malabsorption. Crohn's disease typically waxes and wanes with recurrent attacks over many years, but there are intervening symptom-free periods of remission. Later presentations include bowel obstruction secondary to fibrous stricturing and symptoms related to fistula formation. There is a slight increased risk of colorectal cancer. The features of Crohn's disease are summarised in Figure 43A.

Ulcerative colitis

Ulcerative colitis is also a chronic relapsing inflammatory condition. It is slightly more common than Crohn's disease (incidence of ulcerative colitis is 4–6 per 100 000) but shares peak onset in early adulthood, equal frequency in males

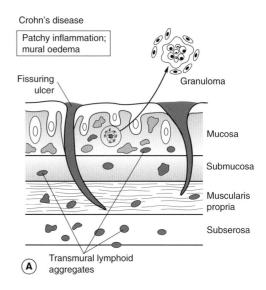

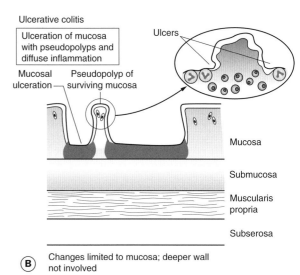

Figure 43 (A) Crohn's disease and (B) ulcerative colitis.

and females and predilection for white people. Unlike Crohn's disease, ulcerative colitis is characterised by continuous disease extending proximally from the rectum, involving a variable distance of colon up to and occasionally including the terminal ileum. Isolated small intestinal disease does not occur in ulcerative colitis. Inflammation is restricted to the colonic mucosa, with occasional involvement of the submucosa. During acute attacks of colitis, there may be extensive mucosal ulceration, from which multiple islands of surviving epithelium stand proud as 'pseudopolyps'. Microscopically the lamina propria of residual mucosa shows diffuse chronic inflammation with lymphocytes and plasma cells, and acute inflammation of mucosal glandular crypts. Granulomas are characteristically absent. With progressive disease the mucosa becomes atrophic, with disruption of glandular architecture and gland loss. There is a risk of epithelial dysplasia and subsequent carcinoma developing in longstanding ulcerative colitis. This risk is greatest in patients having involvement of the entire large intestine (pancolitis). The features of ulcerative colitis are summarised in Figure 43B.

Box 23 Megacolon

Definition: Marked dilatation of colon

Causes:
- toxic megacolon – a complication of severe acute inflammation, most commonly seen in ulcerative colitis
- obstruction – neoplasia, inflammatory stricture
- infection – destruction of enteric nerve plexuses in Chagas' disease
- congenital – Hirschsprung's disease

Clinical course: High risk of gangrene and perforation in toxic megacolon

Ulcerative colitis commonly manifests as recurrent attacks of bloody, mucoid diarrhoea and abdominal pain. Occasionally patients present with severe bleeding and fluid imbalance. Severe acute ulcerative colitis is one of the causes of toxic megacolon (see Box 23). As inflammation is restricted to the mucosa and submucosa, fistulae and strictures do not occur in ulcerative colitis.

Diverticular disease

A diverticulum is essentially a blind pouch, which is lined by epithelium and communicates with the bowel lumen. The wall of a true (congenital) diverticulum contains all layers of the bowel wall (mucosa, submucosa and muscularis propria). Diverticula occur in the small intestine as the solitary Meckel's diverticulum (a remnant of the embryonic vitelline duct) or as multiple jejunal lesions. However, the distal large intestine is the most common site. Approximately half of all adults over 60 have developed (acquired) multiple, small, flask-like or spherical outpouchings in the sigmoid colon. The diverticula extend from the luminal surface into the deep muscularis mucosa and pericolic fat, and are a frequent incidental finding on barium enema examination in elderly patients. Obstruction of a diverticulum by faeces can cause inflammation (diverticulitis), pericolic abscess formation and local or generalised peritonitis. Chronic inflammation and fibrosis may complicate acute diverticulitis, leading to fistula formation and colonic stricture.

Diverticula formation occurs at points of weakness in the colonic wall where vessels and nerves penetrate the muscle coat. Low-fibre diet is thought to contribute to pathogenesis; low stool bulk results in exaggerated peristalsis and increased intraluminal pressure in the affected colon. Symptomatic diverticular disease may present with cramping or continuous lower abdominal pain, constipation or alternating bowel habit, and chronic blood loss.

17.2 Ischaemia and infarction

Learning objective

You should:
- understand the pathogenesis and clinical consequences of intestinal ischaemia.

Intestinal ischaemia can be acute or chronic, and result from both arterial and venous disease. Elderly adults are most frequently affected. Atherosclerosis is often the underlying pathology. Mesenteric arteries supplying the gut may be blocked by thrombosis superimposed on atherosclerosis, or by embolisation of fragments of atheromatous plaque originating from the aorta. Non-occlusive bowel ischaemia can follow hypoperfusion due to, for example, cardiac failure, shock or dehydration. The 'watershed areas' of the colon – splenic flexure and rectum – which lie between the major arterial blood supplies are especially vulnerable. Mesenteric venous thrombosis can complicate sepsis, neoplasia, liver cirrhosis and abdominal surgery. Therapeutic radiotherapy used in the treatment of malignant disease can cause vascular damage with progressive narrowing and occlusion of arteries. Radiation enterocolitis most commonly occurs in the small intestine of patients receiving treatment for carcinoma of the cervix.

Ischaemic injury may be restricted to the mucosa and submucosa of the gut or may involve all layers of the bowel wall. In full-thickness acute bowel infarction, the serosal surface of the gut appears plum coloured due to congestion and reflow of blood into the damaged tissue. The intestinal lumen usually contains blood or blood-stained mucus. Histological changes of infarction (ischaemic necrosis) and oedema are present. Acute small bowel infarction has a high mortality, due to the short time interval between onset of symptoms and development of bowel perforation or septicaemia. The poor prognosis is partly due to coexistent cardiac and vascular disease in the at-risk elderly population. Less severe vascular occlusion which develops gradually can present as chronic ischaemic colitis, with patchy mucosal ulceration. Chronic ischaemia involving the submucosa may heal by fibrosis, causing colonic stricture.

17.3 Immunological disorders

Learning objective

You should:
- understand the pathology of coeliac disease and the reason for excluding gluten from the diet.

Coeliac disease

Coeliac disease is a chronic inflammatory condition of the small intestinal mucosa, in which immunologically mediated injury to the epithelium causes malabsorption. It is also known as coeliac sprue and gluten-sensitive enteropathy. The disease is relatively common in white people of European origin (prevalence of 1:2000–3000). There is evidence of a genetic predisposition to coeliac disease, with family clustering and high frequency of association with certain human leucocyte antigen (HLA) alleles. Affected individuals develop an immune response to gluten, which contains the protein component gliadin in wheat and closely related grains (oat, barley and rye). Gliadin

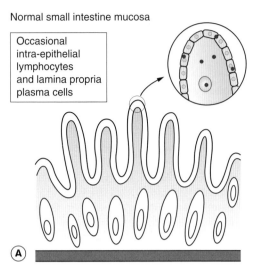

Normal small intestine mucosa

Occasional intra-epithelial lymphocytes and lamina propria plasma cells

Ⓐ

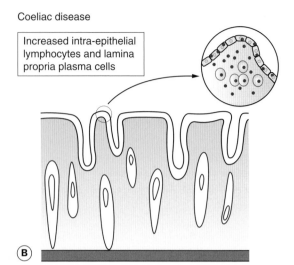

Coeliac disease

Increased intra-epithelial lymphocytes and lamina propria plasma cells

Ⓑ

Figure 44 Coeliac disease.

sensitive B cells accumulate in the small intestinal mucosa on exposure to gluten, and antigliadin antibodies are present in the blood. Characteristically, the small bowel mucosa loses its normal villous architecture and becomes flat. Microscopically there is diffuse chronic inflammation with greatly increased numbers of lymphocytes accumulating within the surface epithelium (Figure 44). The lamina propria contains many plasma cells. These histological abnormalities revert to normal when gluten is excluded from the diet, with subsequent improvement in clinical symptoms. There is a small long-term risk of malignancy (small intestinal lymphoma).

Graft-versus-host disease

Patients treated with donated bone marrow receive an allograft of foreign lymphocytes, which are able to mount an immune response against their new host. Graft-versus-host disease has acute and chronic phases. The acute phase may involve the intestinal mucosa, producing severe watery diarrhoea, intestinal haemorrhage and sepsis.

17.4 Neoplasia

Learning objectives

You should:
- be able to define the terms polyp and adenoma
- be able to explain the adenoma-carcinoma sequence
- understand the risk factors for colorectal cancer, and be able to describe Dukes' staging
- be aware of other types of tumour that occur in the colon and rectum.

The majority of tumours occurring in the lower gastrointestinal tract arise from the glandular epithelium of the large bowel mucosa. Colorectal adenocarcinoma is the second commonest cause of cancer mortality (after lung cancer) in the UK. The jejunum and ileum together make up 75% of the entire intestinal length but are responsible for only 5% of intestinal tumours.

Polyps

Polyps are tissue masses, which protrude into the bowel lumen. They may be described as pedunculated (when there is a recognisable stalk) or sessile (when the polyp has a broad flat base). The word 'polyp' is not synonymous with neoplasia, as polyps may be inflammatory, hyperplastic or hamartomatous in nature, as well as neoplastic (see Box 24). Benign tumours of colonic epithelium are

---

Box 24 Intestinal polyps

Metaplastic (hyperplastic) polyps
- Commonest polyps
- Arise from ?hypermaturation of glandular epithelium
- Very low (if any) malignant potential

Hamartomatous polyps*
- Peutz–Jeghers syndrome
- Juvenile polyps
- Cowden syndrome

Inflammatory polyps
- Ulcerative colitis
- Crohn's disease
- Diverticular disease
- Chronic infections

Neoplastic polyps
- Adenomas
- Adenocarcinomas

*Hamartoma = mass of disorganised but mature tissues, which are native to the site of origin.

Peutz–Jeghers polyps arising in the jejunum and ileum consist of a branching smooth muscle core covered by small intestinal-type epithelium.

often polypoid in structure. Occasionally, masses arising from deeper in the bowel wall (for example, smooth muscle tumours developing in the muscularis propria) may project into the bowel lumen in a polypoid fashion.

Adenomatous polyps

Adenomatous polyps are benign epithelial neoplasms, and very common in the colon. Up to 50% of all adults over the age of 60 in the UK have at least one. They are classified as tubular (>90%), tubulovillous (5–10%) or villous (1%) according to the mixture of tubular glands and villous (finger-like) projections within the polyp (Figure 45). Adenomas are much more common in the large intestine than in the small intestine, and occur more frequently on the left side (rectum and sigmoid) than the right. Histologically, adenomas show mild, moderate or severe dysplasia. Milder degrees of cellular atypia are usual in small, pedunculated tubular adenomas, but large, sessile villous adenomas frequently show high-grade dysplasia, and up to 40% will contain invasive malignancy on microscopic examination. Most adenomas are asymptomatic and first identified on sigmoidoscopy or colonoscopic examination. Occult or overt bleeding, and rarely mucus hypersecretion per rectum can occur.

The adenoma-carcinoma sequence

There is good evidence that many colorectal carcinomas evolve from pre-existing benign adenomas, which subsequently become malignant.

- Populations with high prevalence of colorectal adenomas also have a high incidence of large-bowel adenocarcinoma.
- The distribution of adenomas within the colon and rectum mirrors that of adenocarcinomas (left side greater than right side).
- The peak age incidence of adenomas precedes that of adenocarcinomas.
- Foci of invasive adenocarcinoma can be seen within some adenomatous polyps.
- The risk of developing colorectal adenocarcinoma is related to the number of adenomas the patient has developed.
- Removing adenomas decreases the incidence of colorectal adenocarcinoma.

Progression from the normal colonic epithelial cell to adenoma and then to carcinoma requires accumulation of DNA damage in key genes that control cellular growth, differentiation and apoptosis (Figure 46). However, the

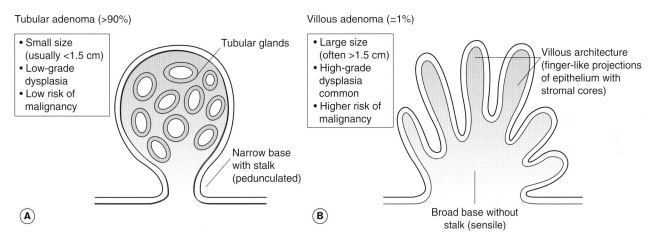

Tubular adenoma (>90%)

- Small size (usually <1.5 cm)
- Low-grade dysplasia
- Low risk of malignancy

Tubular glands

Narrow base with stalk (pedunculated)

(A)

Villous adenoma (≈1%)

- Large size (often >1.5 cm)
- High-grade dysplasia common
- Higher risk of malignancy

Villous architecture (finger-like projections of epithelium with stromal cores)

Broad base without stalk (sensile)

(B)

Figure 45 (A) Tubular and (B) villous adenomas of the large intestine.

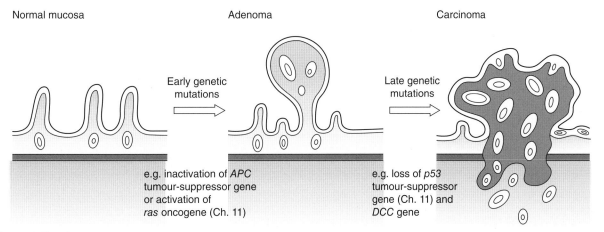

Normal mucosa

Adenoma

Carcinoma

Early genetic mutations

Late genetic mutations

e.g. inactivation of *APC* tumour-suppressor gene or activation of *ras* oncogene (Ch. 11)

e.g. loss of *p53* tumour-suppressor gene (Ch. 11) and *DCC* gene

Figure 46 The adenoma-carcinoma sequence.

precise sequence and nature of these multiple genetic 'hits' probably varies between individual tumours.

Colorectal cancer

Colorectal adenocarcinoma accounts for 98% of all large intestinal malignancies. Although worldwide in distribution, the incidence is much higher in North America, Australia and northern Europe than in Japan, South America and Africa. This geographical distribution suggests that differences in lifestyle have an important aetiological role. The typical Western low fibre, high fat and high refined carbohydrate diet appears associated with higher risk of development of malignancy. Peak incidence of colorectal cancer is between 60 and 70 years of age. Rectal lesions are twice as common in men than women, but colonic tumours occur with equal sex incidence. See Table 29.

As described in the previous section, many colorectal cancers arise from adenomas. Risk of malignant transformation is greatest in large villous adenomas. Although many of these adenomas occur spontaneously, some arise in patients with inherited genetic abnormalities.

Familial adenomatous polyposis (familial polyposis coli)

Familial adenomatous polyposis (FAP, familial polyposis coli) is a rare autosomal dominant disorder in which patients typically develop 500–2500 adenomas within the large intestine before the age of 30. Unless prophylactic colectomy is performed at an early age, virtually all

Table 29 Cancer checklist: colorectal carcinoma

Incidence	Usually over 50, unless associated with inherited genetic condition, e.g. FAP, HNPCC
Risk factors	Adenomas, FAP, HNPCC; slightly increased risk in ulcerative colitis and Crohn's disease
	High fat, low fibre diet
Protective factors	High fibre, low fat diet, ?aspirin
Associated lesions	Colorectal adenomas
Common clinical presentation	Change in bowel habit, rectal bleeding, iron deficiency anaemia
Location	Sigmoid, rectum, caecum (but can occur anywhere in large bowel)
Macroscopic appearance	Usually polypoid, often ulcerated
Histological features	Adenocarcinoma (gland-forming)
Pattern of spread	Lymph nodes, liver (via blood); through peritoneal surface, directly into adjacent bowel loops
	Lower rectal tumours can directly invade bladder and pelvic organs
Prognosis (per cent 5-year survival)	Related to stage; approximately 90% for Dukes' A, 60% Dukes' B, 30% Dukes' C

patients will develop invasive malignancy in at least one of these polyps.

Hereditary non-polyposis colorectal cancer

Another form of familial colorectal cancer accounts for around 10% of all cases, and is also associated with malignancy outside the gut (including ovarian and endometrial cancer).

People with hereditary non-polyposis colorectal cancer (HNPCC) have inherited mutations of DNA repair genes on chromosome 2. DNA damage can accrue unchecked throughout life and when growth-controlling genes are affected, malignancies may develop. Tumours show a preponderance for the right side of the colon, are often mucin-rich and develop 10–20 years before sporadic colorectal cancer. It is important to identify individuals with suspected HNPCC so that they can be regularly examined to exclude extra-intestinal malignancies, and so that family members can be screened for the condition.

Colorectal cancer can not only grow into the bowel lumen as a polypoid mass, but it can also invade into the intestinal wall. Circumferential involvement can cause obstruction, which classically has an 'apple-core' appearance on barium enema examination. Ulceration and bleeding are common. In distal colonic and rectal lesions, fresh blood is often passed per rectum. In more proximal tumours, haemorrhage may be occult – the blood becomes altered on passage through the bowel and may not be recognised in the stool. It is not uncommon for caecal cancers to present with unexplained iron deficiency anaemia. Less specific symptoms of colorectal cancer include abdominal pain and alteration of bowel habit.

Microscopically, colorectal cancers show mucin production. They may be well, moderately or poorly differentiated (tumour grade). The extent of spread (stage) is of great importance in prognosis. The Dukes' staging system is commonly used in the UK (Figure 47).

Carcinoid tumours

The normal intestinal mucosa contains a population of scattered neuroendocrine (NE) cells, which are located in the gland bases (crypts). As their name suggests, these cells show features of both neuronal and endocrine differentiation, and produce a variety of peptide hormones. Tumours arising from NE cells account for approximately 50% of all small intestinal neoplasms, and are often collectively referred to as **carcinoid** tumours. All are potentially malignant, but behaviour depends on site of origin, depth of invasion and tumour size. Gut carcinoids are most commonly seen in the appendix, and often present as an incidental finding in routine appendicectomies. Some carcinoids secrete functional hormones which produce symptoms. Examples include **gastrinomas**, which are associated with multiple gastric and duodenal ulcers (Zollinger–Ellison syndrome) and **insulinomas**, which can present with the effects of hypoglycaemia secondary to tumour production of insulin. The **carcinoid syndrome** is rare and only occurs in malignant tumours that have metastasised to the liver. Patients experience episodes of facial flushing and diarrhoea, related to hormone production by the tumour (probably excess serotonin).

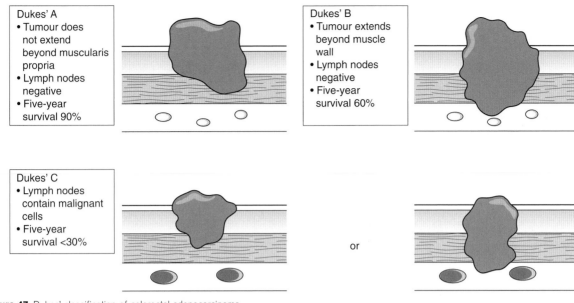

Figure 47 Dukes' classification of colorectal adenocarcinoma.

Lymphoma

Intestinal involvement by malignant lymphoma may occur in widespread node-based disease or as a localised lymphoma arising within the gut itself. Primary bowel lymphomas arise from mucosal associated lymphoid tissue (MALT), and tend to remain localised to the bowel in the early stages. Primary intestinal lymphomas can be associated with immunological disorders including coeliac disease and HIV infection.

Other primary intestinal neoplasms

Mesenchymal neoplasms of the large intestine include benign tumours of fat (lipomas) and gastrointestinal stromal tumours, which may show smooth muscle or neuronal differentiation.

The lower anal canal is lined by squamous epithelium. Most malignancies of the anus resemble the squamous cell carcinomas seen elsewhere in the skin.

17.5 Miscellaneous conditions

Obstruction

Obstruction of the small and large bowel can occur in a number of pathological processes, some of which (Crohn's disease, ischaemic colitis, diverticulitis and malignant neoplasms) have already been described. The following four conditions – hernias, adhesions, intussusception and volvulus – account for around 80% of cases of bowel obstruction (Figure 48).

Hernia

Hernia is the name given to a pouch-like peritoneal-lined sac that protrudes through a defect or weak area in the peritoneal cavity. Common sites for herniation include the inguinal and femoral canals, the umbilicus and surgical scars. The hernial sac often contains loops of small bowel, and sometimes omentum or large bowel, which can become trapped. Pressure at the neck of the hernia can impair venous return, causing stasis and oedema, and eventual infarction. Permanent trapping of bowel within the hernia is known as incarceration.

Fibrous adhesions

Fibrous adhesions between intestinal loops and other peritoneal structures can follow any cause of peritoneal inflammation, and are particularly common after abdominal or pelvic surgery.

Intussusception

Intussusception occurs when one segment of bowel becomes telescoped into the immediately adjacent (distal) segment. Intussusception can arise within previously normal intestine in children, sometimes in relation to hyperplastic lymphoid tissue. In adults, a mass lesion (usually a neoplasm) is often found at the site of intussusception.

Volvulus

Volvulus is the complete twisting of a bowel loop around its mesenteric attachment. This cause of obstruction is most frequent in the sigmoid colon of older adults.

Large intestinal haemorrhage

As mentioned earlier in this chapter, infectious colitis, diverticulitis, ulcerative colitis, Crohn's disease and colonic neoplasms may all present with rectal bleeding. Two further clinically important causes of colonic bleeding are haemorrhoids and angiodysplasia.

Haemorrhoids

Haemorrhoids are common abnormalities, consisting of dilated thick-walled veins in the anus and rectal

Hernia

Adhesions

Intussusception

Serosa

Mucosa

Muscularis

Volvulus

Mesentery

Sigmoid colon

Tumour

Fibrous stricture
(post-inflammatory)

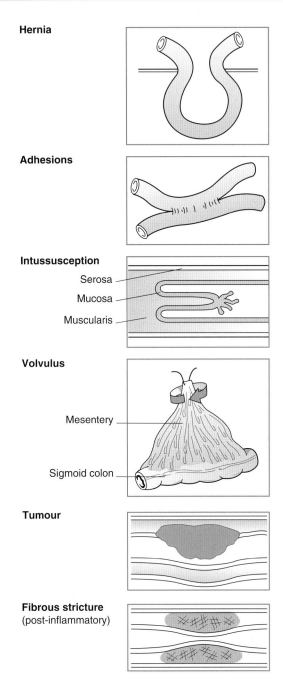

Figure 48 Causes of intestinal obstruction.

submucosa. These abnormal vessels may protrude from the anal orifice and become traumatised, causing haemorrhage and thrombosis. Predisposing factors for developing haemorrhoids include constipation, pregnancy and portal hypertension (see Ch. 18).

Angiodysplasia

Angiodysplasia is a condition of unknown aetiology, characterised by the presence of dilated blood vessels in the mucosa and submucosa of the large intestine. The caecum is the most common site. Angiodysplasia accounts for up to 20% of cases of symptomatic lower intestinal haemorrhage in the elderly.

Self-assessment: questions

One best answer questions

1. An 87-year-old woman is admitted to hospital with pneumonia and treated with antibiotics. Several days later she develops acute onset watery diarrhoea and mild abdominal pain. The most likely diagnosis is:

   a. colorectal cancer
   b. rotavirus infection
   c. *Clostridium difficile* infection
   d. diverticular disease
   e. *Escherichia coli* infection

2. A 7-year-old girl presents with symptoms of acute appendicitis and peritonitis. Her appendix is removed at emergency laparotomy. The most likely microscopic changes on histological examination are:

   a. granulomatous inflammation
   b. neutrophil polymorph inflammation confined to the mucosa
   c. scarring
   d. neutrophil polymorph inflammation involving the muscle coat and the serosa
   e. obstruction by carcinoid tumour

True-false questions

1. The following are correctly paired:

   a. ulcerative colitis – sclerosing cholangitis
   b. diverticular disease – increased risk of malignancy
   c. pseudomembranous colitis – *C. difficile*
   d. coeliac disease – anti-DNA antibodies
   e. Peutz–Jeghers syndrome – hamartomatous polyps

2. Colorectal cancer:

   a. always arises from a pre-existing benign tumour (adenoma)
   b. may present with iron deficiency anaemia
   c. has a 5-year survival of less than 30% in the absence of lymph node involvement
   d. occurs with increased incidence in cigarette smokers
   e. shows squamous differentiation in 20% of cases

3. The following statements are true:

   a. cytotoxin-producing bacteria cause diarrhoea without tissue damage
   b. fibrous strictures occur in ischaemic colitis

c. intussusception is a cause of bowel obstruction in infants
d. coeliac disease is characteristically associated with increased numbers of neutrophil polymorphs in the surface epithelium of the small intestine
e. bowel obstruction is a long-term complication of abdominal surgery

4. Concerning small bowel infarction:

   a. it only occurs in the presence of arterial occlusion
   b. mesenteric artery atherosclerosis is a common predisposing factor
   c. peritonitis is a rare complication
   d. necrosis confined to the mucosa heals by scarring
   e. the mortality rate is low

Case history questions

Case history 1

A 24-year-old woman presents with several weeks' history of diarrhoea, abdominal pain and weight loss. On questioning she admits to having similar symptoms 2 years previously. Clinical examination reveals no abdominal abnormality, but swollen (oedematous) skin tags are noted around the anus. Stool culture is negative. Haematological investigation shows a normochromic, normocytic anaemia. Sigmoidoscopy is performed and a mucosal biopsy is done for histological examination. The pathologist's report states that the appearances are consistent with Crohn's disease.

1. Which pathological features distinguish Crohn's disease from ulcerative colitis?
2. List the complications of Crohn's disease.
3. Why is the patient anaemic?

Case history 2

A 73-year-old man complains of passing blood and mucus per rectum. On sigmoidoscopy, a 4 cm polypoid lesion is seen and part of the polyp is biopsied. The pathologist reports a villous adenoma with severe dysplasia. The sigmoid colon containing the remainder of the polyp is removed. Pathological examination of the surgical resection shows invasive adenocarcinoma.

1. What is meant by dysplasia?
2. Which features of colorectal adenomas are associated with a high risk of developing invasive malignancy?
3. What pathological factors are of prognostic importance in colorectal cancer?
4. Why might postoperative measurement of blood carcinoembryonic antigen (CEA) be useful?

Short note questions

Write short notes on the following:

1. Carcinoid tumour.
2. Bacterial enterocolitis.
3. Colonic polyposis syndromes.

Self-assessment: answers

One best answer

1. c. *C. difficile* infection is a particular risk in hospitalised patients receiving antibiotic treatment, and a low threshold of suspicion is appropriate in these circumstances. Rotavirus enterocolitis predominantly affects young children. Although a change in bowel habit, including diarrhoea, can be a symptom of both diverticular disease and colorectal cancer, acute onset diarrhoea is usually infective in nature.

2. d. Acute appendicitis is a suppurative inflammatory process in which neutrophil polymorphs predominate. Symptoms of peritonitis arise when the inflammation extends to the serosal surface of the appendix. Granulomatous inflammation is a chronic process in which macrophages and lymphocytes usually feature – a granuloma is an aggregate of several enlarged (or 'epithelioid') macrophages. If seen in the large bowel, granulomas suggest a number of conditions including Crohn's disease and certain infections (such as mycobacteria and *Yersinia*). Carcinoid tumour does occur in the appendix and can cause obstruction with subsequent acute inflammation, but the more common initiating cause of acute appendicitis is luminal blockage by a faecolith.

True-false answers

1. a. **True.** Extra-intestinal manifestations of ulcerative colitis include sclerosing cholangitis, an inflammatory disorder of bile ducts leading to multiple areas of fibrous stricture formation in the biliary system. Other associated conditions include arthritis and ocular inflammation.

   b. **False.** Diverticular disease and colonic cancer both occur most frequently in the distal large intestine of older adults, and may coexist in individual patients. However, there is no evidence that diverticular disease increases the risk of developing malignancy (or vice versa).

   c. **True.** Identification of *C. difficile* toxin in the stool of patients with suspected antibiotic-associated diarrhoea is diagnostic of pseudomembranous colitis, even in the absence of characteristic sigmoidoscopic appearances (a reddened, ulcerated colonic mucosa with multiple yellow plaques).

   d. **False.** Coeliac disease is associated with anti-gliadin antibodies. Gliadin is a component of gluten, and treatment of coeliac disease requires removal of the offending antigen by excluding gluten from the diet. Anti-DNA antibodies are found in a number of autoimmune connective tissue diseases, particularly systemic lupus erythematosus (see Ch. 8).

   e. **True.** Peutz–Jeghers syndrome is a rare autosomal dominant disease characterised by multiple intestinal polyps and pigmentation of mucous membranes and skin. The polyps are hamartomas (benign overgrowths of mature tissue) consisting of a smooth muscle core covered by epithelium. They arise most commonly in the small intestine but can also occur in stomach, duodenum, colon and rectum.

2. a. **False.** Many colorectal cancers can be seen to arise within a pre-existing benign tumour, usually a large villous adenoma. However, malignancies occurring in patients with hereditary non-polyposis colorectal cancer or ulcerative colitis often develop within flat mucosa that is macroscopically normal. Patients with ulcerative colitis are followed up with regular colonoscopic investigations, at which random biopsies of the intestinal mucosa can be done for assessment of premalignant histological changes (dysplasia).

   b. **True.** Ulceration of the luminal surface of intestinal tumours can lead to chronic blood loss. This is particularly true for proximal cancers in the caecum and ascending colon, when the blood becomes altered on passage through the bowel and the patient is unaware of the haemorrhage. Tumours arising in the sigmoid colon and rectum are more likely to alert the patient to their existence by way of fresh rectal bleeding on defecation.

   c. **False.** Tumour stage (extent of spread) is one of the most important prognostic factors for malignant disease arising at any site. Metastasis can occur via the lymphatic system, bloodstream or across body cavities. For colorectal cancer, the absence of lymph node spread in a surgical resection specimen predicts at least a 60% chance of long-term survival, provided that local removal of the tumour is complete.

   d. **False.** Risk factors for large intestinal carcinoma include genetic predisposition (hereditary non-polyposis colorectal cancer and familial polyposis coli), inflammatory bowel disease (particularly ulcerative colitis) and environmental factors (diet high in animal fat).

   e. **False.** Over 98% of malignant colorectal neoplasms are adenocarcinomas. Squamous cell carcinoma occurs most frequently in the anal canal.

3. a. **False.** Cytotoxins by definition cause tissue damage. In gut infections, cytotoxins cause epithelial cell death with subsequent loss of normal intestinal absorptive function. In contrast, secretory toxins exert their effects by altering the function of viable cells (e.g. activation of adenylate cyclase by cholera toxin).

   b. **True.** Ischaemic injury to the colon may be restricted to the mucosa or extend beyond into submucosa. Chronic inflammation within the submucosa heals by fibrous scarring, which, if extensive, can lead to stricture formation.

   c. **True.** In infants and children, often no underlying cause is identified. In adults there is a much higher likelihood of a mass lesion (tumour) causing the intussusception.

   d. **False.** Coeliac disease is characterised by increased numbers of intra-epithelial lymphocytes in the small intestine mucosa, along with numerous plasma cells in the lamina propria. Coeliac disease is immunologically mediated, and plasma cells produce antibodies in immune reactions. Neutrophil polymorphs are the characteristic cell of acute inflammation.

   e. **True.** Injury to the peritoneal lining of the intestine or abdominal cavity causes inflammation. The damaged tissue can undergo repair with formation of thin fibrous bands (adhesions) between bowel loops. Adhesions can follow any cause of peritonitis but are most commonly associated with previous surgery. Adhesions are a frequent cause of small intestinal obstruction.

4. a. **False.** It can follow arterial occlusion, venous thrombosis or obstruction, or generalised hypoperfusion (e.g. any cause of shock).

   b. **True.** Atherosclerosis is usually complicated by thrombosis or embolism to cause acute intestinal ischaemia.

   c. **False.** Infarction involving the full thickness of the bowel wall often results in peritonitis and perforation.

   d. **False.** If infarction is restricted to the mucosa, it can heal by regeneration rather than repair/fibrosis (scar tissue).

   e. **False.** Small bowel infarction is a serious condition, and patients are often elderly with pre-existing cardiovascular disease.

Case history answers

Case history 1

1. Crohn's disease is characterised by chronic inflammation involving all layers of the bowel wall. Fissuring ulcers, lymphoid aggregates and non-necrotising granulomas are the classical microscopic features. The disease is segmental in distribution, with intervening areas of normal bowel in between abnormal areas ('skip lesions'). Chronic inflammation in ulcerative colitis is restricted to the mucosa. The large intestine is involved in a continuous fashion, extending proximally from the rectum.

2. Complications of Crohn's disease include abscesses, strictures and fistula formation. Perforation, toxic dilatation and carcinoma are serious but rare complications. The terminal ileum is frequently involved in Crohn's disease, causing diarrhoea, steatorrhoea (fat malabsorption) and general malabsorption. Anal disease (oedematous anal tags, fissure and perianal abscesses) is very common in colonic Crohn's disease. Ulceration is often seen in the mouth. Extra-gastrointestinal manifestations include arthritis, skin lesions, biliary tract inflammation and iritis.

3. Anaemia is common in Crohn's disease and is usually the normochromic normocytic anaemia of chronic disease, due to deficient erythropoiesis. Although the terminal ileum is often involved in Crohn's, megaloblastic anaemia due to vitamin B_{12} deficiency is unusual.

Case history 2

1. Dysplasia means abnormal growth. The term is usually applied to epithelium that shows many of the cytological features of tumour cells, but without evidence of invasive malignancy. These features include hyperchromatic (darkly staining) nuclei, increased nuclear to cytoplasmic ratio, pleomorphism (variation in the size and shape of individual nuclei and cells), increased numbers of mitotic figures (often with abnormal forms), loss of polarity (orientation) of the epithelial cells and lack of maturation of the epithelium. Dysplasia in its early stages may be reversible but many dysplastic lesions if left long enough without treatment will progress to malignancy.

2. High risk features for development of malignancy in colorectal adenomas are large size (especially >2 cm), severe dysplasia and villous architecture. These features often occur together.

3. The most important pathological prognostic features are the tumour grade (the degree of differentiation) and stage (the extent of spread). The depth of invasion into the bowel wall and the presence or absence of local lymph node metastases are factors in all staging systems for colorectal cancer. Pathological assessment of the completeness of excision of a tumour in a surgical resection specimen is also an important predictor of the likelihood of achieving cure.

4. Carcinoembryonic antigen (CEA) is a glycoprotein normally produced by gut, pancreas and liver in the embryo. It can be elevated in the serum of adults with a variety of benign and malignant diseases, including colorectal cancer. Due to the lack of specificity, measurement of blood CEA level is not a useful diagnostic test for colorectal neoplasia.

However, increasing serum levels of CEA after treatment can be used as a biochemical marker of residual or recurrent disease.

Short note answers

1. *Comment*: Begin with a definition – carcinoid tumour is a neoplasm of neuroendocrine cells. Remember that carcinoid tumours do not just occur in the gut but can also arise in other epithelial sites, particularly lung. Many of these tumour-based questions can be approached in a similar way, by considering incidence, age, sex and geographical distribution, risk factors (including any genetic predisposition, environmental factors and occupational associations), tumour site, macroscopic and microscopic appearances, patterns and frequency of local and metastatic spread, clinical manifestations and prognosis. It is impossible (and unnecessary) to retain all this factual information for every tumour, but thinking about diseases systematically in this manner will help you to recall information and construct your answers in a logical and coherent manner.

Carcinoids are uncommon tumours with peak incidence in the sixth decade. In the gut they arise most frequently in the small intestine. Tumours appear as small masses arising in the bowel wall, with a characteristic solid yellow cut-section appearance. Histologically they are formed of uniform epithelial-like cells arranged in a variety of architectural patterns. All carcinoids are potentially malignant but behaviour depends on site of origin, depth of local invasion and tumour size. Local lymph node spread and blood-borne liver metastasis may occur. The latter can produce the carcinoid syndrome – facial flushing, diar-

rhoea, bronchoconstriction, cardiac valve fibrosis – due to the systemic effects of hormones (mainly serotonin) released from tumour cells. Overall 5-year survival is greater than 50%.

2. Key points regarding bacterial enterocolitis:

   - it is common throughout the world, and an important cause of mortality in developing countries
   - pathogenesis may be due to preformed toxins in food or toxins elaborated by bacteria multiplying within the gut
   - toxins may cause symptoms by affecting gut secretion (secretory toxins) or by tissue damage (cytotoxins)
   - non-toxin producing strains of bacteria cause tissue damage by direct invasion of intestinal epithelium
   - common symptoms include fever, pain, diarrhoea and dysentery
   - a large range of organisms may cause enterocolitis. Common examples are *E. coli*, *Salmonella*, *Shigella* and cholera.

3. Colonic polyposis syndromes are rare autosomally inherited diseases, characterised by multiple polyps in the large intestine, sometimes with polyps elsewhere in the gut and/or extra-intestinal manifestations. The polyps may be hamartomas (Peutz–Jeghers syndrome) or adenomas (familial polyposis coli and related conditions). It is important to identify patients with adenomatous polyposis syndromes as they are at very high risk of developing colorectal cancer, and it is necessary to screen other family members for the disease.

Liver, biliary system and exocrine pancreas

Part 1: Liver

Learning objectives

You should:

- understand the definition, causes and clinical consequences of cirrhosis
- know the natural history of hepatitis B and C infections
- know the pathological effects of alcohol on the liver
- understand how therapeutic drugs can cause liver disease
- understand the range of viral, genetic and autoimmune diseases that can cause chronic hepatitis
- know the epidemiology and pathology of hepatocellular carcinoma.

Chapter overview

The liver performs many varied and vital functions. These include: the metabolism of protein, carbohydrate and fat; synthesis of proteins (including albumin, α_1-antitrypsin, transferrin and coagulation factors); detoxification of waste products and ingested chemicals; and participation in the reticuloendothelial system. Chronic liver disease, the causes and consequences of which are discussed in this chapter, most frequently results from viral or alcohol-induced injury. Genetic, autoimmune and vascular diseases also affect the liver. Primary hepatocellular carcinoma is uncommon in the UK but is very common in countries with high rates of hepatitis B infection. The liver is a very common site for metastatic malignancy.

The biliary system functions include digestion of dietary fat and excretion of certain metabolites via the bile. While gall bladder stones and inflammation are very common in the Western world, congenital biliary atresia and malignant disease are unusual but clinically important conditions.

The exocrine pancreas produces digestive enzymes, including lipases, amylases and trypsin. These enzymes have a role in pancreatitis, a disease that is usually precipitated by alcohol ingestion or gallstones. Pancreatic adenocarcinoma is a major cause of cancer mortality.

18.1 Inflammation, fibrosis, cirrhosis and liver failure

The clinical effects of cellular injury in the liver depend on the extent of cell death and the duration of the insult. For example, infection with hepatitis A virus may cause minimal asymptomatic disease, clinically apparent acute hepatitis with jaundice or, very rarely, acute liver failure (Box 25). In virtually every case, liver mass and architecture will be restored once the transient infection is cleared, and there is no residual hepatic damage. However, chronic inflammation in the liver can result in extensive fibrous tissue formation. Scarring may link portal tracts and central veins. Bands of fibrous tissue entrap regenerating nodules of hepatocytes, causing liver cirrhosis (Figure 49). Cirrhosis is the end stage of chronic inflammatory liver disease from numerous causes, including:

- alcohol
- chronic viral hepatitis (B and C)
- biliary disease (primary and secondary biliary cirrhosis)
- haemochromatosis

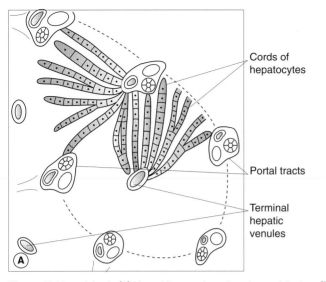 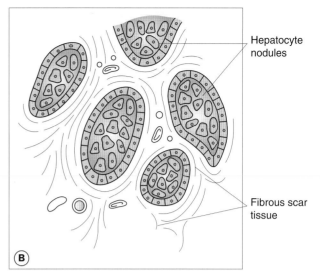

Figure 49 Liver cirrhosis. (A) Normal liver – schematic acinar architecture. (B) Liver cirrhosis – loss of normal architecture.

Box 25 Clinical and laboratory features of liver disease

Hepatic failure
Jaundice
Encephalopathy

- drowsiness, confusion, coma
- coarse hand tremor ('liver flap')
- fetor hepaticus

Hepatorenal syndrome (renal impairment secondary to liver failure)
Ascites/oedema
Chronic liver disease
Bruising
Gynaecomastia
Testicular atrophy
Palmar erythema
Clubbing
Dupuytren's contracture (alcoholic cirrhosis)
Xanthomas (primary biliary cirrhosis)
Spider angiomas (spider naevi)
Ascites/oedema
Hypoalbuminaemia
Raised liver enzymes, coagulopathy, hyponatraemia
Raised serum ammonia in liver failure

- other genetic diseases (α_1-antitrypsin deficiency, Wilson's disease)
- idiopathic.

Cirrhosis

Cirrhosis is a diffuse process and the damage is usually irreversible. The scarring disrupts and impairs blood flow through the liver, elevating the portal venous pressure (portal hypertension). As a consequence, blood flow increasingly bypasses the liver and flows through lower resistance vessels that communicate between the portal and systemic circulations. These anastomoses arise at four main sites:

- gastro-oesophageal junction (oesophageal varices)
- rectum
- retroperitoneum
- anterior abdominal wall (caput medusae).

There are two serious consequences of this vascular shunting:

- life-threatening haemorrhage from rupture of oesophageal varices
- impaired detoxification of noxious chemicals (e.g. ammonia), contributing to hepatic encephalopathy, coma and death.

Portal hypertension also causes splenomegaly and contributes to the development of ascites. Portal hypertension can be caused by other lesions that obstruct hepatic blood flow in the absence of cirrhosis, such as portal vein thrombosis and Budd–Chiari syndrome (see Section 18.3).

Cirrhosis is associated with development of hepatocellular carcinoma, although the degree of risk varies with the underlying disease.

Liver failure

Liver failure can be acute or chronic, and results when hepatic functional impairment is extreme. Mortality exceeds 70%. It is often precipitated by an event such as gastrointestinal haemorrhage or infection in a patient with chronic liver disease. Acute liver failure is uncommon, but may follow viral infection, drug exposure (e.g. paracetamol overdose, halothane), toxin damage (carbon tetrachloride), acute fatty liver of pregnancy and Reye's syndrome (Section 18.3). In acute liver failure without pre-existing hepatic disease, there is extensive liver necrosis with shrinkage of the organ, and clinical features of hepatic failure – clotting deficiencies, jaundice, hepatic encephalopathy – developing over 2–3 weeks. Massive liver destruction may prove fatal without transplantation, or cause irregular scarring in survivors.

Infectious hepatitis

Viral infection of the liver has various clinical manifestations, according to the specific agent involved:

- asymptomatic subclinical infection with complete resolution
- acute hepatitis
- chronic hepatitis
- asymptomatic carrier state
- hepatic failure (acute or chronic)
- cirrhosis
- hepatocellular carcinoma.

Acute hepatitis

In acute viral hepatitis (Box 26) there may be isolated liver cell necrosis or more severe bridging necrosis between portal tracts and central veins. Portal tracts are inflamed and there are increased numbers of Kupffer cells (sinusoidal macrophages). Swelling, necrosis and regeneration of hepatocytes produces architectural distortion called lobular disarray. All of these changes can revert to normal if infection is cleared.

Chronic hepatitis

Chronic hepatitis is defined as abnormal LFTs and/or clinical evidence of continuing hepatic inflammation for >6 months. The severity of inflammation varies within and between individual cases over time. Bile duct injury, fatty change, portal tract lymphoid aggregates and lobular inflammation are typical features of hepatitis C. Hepatocytes infected with hepatitis B may show 'ground glass' pink (eosinophilic) cytoplasm. The fibrosis and hepatocyte regeneration associated with chronic inflammatory damage may develop into cirrhosis.

Chronic hepatitis is not only due to viral infection – drugs, autoimmune disease and certain genetic disorders (see later) can cause very similar histological changes. Reaching the correct diagnosis requires consideration of all the clinical, serological, biochemical and pathological findings.

Carrier state

Disease carriers harbour persistent asymptomatic infection; they may be entirely healthy or have covert subclinical chronic liver disease. A carrier can pass infective virus on to non-immune contacts. Hepatitis B, C and D infections can produce a carrier state.

Hepatic failure, cirrhosis and hepatocellular carcinoma

These have been discussed above. Within the family of specific hepatitis viruses (Table 30), hepatitis B and C are the clinically most important causes.

Hepatitis B

Hepatitis B infection occurs worldwide, but is extremely common in southeast Asia, where the disease is frequently transmitted from mother to fetus. Exposure early in life creates a permanent carrier state in over 90% of patients. Infection in the UK is usually acquired in adult life, through sexual contact, infected needles (drug misusers and healthcare workers) or an unknown source. Needlestick injury from a hepatitis B carrier confers a 30% risk of infection. The virus is present in blood and body fluids during incubation (which can be up to 6 months from inoculation) and during periods of acute liver inflammation. The viral antigens and host antibodies detected in the serum reflect the stage of disease and infectivity of the patient. Core antigen (HbcAg) and the related HBe antigen are infective. The presence of IgM anti-HBc indicates recent infection. As the time period from infection increases, the antibody class switches to IgG. Surface antigen (HbsAg) positivity indicates acute infection or carrier state. HbsAb appears late and indicates immunity.

Hepatitis C

Hepatitis C prevalence is uncertain, but estimated at between 0.1% and 1% of the UK population. There is an estimated 3% risk of transmission from an infected needlestick injury. Acute infection is asymptomatic in the majority. HCV antibodies are found in many patients with previously unexplained cirrhosis and hepatocellular carcinoma. Liver function tests characteristically fluctuate throughout the course of the disease, and HCV RNA is detectable despite anti-HCV antibodies (the latter do not appear to confer immunity). Liver damage in part appears immunologically mediated. Patients may benefit from immune modulation therapy with interferon. Selection for such treatment is based on histological assessment of the degree of active inflammatory damage and the extent of fibrosis in a liver biopsy specimen.

Other causes of infectious hepatitis include:

- bacterial – tuberculosis, leptospirosis
- viral – cytomegalovirus (CMV), infectious mononucleosis (EBV)
- parasitic – malaria, amoebiasis.

Hydatid disease

Hydatid disease is a systemic infection due to the canine tapeworm *Echinococcus*. Although uncommon in the UK,

---

Box 26 Acute viral hepatitis

- Symptoms can include fever, fatigue, nausea, anorexia and right upper quadrant pain.
- Mild hepatomegaly may be detected on examination.
- Liver function tests (LFTs) are abnormal, with raised serum liver enzymes.
- If there is conjugated hyperbilirubinaemia, jaundice develops.
- Increased urinary bilirubin excretion produces dark urine, whereas decreased biliary excretion results in pale stools.
- Bile salt retention in the skin causes itching.

Table 30 Hepatitis viruses

Hepatic virus	Nature of virus	Mode of spread	Clinical disease
A	Single-stranded RNA virus	Faecal–oral spread from contaminated food and water, especially seafood	Usually self-limiting acute infection Acute liver failure occurs in <1% No chronic disease No carrier state
B	Double-stranded DNA virus	Vertical (mother to fetus), sexual contact, blood transfusion, intravenous drug misuse	Very high rate of carrier state if infected in early life, with frequent chronic hepatitis, cirrhosis and hepatocellular carcinoma Risk of chronic disease and malignancy is less if infection is acquired in adult life
C	Single-stranded RNA virus	Blood transfusion (patients with haemophilia) and inoculation (intravenous drug misuse)	Up to 85% develop chronic hepatitis; up to 50% of these progress to cirrhosis ± hepatocellular carcinoma ± hepatic failure
D	Defective RNA virus only infective in association with HBV	Parenteral	Can co-infect with HBV (usually recover normally, but risk of severe acute hepatitis is increased) or super-infect a HBV chronic carrier, with greatly increased risk of chronic hepatitis and cirrhosis
E	Single-stranded RNA virus	Faecal–oral spread from contaminated water	Usually self-limiting but 20% mortality rate in pregnant women

Eighteen

hydatid disease occurs worldwide and incidence is increased in sheep- and cattle-farming areas. The liver is frequently involved with formation of single or multiple infected cysts, causing mass effects. There is a risk of disease dissemination or fatal anaphylactic shock if the cyst contents are liberated and care must be taken during surgical removal.

Liver abscesses

Liver abscess is uncommon in the UK and is usually due to bacterial infection. Organisms reach the liver via the bloodstream, biliary system or direct spread. Abscesses can be single or multiple. Surgical drainage is usually necessary. Parasitic and protozoal abscesses are more common in the developing world.

Autoimmune hepatitis

Autoimmune liver disease typically occurs in young and middle-aged adult females. Patients have a chronic hepatitis, which clinically and histologically resembles viral hepatitis, but serological tests show raised serum IgG and specific autoantibodies. The latter include antinuclear antibodies (ANA), antimitochondrial antibodies (AMA), anti-smooth-muscle and antimicrosomal antibodies. There is often associated extrahepatic autoimmune disease such as thyroiditis or rheumatoid arthritis.

18.2 Alcohol- and drug-related liver disease

Alcohol misuse is the major cause of chronic liver disease in the UK. Excessive alcohol intake can cause:

- fatty change (steatosis)
- alcoholic hepatitis
- cirrhosis, ± hepatocellular carcinoma.

Fatty change

Fatty change is the accumulation of fat droplets within the cytoplasm of hepatocytes, usually as a single large vacuole (macrovesicular steatosis). The change occurs throughout the liver, and may develop in chronic alcohol misuse or following 'binge' drinking in non-habituated individuals. Fatty change is reversible over several days of abstinence, but with repeated attacks, fibrosis can develop.

Alcoholic hepatitis

In alcoholic hepatitis (steatohepatitis) fatty change is accompanied by acute inflammation, with neutrophil polymorph infiltration around degenerate and necrotic hepatocytes. Abnormal liver cells may contain condensed intracytoplasmic proteins, known as Mallory bodies. Alcoholic hepatitis is associated with developing liver fibrosis, which characteristically starts around centrilobular veins. Whereas simple fatty change usually produces no clinical symptoms, patients with alcoholic hepatitis present with right upper quadrant pain and jaundice. Either condition may cause hepatomegaly.

With or without recurrent attacks of alcoholic hepatitis, individuals who maintain a high regular alcohol intake over several years are at risk of progressive fibrosis, cirrhosis and liver failure. Women appear to be at greater risk with a relatively lower alcohol intake. Coexistent liver disease, particularly haemochromatosis and hepatitis C infection, can be important contributory factors in progression to cirrhosis. Current recommendations are for women to drink no more than 14 units of alcohol per week, and men fewer than 21 units. Moderate regular intake seems less harmful than erratic, heavy, binge drinking. Indeed, regular, low ethanol intake seems to have a protective influence in coronary heart disease.

Acute alcohol intoxication

Acute alcohol intoxication causes injury and death through accidents, hypoglycaemia, epilepsy and direct cerebral toxicity. Chronic alcohol misuse can result in pancreatitis, cardiomyopathy, physical dependence, malnutrition and neurological disease (Wernicke–Korsakoff syndrome – confusion, ataxia and ocular disturbances due to thiamine deficiency; if untreated, severe, irreversible amnesia often results).

Hepatic fat accumulation is most frequently seen in association with ethanol but other causes include:

- non-alcoholic steatohepatitis (diabetes mellitus, obesity, drugs)
- hepatitis C infection
- drugs
- Reye's syndrome
- acute fatty liver of pregnancy.

Drugs and the liver

Drugs can cause many morphological changes in the liver; more common examples are shown in Table 31. As the histological features often mimic endogenous liver disease a thorough clinical history is essential. Mechanisms of drug damage are:

- direct toxicity
- conversion of drug to active toxin by liver
- immune-mediated (e.g. drug causes autoantibody production).

Drug damage may be *predictable*, occurring in any individual who ingests a large enough dose, or *idiosyncratic* (host dependent).

Table 31 Drugs and the liver

Liver lesion	Examples of drugs responsible
Fatty change	Methotrexate, tetracycline
Hepatocyte necrosis	Paracetamol, halothane, isoniazid
Hepatitis and fibrosis	Methotrexate, amiodarone
Granulomatous inflammation	Sulphonamide antibiotics
Cholestasis	Chlorpromazine, contraceptive pill
Veno-occlusive disease	Cytotoxic drugs
Venous thrombosis	Cytotoxic drugs, contraceptive pill
Hepatocellular adenoma	Contraceptive pill

18.3 Genetic, metabolic and vascular liver disease

Haemochromatosis

Haemochromatosis is an autosomal recessive disease with excessive iron storage predominantly in the liver, pancreas, myocardium and synovial joints. The gene involved is on chromosome 6. The heterozygote rate is approximately 10% in the white UK population and the homozygote disease state is relatively common (0.5%). Gene testing can confirm suspected clinical cases of haemochromatosis and can be used to screen other family members for the disease. Men are affected more often than women, possibly due to the ameliorating effect of menstruation in reducing total body iron. Presentation is most frequent in middle-aged adults.

The typical clinical triad consists of cirrhosis, diabetes and skin pigmentation ('bronze diabetes'). Depending on the stage of disease, liver biopsy in homozygotes shows fibrosis or cirrhosis with excess iron in hepatocytes and Kupffer cells (liver macrophages). Iron is present in the form of haemosiderin pigment and appears yellow-brown on histological examination. A special stain, known as Perl's stain, gives a bright blue colour to iron deposits and this allows the degree of iron overload to be graded microscopically. Heterozygotes for the abnormal haemochromatosis gene also show increased hepatic iron storage but not sufficient to cause significant tissue damage. The liver shows little inflammation. Cirrhosis occurring in haemochromatosis carries a very high risk of hepatocellular carcinoma, which is the leading cause of death in these patients. Complications of diabetes or of cardiac involvement (arrhythmias, cardiomyopathy) may also prove fatal. Treatment with iron chelators and regular venesection in the precirrhotic phase is successful.

Secondary causes of hepatic iron overload include severe anaemia, repeated blood transfusions and excessive dietary intake linked to use of iron cooking utensils.

α_1-Antitrypsin deficiency

α_1-Antitrypsin deficiency is a rare autosomal recessive disease which causes emphysema (see Ch. 15) and hepatic cirrhosis. Liver biopsy shows variably sized, round intracytoplasmic globules of α_1-antitrypsin within hepatocytes, demonstrated by diastase periodic acid–Schiff (PAS) staining (see Box 27). Depending on the exact nature of the allele mutation, α_1-antitrypsin can present in neonates, children or adult life. In severe disease, liver transplantation is curative.

Wilson's disease

Wilson's disease is a rare autosomal recessive disorder of copper metabolism, which affects the liver, eye and brain. The incidence is approximately 1:200 000. There is a decrease in the serum copper-containing protein caeruloplasmin. Histological examination shows increased hepatic copper, often with quite marked chronic inflammation, fibrosis and fatty change. Presentation can be at any age but is often in adolescents or young adults. Extrahepatic manifestations include a parkinsonian movement

---

Box 27 Special stains

Routine histology slides are stained with haematoxylin and eosin (H&E). Nuclei take up the blue haematoxylin stain while cytoplasmic components show variable pink–red colouration from the eosin. When required, additional stains can be used in any tissues to demonstrate specific cell components and infectious agents. Examples are:

- Periodic acid–Schiff (PAS): stains carbohydrates magenta pink; PAS will stain glycogen in many cell types. Additional treatment with a diastase enzyme (DPAS stain) removes glycogen reactivity but allows demonstration of: mucin in gland-derived tumours (adenocarcinomas); fungi; and intracellular accumulations, such as α_1-antitrypsin.

- Perls' stain: demonstrates iron, for example in haemochromatosis. It can distinguish haemosiderin (iron-containing) pigment from melanin, both of which appear brown on H&E staining.

- Congo red: stains amyloid deposits salmon pink in normal light. When viewed with polarised light, the amyloid appears light green. (See Ch. 13.)

- Ziehl–Neelsen (ZN): stains mycobacteria (acid fast bacilli).

- Giemsa's: demonstrates *Helicobacter pylori* and *Giardia* organisms.

---

disorder, psychiatric symptoms and iris abnormalities (Kayser–Fleischer rings; green-brown copper deposits). If diagnosed early enough, copper chelating drugs are effective. If cirrhosis intervenes, liver transplantation may be considered.

Reye's syndrome

Reye's syndrome is a rare metabolic liver disease, with fatty change and encephalopathy. Reye's syndrome usually arises in young children following a viral illness. Most patients recover but occasionally fulminant liver failure or permanent neurological deficit results. Reye's syndrome is a disease of mitochondrial metabolism and has been associated with aspirin use – because of this association, aspirin is usually contraindicated in children under 12 years of age.

Vascular disease in the liver

Venous congestion

Venous congestion of the liver is very common in cardiac decompensation, both right sided and congestive (biventricular). Cut section of the liver at autopsy resembles the stippled appearance of the cut surface of a nutmeg, hence the pathologist's descriptive phrase, 'nutmeg liver'. This appearance results from more intense congestion of blood around centrilobular veins than around portal tracts. If there has been severe hypoperfusion of the liver, centrilobular necrosis can occur – this central perivenular area is more at risk of ischaemic damage than the better oxygenated periportal zone.

Portal vein thrombosis

Portal vein thrombosis is uncommon. It is associated with local sepsis, liver cirrhosis, malignancy, adjacent lymphadenopathy and the postoperative state. It may present with pain, ascites, oesophageal varices or bowel infarction.

Hepatic vein thrombosis (Budd–Chiari syndrome)

Hepatic vein thrombosis (Budd–Chiari syndrome) occurs in thrombotic conditions (post-partum, pregnancy, polycythaemia, oral contraceptives, malignancy). It can be acute and fatal or chronic. Membranous webs, presumably representing resolved thrombus, may be seen in hepatic veins and inferior vena cava.

Veno-occlusive disease

Veno-occlusive disease in the UK is seen in bone-marrow transplant recipients, as a result of initial chemotherapy and radiotherapy. Intra-hepatic veins are obliterated and there is a high mortality rate, up to 50%.

18.4 Liver tumours

Benign liver tumours

Benign liver tumours include haemangiomas and liver cell adenomas. The latter occur most commonly in women and are associated with oral contraceptive use. There is a risk of tumour rupture with intraperitoneal haemorrhage during pregnancy.

Hepatocellular carcinoma

Hepatocellular carcinoma (HCC) is relatively rare in the UK but represents the commonest visceral carcinoma in countries endemic for viral hepatitis (Table 32). The distribution is linked to hepatitis B infection, especially if acquired by vertical transmission from mother. The incidence of HCC in the Western world is likely to rise in future years due to hepatitis C infection. In the UK over 85% of patients with HCC have cirrhosis (compared to 50% or less in endemic hepatitis B countries), and most patients are over 60. Aflatoxin is a chemical carcinogen associated with HCC. It is produced by the *Aspergillus* fungus growing on mouldy food materials, particularly peanuts.

The majority of patients with HCC have raised serum α-fetoprotein (AFP), although this is not a specific finding. AFP can be raised in yolk-sac tumours of testis and ovary, in cirrhosis and chronic hepatitis without tumour, and in early pregnancy (fetal neural tube defects also cause raised AFP levels in the mother). Patients usually die within a few months of diagnosis of hepatocellular carcinoma due to cachexia, gastrointestinal bleeding, liver failure or tumour rupture and haemorrhage.

Angiosarcoma

Angiosarcoma is a malignant vascular tumour associated with vinyl chloride and Thorotrast (a radiological contrast agent) exposure.

Table 32 Cancer checklist: liver tumours

Incidence	<2% of UK cancers; commonest visceral cancer in parts of Far East with high hepatitis B prevalence
Risk factors	Cirrhosis; hepatitis B infection (especially vertical transmission); hepatitis C; aflatoxin exposure
Protective factors	Prevention of hepatitis B and C infection
Associated lesions	Chronic viral hepatitis, haemochromatosis, cirrhosis from other causes
Common clinical presentation	Abdominal pain or mass, malaise, weight loss
	Raised serum α-fetoprotein on monitoring of high-risk patients
Location	Single mass or multiple lesions anywhere in liver
Macroscopic appearance	Well-defined solid lesion(s) or diffusely infiltrating
Histological features	Varies from well-differentiated lesion resembling normal liver cell plates to anaplastic malignancy
Pattern of spread	Lymph nodes; vascular spread, bones, lung
Prognosis (per cent 5-year survival)	Death usual within 6 months of diagnosis
	Much better prognosis, 60%, for fibrolamellar variant (young adults, no cirrhosis and hepatitis B negative)

Hepatoblastoma

Hepatoblastoma is a malignant liver cell tumour occurring in childhood.

Metastatic malignancy

The liver is a very common site for secondary tumour spread. Breast, lung, colon and other gastrointestinal cancers metastasise most frequently, but virtually any primary site may seed to the liver. Metastases usually form multiple nodules, and may cause massive hepatomegaly.

Part 2: Biliary disease

Learning objectives

You should:
- know the pathology and complications of gallstone disease
- understand primary and secondary biliary cirrhosis
- know about inflammatory and neoplastic disease of the extrahepatic bile ducts.

18.5 Inflammatory and other non-neoplastic biliary disease

Ascending cholangitis

Ascending cholangitis is infection of the biliary tree, usually by Gram-negative gut bacteria. There is often a biliary stone or stricture causing obstruction and stasis, which predispose to infection.

Primary biliary cirrhosis

Primary biliary cirrhosis (PBC) is characterised by granulomatous inflammation and destruction of intrahepatic bile ducts. It is an autoimmune condition with female predominance, which peaks in middle age. Symptoms include itching, jaundice and xanthomas (the latter due to cholesterol retention). LFTs show a marked increase in alkaline phosphatase, and autoantibodies to mitochondria. PBC is associated with other autoimmune diseases including Sjögren's syndrome, thyroiditis and rheumatoid arthritis. Some cases will progress to cirrhosis.

Primary sclerosing cholangitis

Primary sclerosis cholangitis (PSC) describes chronic inflammation with obliterative fibrosis and segmental dilatation of intra- and extrahepatic bile ducts. As with other causes of bile duct damage, serum alkaline phosphatase is increased. Males are most frequently affected and 70% have coexistent ulcerative colitis. The aetiology of PSC is uncertain. Progressive bile duct obstruction leads to secondary biliary cirrhosis.

Secondary biliary cirrhosis

Secondary biliary cirrhosis follows prolonged extrahepatic biliary obstruction, most commonly due to gallstone impaction in the common bile duct.

Bile duct damage can also occur in viral hepatitis, drug injury and liver transplant rejection.

Gallstones

Gallstones occur in 20% of the adult population, but most do not cause symptoms. Female gender, increasing age, obesity, high-fat diet, pregnancy and oral contraceptive use are risk factors for the commonest type of stone (cholesterol rich). Stone formation requires supersaturation of cholesterol in bile. Biliary stasis – due to prolonged fasting, pregnancy, rapid weight loss or parenteral nutrition – is a promoting factor. Gallstones rich in pigment material develop in individuals with haemolytic anaemia. Biliary tract infection induces deconjugation of bilirubin, and the concentration of deconjugated bilirubin can exceed the low solubility. Clinical consequences of gallstones include biliary colic, obstructive jaundice and cholecystitis (Figure 50). Gallstones are a major cause of acute pancreatitis.

Acute cholecystitis

Acute cholecystitis is usually caused by impaction of a stone in the neck of the gall bladder or the cystic duct. Bile outflow obstruction leads to chemical irritation of the gall bladder mucosa. With increasing distension and

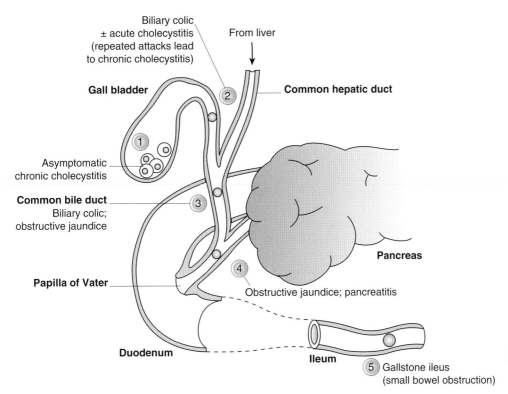

Figure 50 Complications of gallstones.

intraluminal pressure, blood flow to the gall bladder becomes compromised and ischaemia develops. The microscopic changes are typical of acute inflammation, with oedema and neutrophil polymorph infiltration. Complications of acute cholecystitis include:

- secondary bacterial infection
- gall bladder perforation and abscess formation
- rupture with peritonitis and fistula formation between gall bladder and bowel
- gall bladder infarction.

Recurrent attacks of acute cholecystitis can progress to **chronic cholecystitis** with fibrosis and mucosal outpouchings into the muscle layer (Rokitansky–Aschoff sinuses). Acute cholecystitis can also occur in the absence of calculi; precipitating factors include dehydration, gall bladder stasis, bile concentration ('biliary sludge') and bacterial infection. Such patients are often post operative or have suffered severe trauma, burns, sepsis and multiple organ failure.

Extrahepatic biliary atresia

Extrahepatic biliary atresia occurs 1 in 100 000 live births. Bile flow is completely obstructed due to destruction or absence of extrahepatic bile ducts in the neonatal period. The aetiology is uncertain – viral infection, genetic inheritance and anomalous embryological development have been suggested. Untreated, cirrhosis will develop within 6 months. Surgical correction is not often possible as intra-

hepatic ducts are also involved, and transplantation may offer the only chance of survival.

18.6 Bile duct and gall bladder neoplasia

Cholangiocarcinoma

Cholangiocarcinoma is a malignant tumour of either the intrahepatic or extrahepatic bile ducts. Associated factors include:

- Thorotrast
- liver fluke infection (*Clonorchis sinensis*)
- gallstones, ulcerative colitis and choledochal cysts (extrahepatic cholangiocarcinoma).

Cholangiocarcinoma is usually a well-differentiated adenocarcinoma, which induces a large amount of fibrous stroma (desmoplasia), imparting a very hard consistency to the tumour. Prognosis is poor due to local invasion and irresectability.

Carcinoma of the gall bladder

Carcinoma of the gall bladder is rare; it occurs in the elderly, usually associated with gallstones. Extensive local invasion is common at presentation and these unresectable tumours have a very poor prognosis. The vast majority are adenocarcinomas.

Part 3: Exocrine pancreas

You should:
- understand the pathology and complications of pancreatitis
- know the pathology of pancreatic carcinoma.

18.7 Inflammatory disease of the pancreas

Inflammation of the pancreas can occur as a single acute attack or a chronic relapsing condition. Pancreatitis occurs most frequently in middle-aged men. Known precipitating factors of pancreatic inflammation include:

- Common:
  - *gallstones and biliary tract disease*
  - *alcohol misuse (chronic pancreatitis, ?also acute).*
- Rare:
  - *infection (mumps)*
  - *drugs*
  - *trauma*
  - *shock*
  - *localised surgical or endoscopic procedures*
  - *congenital pancreatic abnormalities*
  - *hypercalcaemia.*

Pancreatic duct obstruction and direct injury to acinar cells seem to be involved in the initial insult. Damage to the exocrine pancreas liberates digestive enzymes – lipases, proteases and amylases – which increase the amount of tissue injury within the pancreas and adjacent organs. Raised serum amylase to greater than five times the normal is virtually diagnostic of acute pancreatitis. In severe acute haemorrhagic pancreatitis there is extensive blood vessel damage and abdominal fat necrosis. Systemic effects of enzyme release can include disseminated intravascular coagulation, adult respiratory distress syndrome (ARDS) and shock. Less serious complications are pancreatic abscess and pseudocyst formation. A pseudocyst is a collection of secretions within or outside the pancreas. The pseudocyst has a fibrous capsule but no epithelial lining. (True epithelial-lined pancreatic cysts occur in von Hippel–Lindau disease and adult polycystic kidney disease.)

Table 33 Cancer checklist: pancreatic carcinoma

Incidence	Common visceral cancer; middle-aged and older males, incidence increasing
Risk factors	Not well defined – ?smoking, previous gastric surgery, chronic pancreatitis (alcohol)
Protective factors	Not known
Associated lesions	–
Common clinical presentation	Abdominal and back pain, weight loss, jaundice
	Migratory thrombophlebitis (10%)
Location	60% in head of pancreas, 20% diffusely involve gland
Macroscopic appearance	Hard grey/white mass
Histological features	Gland formation, with reactive, dense, fibrous tissue
	Perineural invasion
Pattern of spread	Extensive local spread to duodenum, bile duct, stomach, retroperitoneal organs, lymph nodes, liver
Prognosis (per cent 5-year survival)	Less than 5%

Repeated, often mild, acute attacks lead to chronic pancreatitis, with marked scarring of the organ and loss of exocrine and endocrine function, with development of steatorrhoea and diabetes in severe cases. Pseudocysts are frequent in chronic pancreatitis. There is an increased risk of pancreatic carcinoma.

18.8 Neoplastic disease of the exocrine pancreas

Benign tumours of the pancreas are often cystic, and may be composed of mucinous or serous glandular epithelium. Malignant pancreatic tumours – adenocarcinomas – almost always derive from the ductal epithelium. Most tumours arise in the proximal organ (Table 33), and cause localising symptoms due to obstruction at the ampulla of Vater or distal common bile duct. The prognosis is poor, death often occurring within months of diagnosis.

Self-assessment: questions

One best answer questions

1. A 56-year-old white man presents with fatigue and arthritis. Following investigations, he is found to have diabetes and liver cirrhosis. He drinks alcohol occasionally. The most likely diagnosis is:
   a. hepatitis C infection
   b. haemochromatosis
   c. alcoholic liver disease
   d. non-alcoholic steatohepatitis
   e. autoimmune hepatitis

True-false questions

1. The following diseases are associated with the development of cirrhosis:
   a. hepatitis C
   b. hepatitis A
   c. haemochromatosis
   d. haemolytic anaemia
   e. alcoholic steatohepatitis

2. Acute liver failure typically occurs in:
   a. paracetamol overdose
   b. acute viral hepatitis
   c. primary biliary cirrhosis
   d. Reye's syndrome
   e. Budd–Chiari syndrome

3. Regarding hepatitis B:
   a. acute infection is usually asymptomatic
   b. infection early in life confers a higher risk of chronic carrier state
   c. the source of infection is always identifiable
   d. HbsAg detection in the blood indicates immunity
   e. co-infection with HDV increases the risk of severe acute hepatitis

4. Complications of cirrhosis include:
   a. gynaecomastia
   b. hepatocellular carcinoma
   c. renal failure
   d. gastrointestinal haemorrhage
   e. confusion

5. The following are correctly paired:
   a. Wilson's disease – abnormal lead metabolism
   b. haemochromatosis – hepatocellular carcinoma
   c. α_1-Antitrypsin deficiency – bronchiectasis
   d. Veno-occlusive disease – cytotoxic chemotherapy
   e. angiosarcoma – vinyl chloride exposure

6. Pancreatic carcinoma:
   a. is increasing in incidence
   b. has a 5-year survival rate of 50%
   c. often presents with painless jaundice
   d. is usually surgically resectable at presentation
   e. histologically is a squamous cell carcinoma

7. Concerning gallstones:
   a. cholesterol is the most frequent stone component
   b. most patients are symptomatic
   c. they are associated with gall bladder adenocarcinoma
   d. stones can develop following prolonged fasting
   e. the incidence is increased in oral contraceptive users

8. The following are causes of extrahepatic bile duct obstruction:
   a. biliary atresia
   b. primary biliary cirrhosis
   c. primary sclerosing cholangitis
   d. gallstones
   e. pancreatic adenocarcinoma

9. Acute cholecystitis:
   a. can occur in the absence of gallstones
   b. is characterised by lymphocytic infiltration of the gall bladder
   c. can be complicated by fistula formation
   d. frequently results in gall bladder infarction
   e. is increased in incidence in postoperative patients

10. The following are associated with primary biliary cirrhosis:
    a. xanthomas
    b. raised serum antimitochondrial antibodies
    c. rheumatoid arthritis
    d. granulomatous inflammation of the portal tracts
    e. decreased serum alkaline phosphatase

Case history questions

Case history 1

A 52-year-old woman presents with abdominal discomfort and increasing girth secondary to ascites. On examination there are additional signs of chronic liver disease.

1. What other physical signs of liver disease would you look for? What specific questions would you ask in the clinical history?

An ultrasound scan shows abnormal liver echogenicity suggestive of cirrhosis.

2. What further investigations would you consider?

3. What information might be provided by a liver biopsy?

4. What are the most important complications of cirrhosis?

Case history 2

You are an occupational health physician and a venesector asks you for advice after sustaining a needlestick injury. The healthcare worker has been immunised against hepatitis B but is anxious about contracting hepatitis C infection.

1. What information could you give regarding the incidence, rate of transmission and rate of progression of hepatitis C infection in this situation?

2. What measures should be taken to reduce the risk of healthcare personnel contracting hepatitis B and C?

Case history 3

A 44-year-old man is admitted to hospital with nausea, vomiting and abdominal pain radiating to the back. He admits to a high alcohol intake. The surgical registrar suspects acute pancreatitis and requests serum amylase, calcium, liver function tests and arterial blood gas measurement.

1. How will these investigations contribute to the patient management?

The patient is confirmed to have acute pancreatitis. He recovers with hospital treatment and is discharged home, but returns 2 weeks later with further pain and vomiting. Ultrasound examination reveals a cystic mass.

2. What is the likely cause of the mass?

Viva questions

1. How would you classify tumours of the liver?

2. How does knowledge of the pathology of haemochromatosis help in the management of patients and their families?

Self-assessment: answers

One best answer

1. b. The combination of cirrhosis, diabetes and arthritis is highly suggestive of haemochromatosis, a relatively common inherited disease in white-skinned races. Women are relatively protected from the effects of iron overload by the effects of menstrual blood loss, such that the disease presents at an earlier age in men. Genetic testing in affected families allows earlier detection and treatment, reducing the risk of certain complications. Diabetes is also associated with non-alcoholic fatty liver disease, which can progress to cirrhosis; investigations including gene analysis and liver biopsy help establish the correct diagnosis. Autoimmune hepatitis is more common in women than men; serological investigations and liver biopsy histology are again used to confirm the correct diagnosis.

True-false answers

1. a. **True.**
   b. **False.** There is no chronic infective state in hepatitis A.
   c. **True.**
   d. **False.**
   e. **True.** If excess alcohol consumption continues.

2. a. **True.**
   b. **True.** Uncommon but can occur in hepatitis A (and E), very rare in B and C.
   c. **False.** Liver failure develops chronically following cirrhosis in severe cases.
   d. **True.**
   e. **True.**

3. a. **True.**
   b. **True.**
   c. **False.** Vertical transmission, sexual contact and inoculation of infected blood are the major methods of transmission but the actual source may not always be identifiable.
   d. **False.** Hepatitis B surface antigen indicates acute infection or carrier state. HbsAb indicates immunity.
   e. **True.** See Table 30.

4. a. **True.** Probably due to altered oestrogen metabolism.
   b. **True.**
   c. **True.** Decompensated cirrhosis can lead to hepatorenal syndrome, in which renal failure occurs secondary to liver failure. The mechanism is thought to involve altered renal blood flow. Kidney dysfunction is reversible if the liver failure can be successfully treated.
   d. **True.** Usually from oesophageal varices, an important complication.
   e. **True.** If hepatic encephalopathy develops.

5. a. **False.** Copper metabolism is deranged in Wilson's disease.
   b. **True.** There is a high risk of liver cancer in patients with haemochromatosis who develop cirrhosis.
   c. **False.** The lung lesion present in α_1-antitrypsin deficiency is emphysema.
   d. **True.**
   e. **True.**

6. a. **True.**
   b. **False.** Five-year survival is less than 5%.
   c. **True.**
   d. **False.**
   e. **False.** Adenocarcinoma.

7. a. **True.**
   b. **False.** Many adults do not complain of symptoms related to their gallstones.
   c. **True.** But the risk to individual patients is very low given the high prevalence of gallstones and rarity of gall bladder cancer.
   d. **True.** Presumably due to increased bile concentration and cholesterol saturation.
   e. **True.**

8. a. **True.**
   b. **False.** This disease is confined to intra-hepatic ducts.
   c. **True.**
   d. **True.**
   e. **True.** Sixty per cent of pancreatic carcinomas arise in the head of the gland and can obstruct the distal common bile duct.

9. a. **True.** But stones are present in >90% of cases, either in the gall bladder neck or cystic duct.
   b. **False.** Neutrophil polymorphs are characteristic of acute inflammation.
   c. **True.** Between the gall bladder and intestine, usually colon.
   d. **False.** Ischaemic necrosis is a rare but serious complication leading to perforation and peritonitis.
   e. **True.**

10. a. **True.**
    b. **True.**
    c. **True.** There is an association between primary biliary cirrhosis and other autoimmune conditions.
    d. **True.**
    e. **False.** Alkaline phosphatase is raised in biliary tract damage, and may be the only abnormality in the liver function tests in primary biliary cirrhosis.

Case history answers

Case history 1

1. The signs of chronic liver disease are shown in Box 25 (page 179). Relevant information from the clinical history would include alcohol consumption (although patients may not give an honest answer!), family history of liver disease (which may point to an inherited disease), possible exposure to hepatitis B and C and any history of autoimmune disease. As many therapeutic drugs can damage the liver in numerous ways, a careful history of recent and long-term prescribed medications is often helpful.

2. Full investigation of chronic liver disease may include:

   - liver function tests – liver enzymes released from damaged cells (γ-glutamyl transferase, aspartate aminotransferase and alkaline phosphatase), and markers of synthetic function, such as albumin
   - coagulation tests (international normalised ratio (INR))
   - viral serology – hepatitis B and C (hepatitis A does not cause chronic disease)
   - autoimmune screen – helpful for diagnosing primary biliary cirrhosis and autoimmune chronic hepatitis
   - ultrasound – to assess liver size, texture (fatty change or cirrhosis) presence of masses/cysts and examine the biliary tree for dilatation (obstruction)
   - gene analysis for haemochromatosis
   - serum protein electrophoresis for α_1-antitrypsin
   - serum caeruloplasmin measurement (Wilson's disease)
   - liver biopsy.

3. Liver biopsy is an invasive procedure which can be helpful in the investigation of:

   - unexplained hepatomegaly or abnormal liver function tests
   - cirrhosis
   - tumours (primary or metastatic)
   - hepatic damage by medications – for example, methotrexate used in psoriasis

   - assessing degree of inflammation and fibrosis in hepatitis C infection, in order to select patients for interferon therapy.

   Percutaneous liver biopsy carries a very small risk of mortality but should not be undertaken in patients with abnormal clotting, obstructive jaundice or ascites. An alternative approach in high-risk patients is to perform a transjugular biopsy, approaching the liver through the inferior vena cava.

4. Important complications of cirrhosis are discussed in the text (Section 18.1) but include:

   - haemorrhage from portal-systemic anastomoses, especially oesophageal varices
   - hepatic encephalopathy
   - development of hepatocellular carcinoma.

Case history 2

1. The incidence of hepatitis C in the UK is probably less than 1% of the general population but there are high-risk factors including intravenous drug misuse and blood transfusion prior to the introduction of hepatitis C screening of blood donations in 1991. There is an approximately 3% risk of contracting hepatitis C via a needlestick injury from an infected patient but the risk may vary according to the stage of the disease and the viral load as assessed by HCV RNA analysis using the polymerase chain reaction. The rate of progression to chronic hepatitis may be as high as 85% and up to 50% of these individuals may develop cirrhosis.

2. All healthcare workers potentially exposed to blood and body fluids should be immunised against hepatitis B for their own and their patients' safety. There is no vaccination for hepatitis C, so minimising the risk of infection is vital, by wearing protective clothing including gloves and eye protection when appropriate. Open wounds must be fully covered with waterproof dressings. Any specimens of blood, body fluid or tissue sent to pathology laboratories with suspected or known infection risk must be clearly labelled as 'high risk' to protect staff – nurses, operating department assistants, porters, laboratory scientists and doctors – who may come into contact with the material. High-risk status applies to any material potentially infected by hepatitis B or C, HIV or tuberculosis. If you need advice, contact your hospital's occupational health department.

Case history 3

1. The clinical history suggests an acute abdomen; the differential diagnosis would include acute pancreatitis, acute cholecystitis and a perforated peptic ulcer. Myocardial infarction must also be excluded. The investigations ordered would be appropriate to confirm a clinical diagnosis of acute pancreatitis and to assess the severity of the attack. Amylase is released from the inflamed pancreas and

a serum rise to greater than five times the normal upper limit usually indicates acute pancreatitis. However, less severe elevation of serum amylase can occur with other conditions including cholecystitis and perforated peptic ulcer. Severe attacks of acute pancreatitis may be associated with decreased serum albumin and calcium, and a lowered arterial oxygen concentration. The mortality rate in poor prognosis cases exceeds 50%.

2. The likely cause is a pancreatic pseudocyst. If large, the cyst may require drainage by aspiration or surgical excision.

Viva answers

1. *Comment*: Remember in viva answers to be logical, structured and emphasise the more common conditions. In the UK, liver metastases are more common than primary tumours. You could classify primary intrahepatic tumours by their cell of origin. The list below is not exhaustive but would be appropriate for this question:

Benign neoplasms

- Epithelial: hepatocellular adenoma.
- Vascular (endothelium): haemangioma.

Primary liver malignancies

- Epithelial: hepatocellular carcinoma; cholangiocarcinoma (arising in intrahepatic bile ducts)

- Vascular (endothelium): angiosarcoma.

Secondary liver tumours

- From many sites, but particularly colon, upper gastrointestinal tract, breast and lung.

2. *Comment*: The question requires you to explain the clinical implications of the pathogenesis, genetics, incidence, progression and complications of haemochromatosis. Points to include are:

- mode of inheritance (autosomal recessive)
- heterozygote carrier and homozygote population frequencies
- subclinical disease in heterozygotes
- the opportunity for familial disease screening and early diagnosis through genetic testing
- prevention of serious complications, cirrhosis and liver cancer, by early treatment aimed at reducing body iron (venesection and chelating agents)
- role of liver biopsy in assessing stage and severity of disease, and response to treatment (reduction in hepatic iron stores and cessation of disease progression).

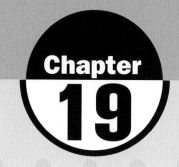

Endocrine system

Chapter overview

The endocrine system is a complex, highly integrated group of organs that have a central role in the maintenance of normal bodily functions. More specifically, the endocrine system plays an important part in the regulation of reproduction, growth and development, maintenance of the internal environment, and energy production, utilisation and storage. Disorders of the endocrine system are therefore important because they have far-reaching and devastating effects, which in some cases can be life-threatening (e.g. addisonian crisis, diabetic ketoacidosis). At the heart of the endocrine system are the endocrine glands, which include the pituitary, adrenals, thyroid, parathyroids and pancreas. Endocrine glands synthesise and secrete hormones into the bloodstream, via which they are carried to distant sites to exert their effects. In this way the endocrine glands are able to influence the function of distant target organs and tissues. Disorders of the endocrine system are usually due to either overproduction or underproduction of a particular hormone, or mass lesions, and to aid understanding, the pathology will be presented in a similar scheme.

Basic principles

The ability of the various organs and tissues in the body to function in an integrated fashion is made possible by extracellular signalling. Signalling is mediated by specialised molecules, which are synthesised within the cell and secreted into the extracellular environment, where they exert their effects on other cells. There are three main signalling modalities:

- **Paracrine**, where molecules secreted by cells exert their effects on neighbouring tissues.
- **Autocrine**, where the secreted molecules exert their effects on the cell of origin.
- **Endocrine**, where the secreted molecules exert their effects at distant sites that can be accessed only by the bloodstream.

Molecules that exert their effects via the endocrine modality are called hormones, and hormones are secreted and synthesised by endocrine glands. The effects of hormones are often complex. A single hormone can have different effects on several tissues, and some target tissues require the interaction of several hormones to carry out their physiological functions.

A distinguishing characteristic of the endocrine system is the feedback control of hormone production. Increased activity of a target organ down-regulates the activity of the endocrine gland, a process known as negative feedback or feedback inhibition.

There are two broad categories of hormones:

- **Peptide or amino acid derivatives** – these types of hormones bind to cell surface receptors and exert their effects by causing an increase in intracellular signalling molecules.
- **Steroid hormones** – steroid hormones are able to diffuse across the lipid cell membrane and bind to intracellular receptors. The hormone/receptor complex then acts directly on the cell DNA.

19.1 The pituitary gland

Learning objectives

You should:
- know the structure and function of the pituitary gland
- know the causes of anterior pituitary hypo- and hyperfunction, and the clinical manifestations
- know the clinical syndromes associated with disorders of antidiuretic hormone (ADH) secretion from the posterior pituitary.

Structure

The pituitary gland is located at the base of the brain within the confines of the sella turcica. It lies beneath the hypothalamus, to which it is attached by means of a stalk, and in close proximity to the optic chiasm. Despite its small size (it measures only ~1 cm across), the pituitary gland has a pivotal role in the regulation of most other endocrine glands. The pituitary gland consists of two parts; the anterior pituitary (or adenohypophysis), and the posterior pituitary (or neurohypophysis) (Figure 51).

The anterior pituitary (adenohypophysis)

The anterior pituitary constitutes 75% of the gland and is derived from an outpouching of the embryonic oral cavity known as the Rathke pouch. This part of the gland secretes six different hormones into the bloodstream. There are five different cell types in the anterior pituitary, each responsible for synthesising and secreting one or more of the six hormones. The synthesis and secretion of anterior pituitary hormones is controlled by the hypothalamus (the hypothalamic-pituitary axis). Hypothalamic neurones in the median eminence release hypothalamic-releasing

hormones, which are then carried to the anterior pituitary via a portal venous system in the pituitary stalk (Figure 51). There are several types of hypothalamic-releasing hormone, each acting on and controlling the functions of a specific cell type within the anterior pituitary (see Table 34). The secretion of hypothalamic-releasing hormones is under neural control from other parts of the central nervous system (CNS) and hormonal control from the levels of anterior pituitary hormones circulating in the blood. If there are high circulating levels of a particular hormone, the secretion of the relevant hypothalamic-releasing hormone is reduced (negative feedback or feedback inhibition).

Hypopituitarism

The most common causes of hypopituitarism are:

- pituitary adenoma (commonest cause)
- craniopharyngioma
- Sheehan's syndrome.

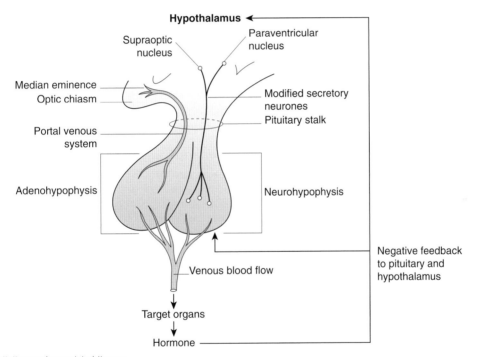

Figure 51 The pituitary and associated tissues.

Table 34 Anterior pituitary cell types, hormone products, and controlling hypothalamic hormones

Pituitary cell type	Hormonal product	Controlling hypothalamic hormone
Somatotroph	Growth hormone (GH)	Growth hormone-releasing hormone (GHRH) Somatostatin (inhibits release of GH)
Corticotroph	Pro-opiomelanocortin (POMC) from which adrenocorticotrophic hormone (ACTH) is a cleavage product	Corticotrophin-releasing hormone (CRH)
Gonadotroph	Follicle stimulating hormone (FSH) and luteinising hormone (LH)	Gonadotrophin-releasing hormone (GRH)
Lactotroph	Prolactin	Prolactin-inhibiting factor (PIF)
Thyrotroph	Thyroid stimulating hormone (TSH)	Thyrotrophin-releasing hormone (TRH)

Nineteen

These conditions can lead to a deficiency in all of the anterior pituitary hormones (panhypopituitarism) leading to hypofunction of one or more of the target endocrine organs under pituitary control, a situation that can be life-threatening.

Non-secretory pituitary adenomas

Non-secretory pituitary adenomas are benign tumours that may arise from any of the hormone secreting cells in the anterior pituitary.

Craniopharyngiomas

Craniopharyngiomas are usually benign tumours that occur most commonly in children, and are thought to arise from squamous cell rests representing the remains of the Rathke pouch.

Clinical presentation of these two types of tumour is related to their local effects on the surrounding tissues, which include:

- compression damage to the adjacent pituitary tissue, leading to underproduction of the adenohypophysis hormones
- compression of the optic chiasm, which leads to abnormalities in the visual fields (bitemporal hemianopia)
- symptoms of raised intracranial pressure.

Sheehan's syndrome (post-partum ischaemic necrosis)

During pregnancy, the pituitary enlarges to almost twice its normal size and becomes highly vascular. Sheehan's syndrome occurs if haemorrhage during childbirth causes a severe fall in blood pressure sufficient to cause ischaemic necrosis of the anterior pituitary, resulting in hypofunction. The posterior pituitary is usually spared. The resultant syndrome associated with anterior pituitary hypofunction is known as Simmond's disease, the first manifestation being failure of lactation due to prolactin deficiency. The effects of the loss of TSH, LH, FSH and ACTH follow.

Clinical manifestations of hypopituitarism

Lack of growth hormone In pre-pubertal children, lack of growth hormone causes symmetrical growth retardation termed pituitary dwarfism. In this condition, sexual development may also be retarded. Lack of growth hormone in adults may cause fasting hypoglycaemia.

Lack of LH and FSH In post-pubertal women, deficiency of LH and FSH induces amenorrhoea, sterility, atrophy of the ovaries and external genitalia, and loss of axillary and pubic hair. In men, deficiency is manifest by decreased libido, sterility, testicular atrophy, and loss of axillary and pubic hair.

Lack of TSH Deficiency of TSH induces hypothyroidism and atrophy of the thyroid gland.

Lack of ACTH Deficiency of ACTH induces hypoadrenalism and atrophy of the adrenals.

Lack of prolactin In affected women who have just given birth there is failure of lactation.

Hyperpituitarism

Hyperfunction of the anterior pituitary is almost always due to a functioning adenoma. Functioning carcinomas are rare. Adenomas may produce any anterior pituitary hormone depending on their cell of origin. Clinical presentation is related to:

- overproduction of a particular hormone
- compression of the optic chiasm, causing visual abnormalities
- raised intracranial pressure.

Somatotrophic adenomas

These adenomas lead to growth hormone overproduction. When the growth hormone excess occurs in children (before the epiphyses have closed) the result is gigantism, which is extremely rare. When the growth hormone excess occurs in adults, the resulting condition is called acromegaly. The excess growth hormone affects the viscera, bones, skin and soft tissues. The main presenting features are enlargement of the hands, feet and head with development of prominent supraorbital ridges, prominent lower jaw (prognathism) and separating of the teeth. Around a third of all acromegalic patients develop cardiac disease, which can be life-threatening.

Corticotrophic adenomas

Excess production of ACTH leads to Cushing's disease (see later section on The adrenal gland).

Gonadotrophic adenomas

These rare tumours tend to secrete the hormones LH and FSH inefficiently and variably. There is often no evidence of increased gonadotroph hormone production, but there may be evidence of underproduction.

Prolactinomas

These are the most common type of pituitary tumour. Hyperprolactinaemia induces galactorrhoea in females, and hypogonadism (infertility) in males and females. Prolactinomas are an important cause of amenorrhoea in women.

Thyrotroph adenomas

These tumours cause hyperthyroidism, but they are extremely uncommon.

The posterior pituitary (neurohypophysis)

The posterior pituitary is derived from a downgrowth of the hypothalamus. Only two hormones are secreted – ADH and oxytocin. These hormones are stored within secretory granules of modified nerve fibres that originate from the supraoptic and paraventricular nuclei. These modified nerve fibres ramify in the pituitary stalk and have their terminal endings in the posterior pituitary. The stored hormones are released in response to hypothalamic stimuli.

ADH is secreted in response to raised plasma osmolarity and induces conservation of body water. It does this by causing an increase in the permeability of the renal collecting ducts, resulting in increased resorption of water and reduced urine output. The urine becomes concentrated. The secretion of oxytocin stimulates uterine smooth muscle to contract during childbirth, and causes the ejection of milk during lactation.

Disorders of the posterior pituitary are rare. The most important disorders are related to the secretion of ADH.

Decreased ADH production

Damage to the hypothalamus, for example by a tumour or trauma, causes a deficiency of ADH, producing a syndrome known as diabetes insipidus, which is characterised by polyuria and hyperosmolarity of the blood leading to compensatory polydipsia (excessive drinking).

Increased or inappropriate ADH production

Inappropriate ADH production implies persistent release of ADH unrelated to the plasma osmolarity. The most common cause is ectopic production of ADH by tumours such as bronchogenic carcinoma (especially the small cell variant), and less commonly thymomas, pancreatic carcinomas and lymphomas. Other causes of inappropriate ADH production include CNS disorders (e.g. head injury, meningitis), non-neoplastic lung disorders (e.g. pneumonia, tuberculosis) and drugs.

19.2 The adrenal gland

> **Learning objectives**
>
> You should:
> * understand the structure and function of the adrenal glands
> * know the common disorders that can affect the adrenal medulla
> * know the disorders that can cause hypo- or hyperfunction of the adrenal cortex.

Structure

The adrenal glands are located in the retroperitoneum, superomedial to the kidneys. Each is composed of two totally separate functional units: the central medulla and the peripheral cortex (Figure 52).

The adrenal medulla

The adrenal medulla, which is derived from the embryonic neural crest, is part of the sympathetic nervous system. It consists of neuroendocrine cells (chromaffin cells) and sympathetic nerve endings. The main function of the chromaffin cells is to synthesise and secrete the catecholamines, adrenaline and noradrenaline. The adrenal medulla is the main source of endogenous adrenaline.

The most significant disorders arising from the adrenal medulla are neoplasms, which include phaeochromocytomas (most common), neuroblastomas and ganglioneuromas.

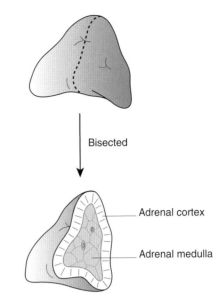

Figure 52 An adrenal gland.

Phaeochromocytoma

This is a functioning tumour derived from the chromaffin cells of the adrenal medulla, and is classified as a paraganglioma. Overproduction of catecholamines produces hypertension (which may be intermittent) associated with headaches, sweating, palpitations, pallor, anxiety and nausea. The presence of a phaeochromocytoma should be suspected in any young hypertensive patient and, although rare, is one of the curable causes of hypertension. Around 10–20% of these tumours are associated with familial syndromes such as multiple endocrine neoplasia (MEN) syndrome, von Hippel–Lindau disease, von Recklinghausen's disease, tuberous sclerosis, and Sturge–Weber syndrome. About half of these familial cases are bilateral. The diagnosis of phaeochromocytoma is based on estimating the urinary excretion of the catecholamine metabolite vanillylmandelic acid (VMA), which is at least doubled when the tumour is present.

The adrenal cortex

The adult cortex constitutes the peripheral 80% of the adrenal gland. The adrenal cortex is derived from mesoderm and synthesises and secretes the three main classes of steroid hormones: mineralocorticoids, glucocorticoids and sex steroids. There are three functional zones of the adrenal cortex:

* zona glomerulosa (10%), which lies beneath the capsule and secretes mineralocorticoids
* zona fasciculata (80%)
* zona reticularis (10%), which corresponds to the middle and inner zones of the adrenal cortex and secretes glucocorticoids and sex steroids.

Glucocorticoids

These hormones have important effects on a wide range of tissues and organs. The effects include:

- increased blood sugar
- increased protein breakdown
- increased fat loss from the extremities, but fat accumulation in the trunk, neck and face
- effects on the immune system, bone, kidneys, CNS, circulatory system, other endocrine glands and connective tissue.

The most important glucocorticoid is cortisol. The synthesis and secretion of glucocorticoids is under negative feedback control by ACTH, which is synthesised by the anterior pituitary.

Mineralocorticoids

Aldosterone is the most important mineralocorticoid. Its function is to maintain intravascular volume. When intravascular volume is decreased, aldosterone acts on renal tubules to increase the reabsorption of sodium and elimination of potassium and hydrogen ions. The retention of sodium leads to retention of water and consequent restoration of the intravascular volume. The synthesis and secretion of the mineralocorticoids is controlled by the renin-angiotensin system and *not* the pituitary (see Figure 53).

Sex steroids

The sex steroids are involved in the development of the male and female sexual characteristics. Most of the body's sex steroids are synthesised in the gonads, but the adrenal sex steroids usually have a role in the development of some of the secondary sexual characteristics.

Adrenocortical hyperfunction (hyperadrenalism)

The clinical syndromes of cortical hyperfunction are due to excess production of one of the adrenal steroids. Cushing's syndrome is due to excess glucocorticoids,

Conn's syndrome is due to excess mineralocorticoids, and adrenogenital syndromes result from excess sex steroids.

Cushing's syndrome

There are four main causes of excess circulating glucocorticoids. The commonest is administration of exogenous glucocorticoids. The three remaining causes are related to the overproduction of endogenous glucocorticoids as follows:

- excess production of ACTH from the anterior pituitary
- oversecretion of cortisol by an adrenal neoplasm
- secretion of ectopic ACTH.

Excess production of ACTH by the anterior pituitary Overproduction of ACTH by an adenoma results in bilateral adrenocortical hyperplasia and hypercortisolism. This form of Cushing's syndrome is known as Cushing's disease. Removal of the pituitary tumour is the treatment of choice. Removal of the adrenals is not advocated because this may result in the development of the Nelson syndrome, which is characterised by marked enlargement of the pituitary adenoma, high ACTH levels and skin pigmentation (due to the overproduction of melanocyte-stimulating hormone (MSH), which, as well as ACTH, is a cleavage product of POMC).

Oversecretion of cortisol by an adrenal neoplasm (ACTH-independent Cushing's syndrome) Adrenal adenomas, carcinomas and cortical hyperplasia may cause autonomous production of cortisol independent of ACTH levels. If the neoplasm is unilateral, the uninvolved adrenal gland undergoes atrophy because of suppression of ACTH.

Production of ectopic ACTH Certain non-pituitary tumours, such as small cell carcinoma of the lung, may secrete ectopic ACTH, producing Cushing's syndrome.

Clinical features of Cushing's syndrome

A wide range of clinical features, which together are termed Cushing's syndrome, result from oversecretion of cortisol, including:

- moon face
- buffalo hump
- hypertension
- hair thinning
- central obesity
- osteoporosis
- hirsutism
- abdominal striae
- hyperglycaemia
- acne
- proximal muscle intolerance
- plethora
- wasting and weakness
- tendency to infections
- menstrual abnormalities.

Diagnosis of Cushing's syndrome

Diagnosis of Cushing's syndrome depends on finding raised circulating or urinary cortisol levels. Establishing

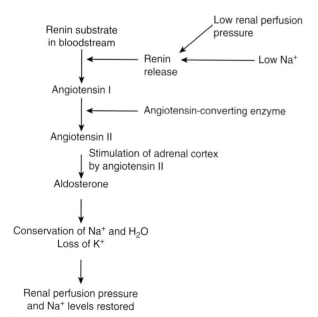

Figure 53 The renin-angiotensin system.

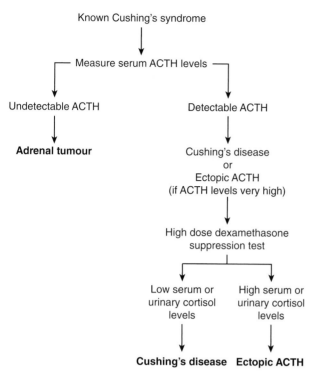

Figure 54 Investigations to determine the cause of Cushing's syndrome.

the cause of the Cushing's syndrome depends on the performance of two tests (Figure 54):

- Levels of serum ACTH
  - *low with adrenal neoplasms*
  - *high with pituitary adenomas and ectopic ACTH production.*
- Measurement of urinary cortisol excretion after administration of high-dose dexamethasone (a potent steroid). This is called the high-dose dexamethasone suppression test.
  - *low with pituitary adenomas*
  - *high with ectopic ACTH production.*

Primary hyperaldosteronism (Conn's syndrome)

In this condition, excess mineralocorticoid production is due to a lesion in the adrenal cortex. The commonest cause is an adenoma of the zona glomerulosa, although bilateral adrenal hyperplasia is sometimes responsible. High levels of aldosterone lead to excessive retention of sodium and water, excessive loss of potassium, and a metabolic alkalosis. The hypokalaemia may lead to muscular weakness, cardiac arrhythmias, paraesthesia and tetany. Diagnosis depends on finding raised levels of circulating aldosterone and low levels of renin (if the renin levels are raised, then the hyperaldosteronism is secondary to raised renin levels and is known as secondary hyperaldosteronism). Adrenal adenomas can be surgically excised, whereas adrenal hyperplasia can be managed medically.

Hypersecretion of the sex steroids

Disorders of sexual differentiation are known collectively as adrenogenital syndromes. There are two main causes of hypersecretion of sex steroids:

- adrenocortical neoplasms
- congenital enzyme deficiency in the pathways of steroid synthesis.

Adrenocortical neoplasm

Adenomas or carcinomas of the adrenal cortex may secrete sex steroids (usually androgens). The effect of these androgens is to cause masculinisation in females and precocious puberty in pre-pubertal males.

Congenital enzyme defects

There is a small group of rare congenital disorders characterised by a deficiency, or total lack, of a particular enzyme involved in the synthesis of steroids. The commonest of these disorders is 21-hydroxylase deficiency. This enzyme is necessary for the synthesis of cortisol and aldosterone. Its absence leads to low levels of cortisol and consequent elevated levels of ACTH resulting in bilateral adrenocortical hyperplasia. The underproduction of mineralocorticoids is life-threatening. Androgens are over-secreted because they are synthesised before the metabolic block, resulting in masculinisation in females and precocious puberty in males.

Adrenocortical hypofunction (adrenocortical insufficiency)

Adrenocortical insufficiency may be due to primary adrenal disease (primary adrenocortical insufficiency) or secondary to decreased stimulation of the adrenals due to a deficiency in ACTH (secondary adrenocortical insufficiency). Insufficiency may be acute or chronic, depending on the speed of onset of the symptoms. The symptoms and signs of adrenocortical hypofunction are related to deficiencies of both mineralocorticoids and glucocorticoids.

Acute adrenocortical insufficiency

Acute primary adrenocortical insufficiency can occur in several circumstances:

- patients with chronic adrenocortical insufficiency may have an acute insufficiency crisis if an event occurs that requires an increased output of steroid hormones by the adrenals
- patients on long-term steroid treatment have suppressed adrenal glands, which are unable to respond adequately if an event occurs that requires an increased output of steroid hormones, or if the steroid treatment is withdrawn too rapidly
- destruction of the adrenal glands by haemorrhage, which can complicate bacterial (e.g. meningococcal) septicaemia (Waterhouse–Friderichsen syndrome) and disseminated intravascular coagulation, and can occur in neonates following a prolonged or difficult delivery.

Affected patients develop hypovolaemic shock due to mineralocorticoid deficiency, and hypoglycaemia due to lack of glucocorticoids.

Primary chronic adrenocortical insufficiency (Addison's disease)

Addison's disease is caused by any destructive process in the adrenal cortex. Previously the commonest cause was tuberculosis of the adrenal cortex, but nowadays autoimmune destruction of the adrenal cortex is commoner. Affected patients may have autoimmune disease at other sites (e.g. diabetes, thyroiditis, pernicious anaemia). The resultant deficiency of mineralocorticoids and glucocorticoids leads to:

- weakness and fatigue
- anorexia, nausea, vomiting and weight loss
- hypotension and dehydration
- hyperpigmentation of the skin (due to excess melanocyte stimulating hormone (MSH)) at pressure points and on sun-exposed skin
- hyponatraemia, hyperkalaemia and hypoglycaemia.

Serum ACTH levels are high. The condition is potentially life-threatening if steroids are not administered. Patients with Addison's disease may also develop an acute addisonian crisis if exposed to any stress requiring an increased output of steroids by the adrenals (e.g. infection), with development of acute insufficiency.

To diagnose Addison's disease, ACTH stimulation tests (Synacthen tests) should be performed (Figure 55). Synacthen is a synthetic ACTH analogue and in a normal individual, administration of Synacthen causes serum cortisol levels to rise. In the short Synacthen test, a rise in serum cortisol levels excludes Addison's disease. If there is no rise in cortisol levels, then the patient has either primary or secondary adrenocortical insufficiency, and the long Synacthen test should then be performed to establish the diagnosis.

Secondary adrenocortical insufficiency

This refers to the underproduction of adrenal steroids due to undersecretion of ACTH by the pituitary. There are two main causes:

- primary lesions of the pituitary
- hypothalamic-pituitary-adrenal suppression as a result of long-term steroid therapy.

There is resultant deficiency of cortisol and sex steroids, but the aldosterone levels are normal, therefore the skin pigmentation and electrolyte disturbances typical of Addison's disease are not seen. Also, unlike the situation in Addison's disease, serum ACTH levels are low. Performance of the long Synacthen test will establish the diagnosis.

19.3 The endocrine pancreas

> **Learning objectives**
>
> You should:
> - understand the structure of the pancreas and have a basic understanding of its function
> - know the various hormones secreted by the pancreas
> - have an understanding of the classification, pathogenesis, clinical features and complications of diabetes mellitus, and have a basic knowledge of the theories of its pathogenesis.

Structure and function

The pancreas consists of two separate functional units – the exocrine pancreas, which secretes digestive enzymes into the duodenum, and the endocrine pancreas, which secretes a number of different hormones.

The endocrine pancreas consists of ~1 million islets of Langerhans, which are scattered throughout the gland. Each islet is composed of a cluster of a number of different cell types, each cell type synthesising and secreting a different hormone (Table 35).

Insulin and glucagon are the hormones responsible for maintaining blood sugar levels; insulin exerts a hypoglycaemic effect and glucagon exerts a hyperglycaemic effect. The two main disorders of the islet cells are diabetes mellitus and islet cell tumours.

Diabetes mellitus

Diabetes mellitus is a condition characterised by an absolute or relative deficiency of insulin and/or insulin resistance, inducing hypoglycaemia.

Classification

There are two main types of diabetes mellitus:

- **Type 1 diabetes** – juvenile-onset diabetes; insulin-dependent diabetes (IDDM), which accounts for 10% of all cases

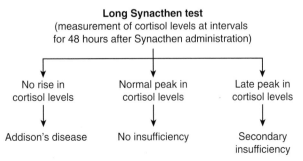

Short Synacthen test
(measurement of cortisol levels for 1 hour after Synacthen administration)

- Plasma cortisol levels increase → Not Addison's disease
- No increase in plasma cortisol levels → Primary insufficiency (Addison's) or Secondary insufficiency

Long Synacthen test
(measurement of cortisol levels at intervals for 48 hours after Synacthen administration)

- No rise in cortisol levels → Addison's disease
- Normal peak in cortisol levels → No insufficiency
- Late peak in cortisol levels → Secondary insufficiency

Figure 55 Diagnosis of Addison's disease.

Table 35 The cell types of the pancreas

Cell type	Hormone synthesised	Action of hormone
β (beta)	Insulin	Increases glucose entry into cells
		Promotes glycogen synthesis and prevents breakdown
		Promotes lipogenesis and prevents lipolysis
α (alpha)	Glucagon	Promotes glycogen breakdown
		Promotes gluconeogenesis
δ (delta)	Somatostatin	Inhibits secretion of insulin and glucagon
PP	Pancreatic polypeptide	Exerts a number of gastrointestinal effects
Enterochromaffin cells	Vasoactive intestinal polypeptide	Stimulates intestinal fluid secretion
D1	Serotonin	Potent vasodilator
		Increases intestinal motility

- **Type 2 diabetes** – adult-onset diabetes; non-insulin-dependent diabetes (NIDDM), which accounts for 80–90% of all cases. Gestational diabetes and maturity-onset diabetes of the young (MODY) are rare causes of diabetes mellitus. MODY is due to a genetic defect in β cell function.

Pathogenesis

Type 1 diabetes

Type 1 diabetes, which typically presents in childhood, is characterised by a complete lack of insulin. Insulin secretion is inadequate because of destruction of the β cells in the islets. Three separate but inter-related mechanisms appear to have a role in this destructive process:

- genetic susceptibility
- autoimmune reaction
- environmental event.

It has been postulated that genetic susceptibility predisposes certain individuals to the development of an autoimmune reaction against the β cells of the islets, and that this autoimmune reaction is triggered by an environmental event (e.g. viral infection, exposure to chemical toxins).

Type 2 diabetes

This type of diabetes usually presents in middle age. The precise pathogenic mechanism is unknown, but obesity and genetic factors are important. Two mechanisms have been postulated:
- defective secretion of insulin by β cells
- resistance of peripheral tissues to the effects of insulin.

Clinical features

Type 1 diabetes

The clinical features are related to increased gluconeogenesis and hyperglycaemia resulting from a lack of insulin.

- Polyuria – due to glycosuria with osmotic diuresis.
- Polydipsia – extracellular hyperosmolarity causes osmotic depletion of intracellular water and triggers osmoreceptors in the brain, with resultant severe thirst.
- Polyphagia – breakdown of proteins and fats for gluconeogenesis causes an increased appetite.
- Weight loss and weakness – despite increased dietary intake, breakdown prevails over storage.

Severe insulin deficiency may lead to diabetic ketoacidosis – lipolysis results in elevated free fatty acids, which are oxidised to produce ketone bodies in the liver. The rate of formation of ketone bodies exceeds the rate at which they are utilised, resulting in ketonuria and ketonaemia. If there is superimposed dehydration, metabolic ketoacidosis results. The condition is life-threatening. Infection, which increases insulin requirements, often precedes development of diabetic ketoacidosis.

Type 2 diabetes

The diagnosis of type 2 diabetes is usually made after routine serum or urine testing in an asymptomatic patient. The metabolic derangements are much less severe than in type 1 diabetes, and metabolic ketoacidosis does not occur. Instead, patients in the decompensated state develop hyperosmolar non-ketotic coma, which results from severe dehydration due to insufficient water intake in the face of polyuria.

Other clinical features of types 1 and 2 diabetes are related to the complications of longstanding diabetes.

Complications of diabetes mellitus

Although the two major types of diabetes have different pathogeneses and clinical presentations, the long-term systemic complications are the same and are the major causes of morbidity and mortality in these patients.

Vascular system

Atherosclerosis There is severe accelerated atherosclerosis in the aorta and large- and medium-sized arteries. Myocardial infarction, stroke, and gangrene of the lower limbs are responsible for ~80% of deaths due to diabetes in adults.

Hyaline arteriolosclerosis Hyaline thickening of the wall of arterioles with narrowing of the lumen.

Diabetic microangiopathy This is characterised by diffuse thickening of the capillary vascular basement membranes. Affected vessels are more leaky to plasma proteins. The change is most evident in the capillaries of the retina and kidney, and may account for some of the changes seen in the peripheral nerves.

Diabetic nephropathy

- Glomerular changes – includes diffuse basement membrane thickening, nodular expansion of mesangial regions and exudative lesions.
- Vascular changes – renal atherosclerosis and arteriolosclerosis.
- Parenchymal changes – pyelonephritis with increased propensity to develop necrotising papillitis.

Diabetic retinopathy

Diabetic retinopathy can be non-proliferative (background) or proliferative. The non-proliferative changes are:

- thickening of the capillary basement membrane (microangiopathy) with development of microaneurysms (dots)
- retinal haemorrhages (blots)
- retinal oedema and exudates (cotton wool spots)
- venous dilatation.

The proliferative changes are neovascularisation and fibrosis, which may lead to retinal detachment and blindness.

Diabetic neuropathy

Neuropathies seen include symmetric peripheral neuropathy, affecting both motor and sensory nerves, and autonomic neuropathy, which may cause impotence, and bladder and bowel dysfunction.

Infections

People with diabetes have an increased tendency to develop infections.

Skin complications

These include necrobiosis lipoidica diabeticorum and granuloma annulare.

Pregnancy

Pregnant women with diabetes are at a higher risk of developing pre-eclampsia and tend to have large babies.

Islet tumours

These tumours are quite rare, and they can arise from any of the cell types present in the islets. The tumours become manifest through hypersecretion of the hormone produced by the cell type from which the tumour is derived. Islet tumours may pursue a benign or malignant course. The various types are as follows:

- insulinoma (the commonest tumour; induces hypoglycaemia)
- glucagonoma (induces diabetes)

- gastrinoma (hypersecretes gastrin, which leads to hypersecretion of gastric acid. The resultant widespread peptic ulceration is known as Zollinger–Ellison syndrome)
- VIPomas (cause watery diarrhoea)
- somatostatinomas.

19.4 The thyroid gland

Learning objectives

You should:
- know the structure and function of the thyroid gland
- know the ways in which thyroid disorders present
- know the major causes of hypo- and hyperthyroidism
- know the causes of a goitre
- know the causes of a solitary nodule in the thyroid
- understand the classification and behaviour of thyroid carcinoma.

Structure and function

The thyroid gland develops from an evagination at the root of the tongue (the foramen caecum), which grows downwards anterior to the trachea to reach its final position in front of the thyroid cartilage. During its descent, the thyroid gland is attached to the root of the tongue by means of a thyroglossal duct, which eventually undergoes atrophy. Persistence of this duct is the basis of thyroglossal cysts.

The adult thyroid gland comprises two lobes connected by an isthmus and consists of follicles lined by cuboidal epithelial cells and filled with colloid. The main function of these epithelial cells is to synthesise and secrete the two thyroid hormones – T_4 (thyroxine) and T_3. The secretion of T_4 and T_3 is under negative feedback control by TSH, which is secreted by the anterior pituitary. Scattered throughout the thyroid are C-cells, which synthesise and secrete the hormone calcitonin. Calcitonin is involved in the regulation of body calcium levels.

Disorders of the thyroid manifest in four main ways:

- hypofunction (hypothyroidism)
- hyperfunction (hyperthyroidism)
- enlargement of the gland (goitre)
- solitary masses.

These groups are not mutually exclusive. For example, goitres can be associated with either hyperfunction or hypofunction of the thyroid gland, and hyperthyroidism may be associated with a goitre.

Hyperthyroidism (thyrotoxicosis)

Excess circulating T_3 and T_4 induce a hypermetabolic state, the resulting clinical syndrome being known as thyrotoxicosis.

Aetiology

The three commonest causes of thyrotoxicosis are as follows:

- Graves' disease (85%)
- functioning adenoma
- toxic nodular goitre.

Graves' disease (Graves' thyroiditis)

Graves' disease typically affects young women who present with the clinical features of thyrotoxicosis and mild goitre. If the patient develops proptosis (protrusion of the eyes) or pretibial myxoedema, the diagnosis of Graves' disease is almost certain since these changes are not seen in thyrotoxicosis due to other causes. Graves' thyroiditis is an 'organ-specific' autoimmune disease; autoantibodies bind to the TSH receptor on thyroid epithelial cells and mimic the stimulatory action of TSH. Histologically, there is an increase in the number of cells lining the follicles and a reduction in the amount of stored colloid.

Functioning adenoma

Rarely, functioning thyroid adenomas have enough secretory activity to induce thyrotoxicosis. Such adenomas may also present as solitary thyroid masses.

Toxic nodular goitre

Rarely, one or more nodules in a multinodular goitre may develop hypersecretory activity, resulting in thyrotoxicosis.

Clinical features of thyrotoxicosis

The systemic features of thyrotoxicosis are as follows:

- eye changes (exophthalmos, lid lag, lid retraction)
- hair loss, weight loss
- anxiety, tremor, diarrhoea, warm moist hands
- cardiac manifestations (tachycardia, palpitations, atrial fibrillation)
- pretibial myxoedema (accumulation of mucopolysaccharides in the skin)
- menorrhagia, osteoporosis
- proximal myopathy.

Exophthalmos and pretibial myxoedema occur only in thyrotoxicosis due to Graves' disease.

Hypothyroidism

Insufficient circulating T_4 and T_3 lead to a hypometabolic state resulting in the clinical syndrome known as hypothyroidism. If hypothyroidism occurs during infancy, it results in a condition known as cretinism, in which mental and physical development is impaired. This condition is now rare. If hypothyroidism occurs in older children or adults it results in a condition known as myxoedema, in which the skin appears oedematous and doughy due to the accumulation of mucopolysaccharides in the dermis.

Aetiology

There are many causes of hypothyroidism, and the commonest cause in adults is Hashimoto's thyroiditis. Most of the remaining cases of hypothyroidism are due to radiotherapy or surgery, or are drug induced.

Hashimoto's thyroiditis

Like Graves' disease, Hashimoto's thyroiditis is an 'organ-specific' autoimmune disease. Antibodies directed against thyroid tissue and thyroglobulin have been detected in patients with this condition. Hashimoto's thyroiditis may present in a number of ways:

- with **goitre**, which after time recedes due to atrophy and fibrosis of the gland as a result of autoimmune destruction
- with **hypothyroidism**
- with **thyrotoxicosis** – in the early stages of the disease, damage to the thyroid follicles may lead to a transient rise in thyroid hormone levels.

Histologically, the gland is infiltrated by lymphocytes and plasma cells. There are lymphoid aggregates, often with germinal centres. The thyroid epithelial cells become eosinophilic and granular, at which time they are termed oncocytes. In advanced cases, the gland is shrunken and fibrotic.

Clinical features of hypothyroidism

The clinical features are as follows:

- myxoedematous face
- loss of the outer third of the eyebrows
- dry hair
- hoarse voice
- slowed physical and mental activity, lethargy, weight gain
- psychosis
- cold intolerance
- constipation, muscle weakness, carpal tunnel syndrome, menstrual irregularities.

Goitre

The term goitre denotes enlargement of the thyroid gland. There are two main causes:

- simple and multinodular goitre
- inflammation of the thyroid (thyroiditis).

Simple and multinodular goitre

Simple goitres are characterised by diffuse hypertrophy and hyperplasia of the thyroid gland, without the production of discrete nodularity. Nearly all longstanding simple goitres develop into multinodular goitres, where tracts of fibrosis separate hyperplastic areas, producing nodularity.

Simple goitres are thought to arise from overstimulation of the thyroid tissue by excess TSH. The oversecretion of TSH is due to a deficiency of the thyroid hormones. The compensatory rise in TSH levels usually renders the individual euthyroid, although hypothyroidism may occur. Goitres can arise in four main settings:

1. endemic goitres due to iodine deficiency. These are usually localised to geographic areas where the soil contains little iodine (e.g. the Derbyshire hills, some mountainous areas). Iodine is necessary for the synthesis of the thyroid hormones

Nineteen

2. ingestion of certain foodstuffs. In individuals whose iodine uptake is suboptimal, ingestion of foodstuffs such as cabbage and turnips may produce a goitre
3. rare inherited defects in thyroid hormone synthesis
4. drug-induced goitres, e.g. amiodarone, lithium.

Thyroiditis

Thyroiditis is a rare cause of goitre. There are four main forms of thyroiditis:

- Hashimoto's thyroiditis (discussed above)
- subacute granulomatous (giant cell or de Quervain) thyroiditis
- Riedel's thyroiditis
- acute bacterial thyroiditis.

Subacute granulomatous thyroiditis

As its name implies, the thyroid in subacute granulomatous thyroiditis is infiltrated by multinucleate giant cells admixed with other inflammatory cells. The cause of the condition is uncertain. Patients usually present with an abrupt onset of thyroid swelling and tenderness on palpation. There may be a fever. The condition is self-limiting.

Riedel's thyroiditis

Riedel's thyroiditis is exceptionally rare. It is characterised by replacement of the thyroid by fibrous tissue, often with involvement of adjacent tissues. The aetiology is unknown. Patients present with an enlarged thyroid, which is hard and immobile on palpation thereby mimicking carcinoma. The condition may be associated with retroperitoneal fibrosis.

Acute bacterial thyroiditis

Acute inflammation of the thyroid can result from direct bacterial spread from adjacent tissues or by blood-borne spread. Patients present with thyroid pain, tenderness and enlargement. There may be systemic features of infection. The condition usually resolves with antibiotic treatment.

Solitary masses

The differential diagnoses of solitary thyroid masses are as follows:

- one dominant nodule in a multinodular goitre
- thyroid cysts
- asymmetrical enlargement due to non-neoplastic diseases (e.g. Hashimoto's thyroiditis)
- thyroid neoplasm.

Thyroid neoplasms

Thyroid neoplasms can be benign or malignant. Most thyroid tumours are non-functioning and therefore appear 'cold' on scintigraphy (i.e. they do not take up radioactive iodine). However, a minority are functioning, appearing 'warm' or 'hot' on scintigraphy and possibly causing thyrotoxicosis.

Benign

Almost all benign tumours of the thyroid gland are follicular adenomas. These tumours are well-encapsulated and have an expansile growth pattern, compressing the adjacent normal thyroid tissue. These features differentiate a follicular adenoma from a dominant nodule in a multinodular goitre. Histologically, they may show a variety of appearances, the most common being a microfollicular architecture comprising multiple closely packed follicles with little colloid.

Malignant

Carcinoma of the thyroid is uncommon, and together with the fact that these tumours often have a good prognosis, they are responsible for less than 1% of all cancer deaths. Thyroid carcinoma is two to three times more common in females than males. The four main types of thyroid carcinoma are as follows:

- papillary carcinoma (75%)
- follicular carcinoma (10–20%)
- anaplastic carcinoma (rare)
- medullary carcinoma (5%).

Papillary carcinoma

Papillary carcinoma typically occurs in women in the third or fourth decade. The tumours are unencapsulated, infiltrative, and may be multifocal. Histologically, papillary carcinomas can exhibit a wide range of appearances. The diagnosis depends on the presence of certain cytological features:

- large hypochromatic nuclei termed 'Orphan Annie' nuclei
- nuclear grooves
- eosinophilic cytoplasmic inclusions
- psammoma bodies (calcified glycoprotein bodies).

Cervical lymph node metastases are present in as many as 50% of cases at presentation. However, because these tumours often pursue an indolent course, the overall prognosis is excellent.

Follicular carcinoma

Follicular carcinoma occurs in older age groups. Histologically, they are solitary encapsulated tumours most commonly consisting of closely packed small follicles, and may therefore be difficult to distinguish from follicular adenomas. Invasion of the capsule or vascular invasion indicate malignancy. Metastatic spread has occurred in 15% of cases at presentation, most commonly involving the lung or bones. The prognosis for these tumours is poorer than for papillary carcinomas.

Anaplastic carcinoma

Anaplastic carcinoma tends to occur in elderly individuals. The tumours are poorly differentiated histologically, have a rapid growth rate, and metastasise widely. The prognosis is very poor.

Medullary carcinomas

Medullary carcinomas are derived from the C-cells within the thyroid, and are therefore neuroendocrine tumours. Most secrete calcitonin but oversecretion of this hormone does not usually produce any clinical effects. Rarely, the tumour may secrete other hormones (e.g. ACTH, or 5-hydroxytryptamine). Histologically, the tumour consists of nests or sheets of tumour cells in a characteristic amyloid stroma. These tumours may pursue an indolent or aggressive course. Most medullary carcinomas are sporadic, but around 20% are hereditary and occur as part of one of the MEN syndromes.

19.5 Parathyroid glands

Structure and function

Most individuals have four parathyroid glands. In the adult, the upper two glands almost always lie close to the upper posterior aspect of the thyroid gland, but the lower two may be found anywhere between the lower posterior aspect of the thyroid gland and the mediastinum. The glands are composed predominantly of chief cells, which secrete parathyroid hormone (PTH). PTH:

- mobilises calcium from bone
- increases renal tubular resorption of calcium
- promotes the production of 1,25-dihydroxyvitamin D_1 (the active form of vitamin D) in the kidney
- enhances phosphate excretion by the kidney.

Overall, serum calcium levels are controlled by the actions of three hormones – PTH, calcitonin and vitamin D. PTH and vitamin D have a hypercalcaemic effect, and calcitonin has a hypocalcaemic effect.

The most important disorders of the parathyroids are hyperparathyroidism, hypoparathyroidism and tumours.

Hyperparathyroidism

Hyperparathyroidism can be divided into primary, secondary and tertiary types:

- primary – hypersecretion of PTH by a parathyroid lesion
- secondary – a physiological increase in PTH in response to hypocalcaemia
- tertiary – development of a hypersecretory parathyroid adenoma in an individual with longstanding secondary hyperparathyroidism.

Primary hyperparathyroidism

This condition can be caused by the following:

- an adenoma in one of the parathyroid glands (75–80%)
- hyperplasia of all of the parathyroid glands (10–15%)
- parathyroid carcinoma (<5%).

The clinical features, with the exception of the bone changes, are due to hypercalcaemia, and are commonly summed up as 'bones, stones, abdominal groans and psychic moans'.

Bone:

- osteitis fibrosa cystica (brown tumour), due to excess PTH.

Renal:

- formation of calcium-containing renal stones
- nephrocalcinosis.

Gastrointestinal:

- peptic ulcer
- pancreatitis
- vomiting
- abdominal pain.

Neuromuscular:

- generalised weakness.

Psychiatric:

- depression
- impaired memory
- emotional lability.

Secondary hyperparathyroidism (and renal osteodystrophy)

This most commonly arises in the setting of renal failure or vitamin D deficiency. In renal failure, there is loss of calcium and reduced synthesis of 1,25-dihydroxy-vitamin D_1 leading to hypocalcaemia and secondary hyperparathyroidism, and there is retention of phosphate, which also induces secondary hyperparathyroidism. The result is hyperplasia of the parathyroid glands and skeletal changes comprising a mixture of osteitis fibrosa cystica (due to increased PTH-dependent osteoclastic resorption of bone) and osteomalacia (due to lack of vitamin D). The skeletal changes are referred to as renal osteodystrophy.

Hypoparathyroidism

The most common causes of hypoparathyroidism are:

- surgical removal or ablation of the parathyroid glands during thyroidectomy
- congenital absence of all of the parathyroid glands (di George syndrome)
- autoimmune destruction of the glands.

The clinical manifestations, which are due to hypocalcaemia, are:

- increased neuromuscular excitability – this is manifest by the Chvostek sign (tapping along the course of the facial nerve causes the facial muscles to twitch), Trousseau sign (occlusion of the arteries in the forearm by inflating a blood pressure cuff induces carpal spasm), perioral paraesthesia, and, if severely hypocalcaemic, overt tetany

Nineteen

- psychiatric disturbances, e.g. irritability, depression or psychosis
- cardiac conduction abnormalities, e.g. prolonged Q-T interval or heart block.

19.6 The multiple endocrine neoplasia (MEN) syndromes

MEN syndromes refers to a group of rare inherited disorders that are characterised by hyperplasia or tumours in several endocrine glands simultaneously. There are three MEN syndromes:

- **MEN I** – characterised by parathyroid, pancreatic and pituitary involvement.
- **MEN II (or IIa)** – characterised by phaeochromocytoma and medullary carcinoma, with or without parathyroid involvement.
- **MEN III (or IIb)** – characterised by phaeochromocytoma, medullary carcinoma and mucocutaneous ganglioneuromas, with or without parathyroid hyperplasia or a marfanoid habitus.

Self-assessment: questions

One best answer questions

1. Which of the following is not a feature of Cushing's syndrome?

   a. osteoporosis

   b. hypotension

   c. hirsutism

   d. proximal muscle wasting

   e. central obesity

2. A 48-year-old woman presents complaining of lack of energy and weakness. She has recently put on weight and 'feels the cold' more than usual. She is also troubled by constipation. The most likely diagnosis is:

   a. hyperthyroidism

   b. Conn's syndrome

   c. Addison's disease

   d. hypothyroidism

   e. hyperparathyroidism

True-false questions

1. The following statements are correct:

   a. the anterior pituitary is derived from a downgrowth of the hypothalamus

   b. pituitary adenomas always cause overproduction of one (or more) hormone

   c. acromegaly is caused by overproduction of ACTH

   d. anti-diuretic hormone is secreted from the posterior pituitary

   e. anti-diuretic hormone may be inappropriately secreted in patients with bronchogenic carcinoma

2. The following are associated with pituitary adenomas:

   a. visual disturbances

   b. headache

   c. nausea and vomiting

   d. MEN I

   e. Sheehan's syndrome

3. The following statements are correct:

   a. Graves' disease is the most frequent cause of hyperthyroidism

   b. Graves' disease is caused by autoantibodies directed against the TSH receptor

   c. Hashimoto's thyroiditis is associated with autoantibodies directed against the C-cells of the thyroid

   d. simple and multinodular goitre are almost always associated with hyperthyroidism

   e. ionising radiation is a major risk factor for the development of thyroid cancer

4. The following statements are correct:

   a. parathyroid hormone has a hypercalcaemic effect

   b. primary hyperparathyroidism is induced by hypocalcaemia

   c. renal failure is a common cause of secondary hyperparathyroidism

   d. hypoparathyroidism may follow total thyroidectomy

   e. primary hyperparathyroidism may be associated with MEN syndrome

5. The following statements are correct:

   a. the adrenal medulla is part of the parasympathetic nervous system

   b. phaeochromocytomas may cause secondary hypertension

   c. the most common cause of Cushing's syndrome is administration of exogenous glucocorticoids

   d. Addison's disease is associated with hyperkalaemia

   e. secondary hyperaldosteronism may be seen in congestive cardiac failure

6. The following statements regarding the endocrine pancreas are correct:

   a. the islets of Langerhans are the functional unit of the endocrine pancreas

   b. type 1 diabetes mellitus is more common than type 2 diabetes mellitus

   c. myocardial infarction is the most common cause of death in people with diabetes

   d. diabetic microangiopathy is characterised by thickened vascular basement membranes, which renders the vessels less leaky to plasma proteins

   e. diabetic retinopathy may cause blindness

7. The following statements are true:

   a. untreated Cushing's syndrome can be fatal

   b. skin pigmentation occurs only in Cushing's syndrome that is ACTH-dependent

   c. hyperpigmentation in Addison's disease may be seen in the mouth and recent scars

   d. steroids should not be given to patients who develop an acute addisonian crisis

   e. a pituitary tumour can cause Addison's disease

8. The following symptoms can be associated with the onset of diabetes mellitus:

   a. decreased urine output

   b. weight loss

   c. feeling tired all the time

d. pruritus vulvae or balanitis

e. loss of appetite

Case history questions

Case history 1

A 40-year-old woman presents to her general practitioner with a lump in the right side of her neck. The lump has been increasing in size over the past 2 months. On examination, a hard nodule was felt in the right thyroid lobe and there was adjacent right-sided cervical lymphadenopathy.

1. What is the differential diagnosis of a thyroid nodule?

2. What features here are suggestive of carcinoma?

3. What investigations could be performed to help establish the diagnosis?

Case history 2

A 68-year-old woman with diabetes, who is a frequent non-attender, attends an outpatient clinic for a routine check-up. She has been a diabetic for 16 years and requires insulin to control her diabetes. On questioning, she reveals that she is getting pain in her left calf muscles on walking. The pain comes on after a certain distance and is relieved by rest. She has also noticed some reduced visual acuity. On examination, she has an absent left dorsalis pedis pulse and the left posterior tibial and left popliteal pulses were present but weak. Routine ophthalmoscopy reveals background and proliferative retinopathy. Routine urinalysis shows moderate proteinuria.

1. What is the pathogenesis of this type of diabetes?

2. What is the cause of her leg symptoms?

3. What is proliferative retinopathy, and why is it important?

4. What are the possible causes of the proteinuria in this case?

Short note questions

Write short notes on:

1. The concept of negative feedback.

2. The major causes of Cushing's syndrome and the tests you might perform to establish the cause in any individual case.

3. Hyperparathyroidism.

Viva questions

1. What is a hormone?

2. What is Waterhouse–Friderichsen syndrome?

3. What is Graves' disease?

Self-assessment: answers

One best answer

1. b. Glucocorticoid excess in Cushing's syndrome causes hypertension.
2. d.

True-false answers

1. a. **False.**
   b. **False.** Some adenomas are non-functioning.
   c. **False.**
   d. **True.**
   e. **True.**

2. a. **True.**
   b. **True.**
   c. **True.**
   d. **True.**
   e. **False.**

3. a. **True.**
   b. **True.**
   c. **False.**
   d. **False.**
   e. **True.**

4. a. **True.**
   b. **False.**
   c. **True.**
   d. **True.** The parathyroid glands lie close to the thyroid gland and may also be removed during surgery.
   e. **True.**

5. a. **False.** It is part of the sympathetic nervous system.
   b. **True.**
   c. **True.**
   d. **True.**
   e. **True.** In congestive cardiac failure, reduced renal perfusion causes increased renin secretion leading to secondary hyperaldosteronism.

6. a. **True.**
   b. **False.**
   c. **True.**
   d. **False.** Affected vessels are more leaky to plasma proteins.
   e. **True.**

7. a. **True.** Death can occur through hypertension or infection.
   b. **True.**
   c. **True.**
   d. **False.**
   e. **False.** Pituitary tumours can cause secondary adrenocortical insufficiency (Addison's is the term reserved only for *primary* insufficiency).

8. a. **False.** Urine output is usually increased (polyuria).
   b. **True.**
   c. **True.**
   d. **True.**
   e. **False.**

Case history answers

Case history 1

1. The differential diagnosis of a thyroid nodule is a dominant nodule in a multinodular goitre, thyroid cyst, asymmetrical enlargement due to non-neoplastic diseases and thyroid neoplasm.

2. The recent increase in the size and the presence of a hard nodule are both suggestive of carcinoma over a benign process. The presence of ipsilateral cervical lymphadenopathy suggests lymph node spread, which can be present at presentation of a thyroid carcinoma.

3. *Comment*: Thyroid function tests (TFTs) may be performed to establish thyroid status, which may aid diagnosis. An ultrasound scan will tell you if the mass is cystic or solid. Solid masses are more suspicious of carcinoma, but be aware that carcinoma can arise within cysts. A radioactive iodine scan will establish whether the mass is functioning ('hot' nodule) or non-functioning ('cold' nodule). Almost all thyroid carcinomas are non-functioning. Lastly, a fine-needle aspiration may be performed. This involves using a needle to aspirate the mass extracting cells, which can then be examined under the microscope for any features of malignancy.

Case history 2

1. The history indicates that this is type 2 diabetes, because of the adult onset. Remember that some patients with type 2 diabetes inject insulin to control their diabetes. The pathogenesis is poorly understood, but obesity and genetic factors are important.

2. Cramp-like pain in the calf muscles on walking, which comes on after a certain distance and is relieved by rest, are the classic symptoms of intermittent claudication and they indicate ischaemia of the limb. Diabetic patients are predisposed to accelerated atherosclerosis in all large- and medium-sized arteries. When the arteries

supplying the limbs are affected, blood flow through them is restricted and cannot be significantly increased when demand is increased (e.g. during exercise). Hence, during exercise the limb becomes ischaemic, leading to pain. The pain is then relieved by rest.

3. The proliferative changes of diabetic retinopathy are neovascularisation and fibrosis. Proliferative retinopathy is important because it can lead to retinal detachment and cause blindness.

4. The proteinuria may be due to:

- a urinary tract infection (to which diabetic patients are predisposed)
- glomerular lesions associated with diabetic nephropathy (basement membrane thickening, expansion of mesangial regions and exudative lesions)
- glomerular damage secondary to chronic ischaemia caused by renal vascular lesions.

Short note answers

1. Negative feedback is a common means of controlling an endocrine gland's production of a hormone. As the plasma concentration of the hormone (or a substance that it regulates) rises, it increasingly inhibits its own production. An example is the hypothalamic-pituitary-thyroid axis. The initial stimulus for the production of thyroxine in the thyroid gland is secretion of thyrotrophin-releasing hormone (TRH) from the hypothalamus. The trigger for TRH secretion is a reduction in the circulating levels of thyroxine. TRH stimulates the release of thyroid-stimulating hormone (TSH) from the anterior pituitary, which in turn stimulates thyroid follicular cells to produce thyroxine. As the levels of thyroxine in the blood rise, the stimulus for TRH secretion is reduced, leading to less thyroxine production by the thyroid. Another example is the β cells of the pancreas, which secrete insulin, the actions of which remove glucose from the blood. The stimulus for insulin secretion is a rise in blood glucose levels. As the blood sugar levels drop as a consequence of the actions of insulin, the stimulus is reduced and less insulin is released.

2. Cushing's syndrome is due to excess glucocorticoids and there are a number of situations in which this can arise. The main causes are administration of exogenous glucocorticoids (e.g. people on long-term steroid treatment for chronic inflammatory conditions), overproduction of ACTH from the anterior pituitary, overproduction of cortisol by an adrenal neoplasm, and secretion of ectopic ACTH (usually by a tumour). If exogenous administration of steroids is the cause, this can usually be elicited from the drug history. To distinguish between the other three causes, a serum ACTH should be performed followed by a high-dose dexamethasone test if necessary.

3. *Comment*: Start by describing the function of the parathyroid glands. They are the sites of production of parathyroid hormone, which is involved in the regulation of serum calcium levels. Hyperparathyroidism denotes overproduction of parathyroid hormone, and it is divided into primary, secondary and tertiary types. Be able to describe each of these. A brief account of the consequences of hyperparathyroidism is also needed – remember 'bones, stones, abdominal groans and psychic moans'.

Viva answers

1. Hormones are substances that are synthesised and secreted by endocrine glands. Hormones exert their effects at distant sites that can be accessed only by the bloodstream.

2. This is a catastrophic condition characterised by an overwhelming bacterial infection (classically *Neisseria meningitidis* septicaemia) associated with shock, disseminated intravascular coagulation, and rapidly progressive adrenocortical deficiency with massive bilateral adrenal haemorrhages. The condition is rapidly fatal if appropriate treatment is not given immediately.

3. Graves' disease is the most common cause of hyperthyroidism. It is an 'organ-specific' autoimmune disease produced by autoantibodies to the TSH receptor on thyroid follicular cells. Binding of the autoantibody stimulates the receptor and leads to increased synthesis and secretion of thyroxine. This account of the pathogenesis should be followed by a description of the clinical findings, remembering to include the presence of goitre, and that pre-tibial myxoedema and proptosis are seen only in hyperthyroidism due to Graves' disease.

Female breast

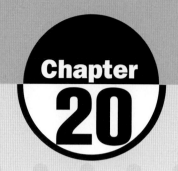

Chapter overview

The female breast is a complex glandular structure, which is extremely sensitive to hormonal influences and can be affected by a number of pathological processes. Breast cancer is one of the most dreaded diseases of women and is the second most common cause of cancer death in women. Hence, malignant and premalignant breast conditions deserve considerable attention. Benign breast conditions, such as inflammatory and fibrocystic changes, are extremely common and frequently receive medical attention because they may mimic breast cancer in their clinical presentation. For these reasons, awareness of benign breast diseases is also important. The male breast is a rudimentary structure and pathological conditions are rare.

20.1 The normal female breast

Learning objectives

You should:
- understand the structure and function of the female breast
- understand hormonal influences on breast tissue.

Structure and function

The function of the female breast is to produce and express milk. The functional unit of the breast is called a lobule (Figure 56) and there are numerous lobules within each breast. A lobule consists of a variable number of acini (glands) lined by secretory epithelium. The acini connect to, and drain into, a terminal duct. Each terminal duct and its acini are together referred to as the terminal duct lobular unit. The terminal ducts drain via a series of larger ducts into the lactiferous ducts and sinuses. The lactiferous ducts

open onto the skin surface at the nipple. The nipple and areola are covered by stratified squamous epithelium, and the areolar skin is pigmented. Areolar glands of Montgomery produce secretions to lubricate the nipple during lactation.

The ducts and acini are lined by two cell types – an inner layer of secretory epithelium and an outer layer of myoepithelial cells. Surrounding and supporting the ducts and acini is breast stroma, which consists of loose connective tissue.

Hormonal influences on the breast

Breast tissue is sensitive to many different hormones. The breast undergoes minor changes with the menstrual cycle, more significant changes during pregnancy and lactation, and undergoes involution when hormone stimulation is withdrawn (menopausal and postmenopausal period).

Changes with the menstrual cycle

After ovulation, there is epithelial proliferation and an increase in the number of acini, and the breast stroma becomes oedematous. These changes occur under the influence of oestrogen and rising levels of progesterone. With menstruation, there is a drop in the levels of these sex steroids with consequent apoptosis of epithelial cells and disappearance of the stromal oedema. The breast becomes quiescent again until the next ovulation.

Pregnancy and lactation

A number of hormones, including oestrogen, progesterone, prolactin and growth hormone, are important in the development of the breast during pregnancy. During pregnancy, there is a marked increase in the number of acini and lobules within the breast at the expense of the stroma. The epithelial cells begin to synthesise milk, which is stored in secretory vacuoles in the cell cytoplasm. With delivery of the baby, the levels of oestrogen and progesterone fall, and the activity of prolactin causes the secretion of milk (lactation).

When breastfeeding ceases, the breast tissue regresses back towards the pre-pregnancy state.

Involution

With increasing age and the reduction in the levels of circulating sex steroids, the ducts and acini begin to atrophy and the amount of breast stroma decreases. In the very

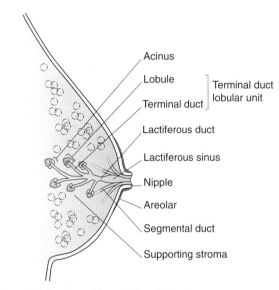

Acinus

Lobule

Terminal duct | Terminal duct lobular unit

Lactiferous duct

Lactiferous sinus

Nipple

Areolar

Segmental duct

Supporting stroma

Figure 56 Structure of the adult female breast.

elderly, the acini may be completely lost, leaving only breast ducts in a little stroma.

20.2 Benign breast conditions

Inflammation

Acute mastitis

Acute mastitis is the most common inflammatory disorder of the breast, and is usually confined to the lactation period. During breastfeeding, the nipple can develop fissures and cracks. Via these cracks, bacteria (usually *Staphylococcus aureus*) gain access to the breast tissue. The infection is usually confined to one segment of the breast, and is manifest by oedema and erythema of the overlying skin.

If severe and untreated, the acute inflammation may progress to abscess formation.

Mammary duct ectasia

This term is used to refer to dilatation of the breast ducts. The ducts become filled with inspissated breast secretions and there is associated inflammation and fibrosis. If there is an unusually heavy infiltrate of plasma cells, the term 'plasma cell mastitis' is sometimes applied. The aetiology of mammary duct ectasia is unknown. Affected women

can present with a palpable mass, skin retraction or nipple discharge, which can occasionally be blood-stained. The lesion is of clinical importance because it can be mistaken for carcinoma clinically, grossly and mammographically.

Fat necrosis

This lesion is usually related to previous trauma to the breast, although a history of trauma may not always be obtained. Histologically, there is an initial focus of necrotic fat cells and acute inflammation, which then becomes heavily infiltrated by macrophages that engulf the debris and hence develop a lipid-laden 'foamy' appearance. With healing, the focus often becomes replaced by fibrous tissue and there may be (dystrophic) calcification. Affected women present with a palpable breast lump or nipple retraction, raising the suspicion of carcinoma. If there is calcium deposition, lesions may also mimic carcinoma mammographically.

Granulomatous mastitis

This condition is rare. Causes include infections (e.g. tuberculosis, deep-seated fungal infections) and systemic disorders (e.g. Wegener's granulomatosis, sarcoid).

Fibrocystic changes

This term is used to refer to a wide range of morphological changes to the breast. Fibrocystic change is the commonest disorder of the breast. The exact pathogenesis remains obscure but hormonal imbalances are thought to be important. Affected women are usually aged between 30 and 55 with a marked decrease in incidence after the menopause. The clinical features vary depending on the underlying morphological changes but, in general, fibrocystic change can mimic carcinoma clinically by producing palpable lumps, nipple discharge and mammographic densities. Evidence indicates that some of these conditions are associated with an increased risk of developing carcinoma of the breast (see later).

The morphological subtypes of fibrocystic disease are listed below:

- adenosis
- cysts
- apocrine metaplasia
- fibrosis
- epithelial hyperplasia
- sclerosing adenosis
- radial scars and complex sclerosing lesions.

An individual may show one, or some, or a combination of all of these changes.

Adenosis

This term denotes an increase in the number of acini within a lobule. The gland lumina in adenosis occasionally contain calcium deposits.

Cysts

This term refers to cystic dilatation of acini or terminal ducts. Some cysts may reach a very large size (up to 2–3 cm across). The secretions within cysts may calcify.

Apocrine metaplasia

This term refers to cysts that are lined by epithelium that resembles that of apocrine sweat glands.

Fibrosis

This is probably a secondary event to rupture of cysts and it may proceed to hyalinisation.

Sclerosing adenosis

In this condition, there is an increased number of acini and increased intralobular fibrosis. The fibrosis causes marked distortion of the acini. The lesion can present as a mammographic density or a palpable mass, therefore mimicking carcinoma. Sclerosing adenosis may be mistaken for carcinoma histologically also. Radial scars and complex sclerosing lesions are morphological variants of sclerosing adenosis, and are characterised by:

- a stellate shape
- a central area of fibrosis and elastosis
- a variable degree of adenosis and distortion of acini.

Radial scar is the term reserved for lesions less than 10 mm in diameter, whereas larger lesions are called complex sclerosing lesions. They can mimic carcinoma clinically, mammographically and histologically.

Epithelial hyperplasia

Epithelial hyperplasia is defined as an increase in the number of layers of cells lining the acini or ducts, often resulting in the obliteration of their lumen. Epithelial hyperplasia is classified as being either of usual type or atypical.

Usual-type epithelial hyperplasia (mild, moderate, florid)

In this type, the proliferating epithelial cells show no atypical features. Epithelial hyperplasia is considered *mild* if the epithelium is three to four cell layers thick, *moderate* if the epithelium is more than five layers thick, and *florid* if the lumina are nearly or completely filled by epithelium.

Atypical hyperplasia

In this type, the epithelial proliferations display various degrees of cellular and architectural atypia. There are two subtypes:

- atypical ductal hyperplasia
- atypical lobular hyperplasia.

Benign breast tumours

Fibroadenomas

Fibroadenomas are the most common benign tumour of the breast. The tumours are composed of both glandular and stromal tissue. These benign neoplasms can occur at any age, but they are most commonly seen in women under 35 years of age. Fibroadenomas are usually solitary, although in some women they may be multiple and bilateral. In younger women they present as palpable lumps (often freely mobile), and in older women they may present as mammographic densities. They can therefore mimic carcinoma clinically.

Pathology

Fibroadenomas grow within the breast as sharply circumscribed soft to firm nodules, and are usually easily enucleated at surgery. They vary in size from less than 1 cm to around 4 cm in diameter, although rarely they can reach up to 15 cm in diameter (juvenile fibroadenoma/giant fibroadenoma – see below). The cut surface is grey-white and sometimes glistening, and contains slit-like spaces. In older women, fibroadenomas can become calcified. Histologically, these tumours are well-circumscribed nodules consisting of loose cellular stroma associated with breast ducts that, in longitudinal section, appear as compressed and elongated clefts.

The vast majority of fibroadenomas are benign. However, those containing cysts, sclerosing adenosis, epithelial calcification or papillary apocrine change (so-called complex fibroadenomas) are associated with an increased risk of developing breast cancer.

Juvenile fibroadenoma/giant fibroadenoma

These terms are interchangeable and are used to refer to a reasonably distinct type of fibroadenoma that tends to occur in adolescents (often black girls) and reaches a large size (over 10 cm in diameter). Histologically, they also tend to be rather hypercellular, but cellular atypia is not a feature.

Duct papillomas

Duct papillomas are uncommon and are usually seen in middle-aged women. They appear as outgrowths projecting into the duct lumen and consist of a fibrovascular core covered by benign breast duct epithelium. There are two types of duct papilloma:

- **Large duct papillomas** – these arise within the large central breast ducts and are usually solitary. Presentation is usually with a bloodstained nipple discharge, although some present as palpable lumps or mammographic densities. They are associated with an increased risk of developing carcinoma.
- **Small duct papillomas** – these arise in the smaller peripheral ducts, are often asymptomatic, and may be multiple. Multiple small duct papillomas are seen in younger patients, and are associated with an increased risk of developing breast cancer.

Adenomas

Adenomas of the breast are rare. There are three main subtypes:

- **Tubular adenomas** – these are sharply circumscribed nodules composed of closely packed ductal structures with little intervening stroma.
- **Lactating adenomas** – these are adenomas that arise during pregnancy and lactation.
- **Nipple adenomas** – these present as nodules just under the nipple. Microscopically, they consist of proliferating ductal structures and show a variety of growth patterns. The overlying skin may become ulcerated, mimicking Paget's disease of the nipple (see below).

Twenty

Benign connective tissue tumours

Any type of benign connective tissue tumour can occur in the breast, e.g. lipoma, haemangioma, leiomyoma.

Risk of invasive breast carcinoma in women with benign breast disease

Several large case–control studies have now clarified the association between benign breast abnormalities and breast cancer risk.

There is no increased risk in the presence of:

- mastitis
- duct ectasia
- ordinary cysts
- apocrine metaplasia
- adenosis
- fibrosis
- mild usual-type epithelial hyperplasia without atypia
- fibroadenoma without complex features.

There is slightly increased risk (1.5–3 times) in the presence of:

- moderate or florid usual-type epithelial hyperplasia without atypia
- radial scars/complex sclerosing lesions
- fibroadenoma with complex features
- duct papilloma.

There is moderately increased risk (4–5 times) in the presence of:

- atypical ductal hyperplasia
- atypical lobular hyperplasia.

A family history of breast cancer increases the risk in all categories.

Some researchers have advocated a new classification system for benign breast disease that reflects the above observations. Three main categories of disease are defined in this system:

- non-proliferative diseases – this category includes the entities that are associated with no increased risk of developing breast cancer
- proliferative diseases without atypia – this category includes entities that are associated with a slightly increased risk of developing breast cancer
- proliferative diseases with atypia – this category includes atypical hyperplasia.

20.3 Breast cancer

Learning objectives

You should:

- know the risk factors for the development of breast cancer
- know the classification of breast cancer
- understand the behaviour and spread of breast cancer
- know the prognostic indicators.

Breast cancer is a major cause of cancer morbidity. One woman in eight will develop breast cancer in her lifetime and, of these, a third will die from the disease.

Risk factors

The cause of breast cancer is still uncertain, but a number of factors that increase the risk of developing breast cancer have been identified.

Genetic predisposition

It has long been known that there is a familial aggregation of breast cancer, and at least four genes that convey increasing susceptibility to breast cancer have been identified. These are:

- *BRCA1*
- *BRCA2*
- *p53*
- ATM gene (responsible for ataxia telangiectasia).

Genetic predisposition is responsible for only 5–10% of breast cancer cases.

Age

Breast cancer is uncommon before the age of 25 years, but the incidence increases steeply with age, doubling about every 10 years until the menopause. The rise slows in the postmenopausal period.

Factors related to menses

Early age at menarche and late age at menopause are associated with an increased risk of breast cancer. These findings indicate that hormones may have an important role in the development of carcinoma of the breast.

Factors related to pregnancy

An early age at first pregnancy is associated with a decreased risk of developing breast cancer.

Demographic influences

The incidence of breast cancer in Western countries is around five times higher than that in Far Eastern countries. Also, the rate of breast cancer is higher in women of high socioeconomic status. These differences are thought to be related to differing reproductive patterns, such as age at first birth, age at menarche and age at menopause.

Radiation

Exposure to ionising radiation increases the risk of breast cancer. The greatest risk has been found among women exposed to radiation around the menarche.

Benign breast disease

The risk of breast cancer varies according to the type of benign breast disease (see above).

Previous breast cancer

Women with breast cancer have an increased risk of developing a new primary lesion in the contralateral breast or the conserved ipsilateral breast.

Hormones

Women who take hormone replacement therapy (HRT) are at an increased risk of developing breast cancer. At present, there is conflicting data as to whether taking the contraceptive pill increases the risk of breast cancer.

Dubious risk factors

The role of obesity, diet and alcohol as risk factors for the development of breast cancer remains controversial and unresolved.

Distribution

Most cancers (50%) arise in the upper outer quadrant of the breast, 10% occur in each of the remaining three quadrants, and 20% occur in the central or subareolar region. Bilaterality of breast cancer occurs in 4% of cases.

Classification

Nearly all breast cancers are adenocarcinomas. Breast cancer is traditionally divided into non-invasive (in situ) carcinoma and invasive carcinoma.

Non-invasive (in situ) carcinoma

This term is used to refer to the situation where the malignant cells are confined to the ducts or acini, with no evidence of invasion by the tumour cells through the basement membrane and into the breast stroma. Women with these lesions have a markedly increased risk (8–10 times) of developing breast cancer. There are two types of non-invasive carcinoma:

- ductal carcinoma in situ (DCIS)
- lobular carcinoma in situ (LCIS).

Ductal carcinoma in situ

In this type of non-invasive carcinoma, the breast ducts contain a malignant population of cells. DCIS is usually unilateral. Presentation can be as a nipple discharge or Paget's disease of the nipple (see later), although DCIS may present as mammographic densities because the involved ducts often contain calcifications. Around half of all mammographically detected cancers subsequently turn out to be DCIS.

Pathology Histologically, DCIS can be divided into five architectural subtypes:

- **Comedocarcinoma** – characterised by the presence of solid sheets of high-grade malignant cells within the ducts with central necrosis. The necrosis commonly calcifies and this calcification is detected on mammography.
- **Solid** – denotes the presence of solid sheets of malignant cells within the ducts.
- **Cribriform** – this type is characterised by numerous gland-like structures within the sheets of malignant cells within ducts.
- **Papillary**.
- **Micropapillary**.

Classification of DCIS for patient management is usually based on the degree of cytological atypia. DCIS is graded by the pathologist as low, intermediate or high grade.

Risk of subsequent invasive cancer Evidence now indicates that many cases of low grade DCIS and most cases of high grade DCIS may progress to invasive carcinoma.

Lobular carcinoma in situ

In this type of non-invasive carcinoma, the malignant cells are found in the acini, although the changes seen may extend into the ducts. LCIS is often multifocal within one breast and frequently bilateral. The lesions do not present as palpable lumps and calcifications rarely occur, which means that they are rarely detected by mammography. Hence, the lesions are usually identified incidentally in biopsies for other breast abnormalities.

Risk of subsequent invasive cancer

Around a quarter to a third of women with LCIS go on to develop invasive carcinoma, but unlike DCIS, both breasts are equally at risk irrespective of which side the LCIS was originally identified.

Invasive carcinoma

With invasive carcinoma, the malignant cells have breached the basement membrane of the ducts or acini, and have spread into the surrounding stromal tissue.

Classification

Invasive breast carcinoma is classified according to overall histological appearance. The various histological subtypes are listed below:

- infiltrating ductal carcinoma (85%)
- infiltrating lobular carcinoma (10%)
- mucinous carcinoma (2%)
- tubular carcinoma (2%)
- medullary carcinoma (<1%)
- papillary carcinoma (<1%)
- others, e.g. apocrine carcinoma, metaplastic carcinoma, neuroendocrine tumours, adenoid cystic carcinomas and squamous cell carcinoma (<1%).

Invasive ductal carcinoma of no special type (NST) Carcinomas that cannot be classified as any other subtype are designated invasive ductal carcinoma NST. Most breast carcinomas fall into this category. Macroscopically, these tumours appear as hard grey-white nodules (scirrhous carcinoma) imparted by their densely fibrous stroma. Histologically, the stroma is infiltrated by malignant cells that can be arranged in cords, nests, tubules or irregular masses – ductal carcinomas do not display any distinctive morphological features.

Invasive lobular carcinoma These tumours can have a scirrhous macroscopic appearance, but they are often softer and have an ill-defined infiltrating outline. Histologically, linear cords of malignant cells infiltrate a densely fibrous stroma. This linear arrangement of cells is often referred to as an 'Indian file' pattern. Carcinoma cells often form concentric rings around ducts. Signet-ring cells are common. It is important to distinguish lobular carcinoma from other types of carcinoma for the following reasons:

- invasive lobular carcinomas tend to be multicentric within the same breast

- around 20% of women with invasive lobular carcinoma in one breast are likely to have bilateral disease
- these tumours metastasise more frequently to serosal surfaces, bone marrow, cerebrospinal fluid (CSF), and the uterus and ovaries compared to other subtypes.

Mucinous carcinoma These tumours typically arise in older women and grow slowly over a number of years. Macroscopically, mucinous carcinomas have a soft, grey, gelatinous cut surface and are well-circumscribed. Histologically, the tumour is composed of small nests and cords of tumour cells lying in lakes of mucin. Because of the absence of densely fibrous stroma, and the fact that this type of carcinoma does not cause skin tethering or nipple retraction, mucinous carcinomas can be mistaken for benign breast lesions clinically. The prognosis for women with this type of breast cancer is better than that for invasive ductal or lobular carcinoma.

Tubular carcinoma These tumours tend to be small (<1 cm in diameter) and are usually detected by mammography. Affected women are younger on average. Macroscopically, tubular carcinomas are small, firm, gritty tumours with irregular outlines. Histologically, they are composed of well-formed tubules in a desmoplastic stroma. The tubules lack a myoepithelial layer, a feature that distinguishes these malignant tumours from benign breast lesions. The prognosis for patients with tubular carcinoma is excellent.

Medullary carcinoma Macroscopically, these tumours tend to have a soft, fleshy consistency and are typically well-circumscribed. Histologically, medullary carcinomas are characterised by syncytial (fused) masses of large cells with pleomorphic nuclei, numerous mitotic figures, a conspicuous lymphoplasmocytic infiltrate, and a pushing (non-infiltrating) border. Gland formation is not seen. Despite the aggressive cytological features of the tumour cells, the prognosis for patients with this type of breast cancer is significantly better than that for many of the other subtypes.

Papillary carcinoma These tumours are rare. Microscopically, they show a papillary architecture. The prognosis is better than that of invasive ductal carcinoma.

Paget's disease of the nipple

This condition presents as roughening and reddening of the skin of the nipple and areola, the appearances resembling eczema. Ulceration may occur. The condition is important to recognise because it is associated with underlying in situ or invasive carcinoma of the breast. Histologically, the epidermis is infiltrated by malignant cells.

Spread of breast carcinomas

Breast carcinomas can infiltrate locally or spread via the lymphatics or bloodstream to distant sites.

Direct spread

Breast carcinomas spread locally in all directions, becoming adherent to the underlying muscle fascia of the breast or tethered to the overlying skin. The latter manifests by dimpling of the skin and nipple retraction.

Spread via lymphatics

Involvement of the breast lymphatics by carcinoma causes blockage of the lymphatic drainage with consequent lymphoedema and thickening of the overlying skin, an appearance referred to clinically as peau d'orange. Several groups of lymph nodes drain lymph from the breast, but the axillary lymph nodes are the commonest initial site of lymph node metastases. Around a third of women with breast cancer will have lymph node metastases at the time of diagnosis.

Spread via the bloodstream

Once the malignant cells have developed the ability to enter the bloodstream, they can reach virtually any organ in the body, but the most frequently affected sites are the lungs, bones, liver, adrenals and brain.

Staging of breast cancer

Two main systems are used to stage breast cancer. These are the International Classification of Staging of Breast Cancer, and the TNM (tumour, node, metastasis) system. The management of the patient will depend on the stage of the disease (Table 36).

Prognostic factors

A number of factors influence the prognosis of breast cancer.

Table 36 Staging of breast cancer

Stage	Extent of spread
International Classification of Staging of Breast Cancer (ICSBC)	
I	Lump with slight tethering to skin, but node negative
II	Lump with lymph node metastases or skin tethering
III	Tumour that is extensively adherent to the skin and/or underlying muscles, or ulcerating or lymph nodes are fixed
IV	Distant metastases
Tumour, Node, Metastases (TNM) classification	
T1	Tumour 20 mm or less, no fixation or nipple retraction Includes Paget's disease
T2	Tumour 20–50 mm, or less than 20 mm but with tethering
T3	Tumour greater than 50 mm but less than 100 mm; or less than 50 mm but with infiltration, ulceration or fixation
T4	Any tumour with ulceration or infiltration wide of it, or chest wall fixation, or greater than 100 mm in diameter
N0	Node-negative
N1	Axillary nodes mobile
N2	Axillary nodes fixed
N3	Supraclavicular nodes or oedema of arm
M0	No distant metastases
M1	Distant metastases

Axillary lymph node status

At present, the best prognostic indicator in patients with breast cancer is the presence or absence of metastatic tumour in the axillary lymph nodes. The prognosis is significantly worse for those who have evidence of lymph node metastases.

Tumour size

Small tumours are associated with a more favourable prognosis.

Histological grade

Many studies have shown the value of histological grade in predicting survival in breast cancer, low-grade cancers being associated with a more favourable prognosis.

Histological subtype

Certain types of breast carcinoma have a better prognosis than others, although the significance is less important than histological grade. Tubular carcinoma (and probably mucinous, medullary and papillary carcinoma) have a more favourable prognosis than invasive ductal carcinoma of no special type.

Oestrogen and progesterone receptors

Women with oestrogen receptor-positive (ER+ve), node-negative breast cancer have a better prognosis than those who have oestrogen receptor-negative (ER–ve) tumours. This is probably because tumours that express oestrogen receptors respond well to hormonal manipulation. The progesterone receptor status of a tumour is less important than the oestrogen receptor status, but it may have a small effect on the overall responsiveness of a tumour to hormonal manipulation in that women with ER+ve tumours which are also progesterone receptor positive (PR+ve) have a slightly increased chance of benefiting while those with tumours that are ER+ve and PR–ve have a slightly decreased chance of benefiting. Tumours that are both ER–ve and PR–ve are less likely to respond to hormonal manipulation than tumours which are ER–ve and PR+ve.

Other molecular markers (including HER2)

It has been proposed that tumour differentiation, invasion, metastasis, and growth can be inferred by measuring certain cellular markers, e.g. expression of growth factor receptors, proteinases, cell-adhesion molecules, and other products of oncogenes and tumour suppressor genes. Much of the research in this field has focused on the onco-gene HER2 (also known a HER2/NEU and c-ERB-B2), the protein product of which is a cell-surface growth factor receptor. Research using molecular techniques indicates that 1 in 4 breast carcinomas show amplification of the HER2 gene and such cancers are referred to as 'HER2-positive'. Studies have shown that HER2-positive cancers have a poorer prognosis, shorter survival, shorter relapse time, tend to be more aggressive and respond poorly to conventional therapies. However, it has now been possible to develop a treatment strategy that employs the use of a monoclonal antibody called trastuzumab (Herceptin), which can block the HER2 receptor and hence reduce tumour growth. Evidence indicates that administration of this antibody to women with HER2-positive breast cancers may significantly improve survival.

Other malignant breast conditions

Phyllodes tumour

Like fibroadenomas, phyllodes tumours are composed of both glandular and stromal tissue, are usually solitary, and can present as palpable lumps or mammographic densities. They can occur at any age but the median age at presentation is 45 years, some 10–20 years later than that for fibroadenomas. Phyllodes tumours can only be differentiated from fibroadenomas by their microscopic appearance.

Pathology

Phyllodes tumours vary greatly in size, and they have been reported to reach up to 450 mm in diameter. They often grow as lobulated masses within the breast tissue. Microscopically, phyllodes tumours can be differentiated from fibroadenomas by the presence of stromal cellularity, mitotic figures and nuclear pleomorphism. Most are low-grade tumours, when the major problem is local recurrence. Rare high-grade tumours can behave aggressively, metastasising via the bloodstream.

Sarcomas

Sarcomas such as angiosarcoma, fibrosarcoma, liposarcoma and leiomyosarcoma are all rare.

Lymphomas

Lymphomas in the breast may be primary, but are more usually secondary to disease elsewhere in the body.

Secondary tumours

Secondary tumours to the breast are rare. Those most commonly encountered are metastases from the lung, the contralateral breast and malignant melanoma.

20.4 Diagnosis of breast lesions

When a breast lesion is suspected on clinical grounds (history and physical examination) or detected by mammography, a number of investigation methods can be used to gain further information about the lesion and lead to a diagnosis. These are:

- ultrasonography
- fine-needle aspiration cytology
- core biopsy
- excision biopsy.

Often, a combination of modalities is used. The value of these methods is that benign and malignant conditions may be diagnosed without the need for removal of the breast (mastectomy). In malignant cases, prognostic information may also be provided (e.g. oestrogen receptor

Twenty

status). Appropriate management plans can then be formulated.

20.5 The male breast

Structure

It is not necessary for the male breast to have secretory capability. Hence, it consists of ductular structures surrounded by a small amount of supporting connective tissue, but there are no acini.

Two main conditions can affect the male breast:

- gynaecomastia
- carcinoma.

Gynaecomastia

This benign condition is defined as enlargement of the male breast due to hypertrophy and hyperplasia of both ductal and stromal elements. Most cases are unilateral, but around 25% of patients show bilateral involvement.

Aetiology

Gynaecomastia is thought to occur as a result of an imbalance between oestrogens (which stimulate the breast) and androgens. The condition can occur as a normal phenomenon in adolescents and very elderly men, but it can also occur in the following situations:

- drug-induced (most common cause):
  - *oestrogens (in the treatment of prostate cancer)*
  - *digitalis*
  - *cimetidine*
  - *spironolactone*
- conditions causing high oestrogen levels:
  - *tumours of the adrenal glands*
  - *tumours of the testis*
  - *chronic liver disease*
- syndromes of androgen deficiency, e.g. Klinefelter's syndrome
- other endocrine disorders:
  - *hyperthyroidism*
  - *pituitary disorders.*

Carcinoma

In situ and invasive carcinoma of the male breast is very rare, accounting for only 1% of all breast cancers. Risk factors (except those functionally confined to women), presentation, spread, histological subtypes and prognostic factors are similar to those seen in women. With regard to prognosis, evidence suggests that when male and female breast cancers are matched for grade and stage, the overall prognosis for men and women is the same. However, men often present at more advanced stages than women.

Self-assessment: questions

One best answer questions

1. A 24-year-old nulliparous woman presents to her general practitioner (GP) with a discrete lump in the breast. There is no history of pain, nipple discharge, nipple retraction or skin changes. On examination, the lump is approximately 20 mm in diameter and is freely mobile. The most likely diagnosis is:
   a. invasive carcinoma
   b. in situ carcinoma
   c. fibroadenoma
   d. fibrocystic change
   e. abscess

2. A 52-year-old smoker presents to her GP with a mass in the left breast. The subsequent ultrasound, fine-needle aspiration cytology and core biopsy confirmed that this was an invasive carcinoma. The hormone receptor status of the tumour was determined on the core biopsy. The patient was given hormone therapy and underwent excision of the breast lesion and the axillary lymph nodes. Six months later, she saw her GP because she was feeling generally unwell and had been experiencing some pain in her left chest. An X-ray showed a lytic lesion in one of the ribs on the left side and a left pleural effusion. The most likely diagnosis is:
   a. bronchopneumonia
   b. pulmonary thromboembolism
   c. metastatic carcinoma of the breast
   d. bronchogenic carcinoma
   e. osteosarcoma

True-false questions

1. The following statements are correct:
   a. acute mastitis is most frequently seen in the early weeks of breastfeeding
   b. mammary duct ectasia may present with a breast mass and nipple discharge
   c. early age at first pregnancy increases the risk of developing breast cancer
   d. breast cancer is more frequent in multiparous women than nulliparous women
   e. men never develop breast cancer

2. The following breast conditions are associated with an increased risk of developing breast cancer:
   a. apocrine metaplasia
   b. atypical hyperplasia
   c. radial scar
   d. duct papilloma
   e. complex fibroadenoma

3. The following statements are true:
   a. most breast cancers arise in the upper outer quadrant of the breast
   b. in situ carcinoma usually presents as a breast mass
   c. lobular carcinoma in situ is frequently multifocal and bilateral
   d. tumour size is the most important prognostic indicator in women with breast cancer
   e. carcinomas that are oestrogen receptor positive have a poorer prognosis than those that are oestrogen receptor negative

4. Invasive breast cancer:
   a. can be genetically inherited
   b. always presents as a breast mass
   c. most commonly metastasises to the mediastinal lymph nodes
   d. may be associated with Paget's disease of the nipple
   e. is most frequently of ductal type histologically

5. The following can be associated with breast cancer:
   a. axillary mass
   b. nipple inversion
   c. roughening and reddening of the skin of the nipple
   d. bone fracture
   e. pleural effusion

6. The following conditions can present with a discrete breast mass
   a. fat necrosis
   b. fibrocystic change
   c. fibroadenoma
   d. gynaecomastia
   e. breast cancer

Case history questions

Case history 1

A 29-year-old women presents to her GP with a lump in the right breast.

1. What is the differential diagnosis?
2. Which of these diagnoses do you think are least likely in this case, and why?
3. What further information would you seek in the history and examination in order to help determine the diagnosis?

Case history 2

A 68-year-old women presents to her GP with a lump in the right breast. She first felt the lump after she fell over a chair sustaining a blunt injury to the right breast. On examination, the right nipple is retracted and the skin of the right breast shows peau d'orange. The breast lump itself is firm and immobile. The right axillary lymph nodes are enlarged and firm.

1. What is the most likely diagnosis?
2. Describe the pathological basis of each of the examination findings?
3. What further tests might you perform?

Short note questions

Write short notes on:

1. The diagnosis of breast cancer.
2. The association between benign breast abnormalities and breast cancer risk.
3. Risk factors for the development of breast cancer.

Viva questions

1. What conditions may affect the male breast?
2. What is the rationale behind mammographic breast screening?
3. What factors influence the prognosis of women with breast cancer?

Self-assessment: answers

One best answer

1. c. Fibroadenoma. The most likely diagnosis is a
        fibroadenoma. This is a benign tumour. Invasive
        and in situ carcinoma are very unusual in
        patients of this age, but should always be
        considered and excluded, even in the absence of
        other symptoms such as nipple retraction or skin
        changes. Fibrocystic change is a possibility, but
        usually causes diffuse lumpiness of the breast
        rather than a discrete lump. An abscess would be
        painful and is most commonly seen in the
        lactation period (this woman is nulliparous). The
        clinical diagnosis can be confirmed using other
        investigative tools including ultrasonography,
        fine-needle aspiration cytology, core biopsy or, if
        necessary, excision biopsy.

2. c. Metastatic carcinoma of the breast. The most
        likely diagnosis is metastatic carcinoma of the
        breast. The lytic lesion in the rib most likely
        represents a metastatic tumour deposit, and the
        pleural effusion is probably due to involvement
        of the pleura, either by direct spread through the
        chest wall or indirect spread to the lung and
        pleura. Bronchogenic carcinoma is a distinct
        possibility, but given the recent history of breast
        cancer this is the more likely diagnosis. The
        diagnosis could be confirmed by performing a
        diagnostic aspiration of the pleural fluid. The
        fluid can be examined under the microscope for
        the presence of malignant cells, and it may be
        possible to determine whether these are likely to
        have originated from a breast or lung primary
        site. Bronchopneumonia and pulmonary
        thromboembolism are possibilities, but the lytic
        lesion in the rib does not fit for these.
        Osteosarcomas are rare and are usually seen in
        younger people. Remember that metastatic
        carcinoma is by far the most common malignant
        tumour in bone.

True-false answers

1. a. **True.**
    b. **True.**
    c. **False.** This is associated with a *decreased* risk.
    d. **False.** Breast cancer is more frequent in
        nulliparous than multiparous women.
    e. **False.**

2. a. **False.**
    b. **True.**
    c. **True.**
    d. **True.**

e. **True.** But fibroadenomas that do not show
    complex features are not associated with an
    increased risk.

3. a. **True.**
    b. **False.**
    c. **True.**
    d. **False.** Lymph node status is the most important
        prognostic factor.
    e. **False.** Oestrogen receptor positive tumours have
        a *better* prognosis.

4. a. **True.** Five to ten per cent of breast cancers are
        due to inheritance of an autosomal dominant
        gene. The genes *BRCA1* and *BRCA2* account for
        most of these cases.
    b. **False.**
    c. **False.** Breast tumours most commonly
        metastasise to the *axillary* lymph nodes.
    d. **True.**
    e. **True.**

5. a. **True.** This may indicate lymph node metastasis.
    b. **True**
    c. **True.** This may represent Paget's disease of the
        nipple.
    d. **True.** This may represent a pathological fracture
        due to bony metastasis.
    e. **True.** Due to spread of the tumour to the pleura.

6. a. **True.**
    b. **True.**
    c. **True.**
    d. **True.**
    e. **True.**

Case history answers

Case history 1

1. *Comment*: It is important to realise that the
    differential diagnosis for a lump in the breast
    includes almost the entire spectrum of breast
    disorders. Inflammatory lesions, fibrocystic disease,
    benign tumours and malignant tumours (principally
    invasive carcinoma) may all present as breast
    lumps. Remember that in situ carcinoma does not
    present as a breast lump (unless it is associated with
    another breast lesion).

2. *Comment*: Taking note of the patient's age is often
    helpful in determining which of the differential
    diagnoses are more likely and which are less likely.
    In this case, the patient is 29 years old. Carcinoma is
    therefore the least likely diagnosis, although young
    patients may develop breast cancer, especially if
    there is a strong family history.

3. Acute mastitis is painful and there would usually be a history of breastfeeding. The skin of the nipple is often cracked. Mammary duct ectasia is usually seen in older women and a history of nipple discharge is common. A history of nipple discharge would also raise the possibility of a duct papilloma. Fat necrosis would follow trauma to the breast tissue. Fibrocystic disease usually causes breast 'lumpiness', and although one lump may be dominant, the lumpiness is often revealed on clinical examination. Fibroadenomas are usually solitary palpable masses, which are freely mobile. Nipple adenomas usually cause a subareolar mass. Breast cancers produce firm masses, which may be immobile due to tethering. The overlying skin may show dimpling or peau d'orange and there may be features of Paget's disease of the nipple. The axillary lymph nodes may be enlarged due to spread of the disease. A family history of breast cancer may alert you to the possibility of carcinoma in young patients presenting with breast lumps.

Case history 2

1. The fact that this woman first felt the breast lump after she sustained an injury to the breast raises the possibility of fat necrosis. However, the clinical findings of a retracted nipple, peau d'orange, a firm immobile mass, and enlarged axillary lymph nodes are all highly suggestive of breast cancer. The preceding trauma may simply have drawn the patient's attention to her breast, and in the ensuing self-examination the lump would have been revealed.

2. Most of the features on physical examination can be explained in terms of the way that breast cancer spreads. Extension into the overlying skin causes retraction and dimpling, and tumours that have become adherent to the deep fascia of the chest wall become fixed in position (immobile). Involvement of the lymphatic channels around the tumour blocks drainage of the overlying skin, causing localised lymphoedema and skin thickening, referred to as peau d'orange. The axillary lymph nodes become enlarged and firm when there are lymph node metastases.

3. Initial further investigations are directed towards establishing a diagnosis of cancer. Several techniques may be employed, but a combination of different modalities is often necessary to make the diagnosis. These include ultrasonography, fine-needle aspiration cytology (FNA), core biopsy and, if necessary, excision biopsy. Further investigations, e.g. computed tomography (CT) scan, are usually aimed at determining the stage of the disease.

Short note answers

1. Whenever you are asked how you might diagnose any condition, your answer must always include the three most important tools, namely: history;

physical examination; and further investigations (or tests). Focus on the most important features that you would want to elicit from the history and examination, i.e. family history, the appearance of the affected breast, the nature of any breast mass and the axillary contents, and the nature of any nipple discharge. Then discuss the further tests that you might use to establish the diagnosis, i.e. ultrasonography, FNA, core biopsy and excision biopsy. Remember that some breast cancers are detected by mammography in the National Breast Screening Programme.

2. What is wanted here is an awareness that there are certain benign breast conditions that are associated with an increased risk of developing breast cancer. Radial scars/complex sclerosing lesions, moderate to florid usual-type epithelial hyperplasia, fibroadenomas with complex features, and duct papillomas are all associated with a slightly increased risk, while atypical hyperplasia is associated with a moderately increased risk.

3. Risk factors for breast cancer include genetic predisposition, age, factors related to the menses and pregnancy, demographic influences, radiation, certain benign breast diseases and previous breast cancer.

Viva answers

1. The two main intrinsic breast conditions that may affect the male breast are gynaecomastia and carcinoma. Try to give an account of the various causes of gynaecomastia. Carcinoma of the male breast is uncommon. However, when it occurs it usually presents at a higher stage and therefore generally has a poorer prognosis. Remember that the male breast may also be affected by pathology of the skin and soft tissue (as may the female breast).

2. Screening implies performing a test in order to detect a particular disease (most commonly cancer) in an asymptomatic but at-risk population. With cancer, the idea is to detect the disease either at its pre-invasive stage, when treatment of the lesion would prevent cancer from developing, or at a stage when the cancer is small and therefore potentially curable. With breast cancer, there is a pre-invasive stage (in situ carcinoma) and small invasive tumours do have a better prognosis. Both in situ and invasive carcinoma can be detected on mammography because they induce densities, calcifications and areas of architectural distortion that can be visualised. Mammography is both sensitive and specific, but it is also acceptable, and it is, therefore, the principal investigative modality in the National Breast Screening Programme.

3. Several factors influence the prognosis of breast cancer. These include lymph node status, tumour size, histological grade, histological subtype and oestrogen receptor status.

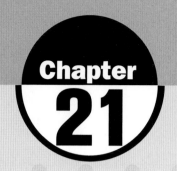

Female genital tract

Chapter 21

Chapter overview

The female genital tract comprises the vulva, vagina, uterus, cervix, fallopian tubes and ovaries. Infections in this region are common. Many are relatively trivial, but pelvic inflammatory disease can cause infertility or serious intra-abdominal sepsis. Infection with certain subtypes of human papilloma virus (HPV) predisposes to dysplasia and malignancy in the cervix. Carcinoma of the ovary is the fifth most frequent cause of female cancer mortality in the UK, and often presents at an advanced state. In contrast, the cervical cytology screening programme has allowed early diagnosis of premalignant and invasive cervical carcinomas in many cases, with a consequential fall in mortality from cervical cancer of approximately 40%. Disorders relating specifically to reproductive function include endometriosis, ectopic pregnancy and hydatidiform mole.

21.1 Inflammation, infection and non-neoplastic disease

Learning objectives

You should:
- know the common female genital tract infections
- know about human papilloma viruses (HPV)-associated diseases
- understand the pathology of endometriosis.

Genital tract infection

Common causes include:

- bacteria – *Gardnerella, Neisseria gonorrhoeae, Chlamydia*
- viruses – HPV, herpes simplex type 2
- fungi – *Candida albicans*
- protozoa – *Trichomonas vaginalis*.

Gardnerella

Gardnerella is a common cause of vaginitis.

Neisseria gonorrhoeae

N. gonorrhoeae can infect the cervix, endometrium, fallopian tubes and ovaries.

Chlamydia trachomatis

C. trachomatis is an intracellular pathogen that causes urethritis, cervicitis and lymphogranuloma venereum (genital ulceration with suppurative and granulomatous inflammation of pelvic, inguinal and rectal lymph nodes). Transmission to neonates during vaginal delivery can cause conjunctivitis and pneumonia.

Staphylococcus

Toxic shock syndrome is a rare but serious infection caused by exotoxins produced by *Staphylococcus aureus*. It is associated with tampon use and presents with fever, diarrhoea and vomiting, rash and shock. Occasionally it can be fatal.

Human papilloma virus

This infects squamous epithelia at many body sites (see Table 37). Low-risk subtypes cause genital warts (condylomata acuminata); high-risk subtypes are associated with the development of cervical carcinoma. HPV changes are frequently seen in association with cervical dysplasia on tissue biopsy. HPV serotyping using the polymerase chain reaction is likely to play an important part in future cervical cancer screening programmes. Cytological features associated with HPV infection include irregular enlarged hyperchromatic nuclei surrounded by poorly staining cytoplasm (these features are known as koilocytosis), multinucleation and abnormal keratinisation.

Herpes simplex type 2

Infection is relatively common in young women. Ulcerating vesicles develop on the vulva, vagina or cervix several days after sexual contact. Spontaneous healing occurs but latent infection leads to recurrent attacks. Neonatal transmission during vaginal delivery can cause severe systemic infection and neonatal death. Herpes simplex 2 is also associated with cervical carcinogenesis.

Table 37 HPV subtype disease associations

HPV subtype	Associated lesions
1, 2, 4, 7	Benign squamous cell papillomas (viral warts)
5, 8	Cutaneous squamous cell carcinoma
6, 11	Benign anogenital warts (condylomata acuminatum)
16, 18 (31, 33, 35)	High-grade cervical epithelial dysplasia (CIN) and squamous carcinoma

Box 28 Clinical notes: endometriosis

Symptoms related to cyclical bleeding and subsequent inflammation:

* pain, often dyspareunia or dysmenorrhoea
* ovarian cysts ('chocolate cysts' containing altered blood)
* infertility (fallopian tube involvement)
* haematuria (bladder endometriosis)
* intestinal obstruction
* endometriotic nodules in abdominal surgical scars.

Candida

This commonly causes vulvovaginitis, with intense itching and a thick white discharge. Infection is associated with diabetes, oral contraceptives, immunosuppression and pregnancy.

Trichomonas vaginalis

Trichomatosis is a sexually transmitted infection and causes a foamy discharge, itching, dysuria and dyspareunia. *Trichomonas*, *Candida* and herpes virus infections may be identified incidentally on cytological examination of routine cervical screening smears (see below).

Pelvic inflammatory disease

Pelvic inflammatory disease (PID) describes a chronic upper genital tract infection that presents as pelvic pain, fever and vaginal discharge. Causative organisms include gonococci and *Chlamydia*, although other bacteria can cause PID following termination of pregnancy or spontaneous vaginal delivery. Actinomycosis is a common infection in users of contraceptive coils. Infection spreads from the lower genital tract to the fallopian tubes and ovaries. Complications include tubo-ovarian abscess, pyosalpinx, peritonitis, intestinal obstruction and infertility.

Chronic endometritis

Chronic endometritis is identified microscopically by the presence of plasma cells in the endometrium. Chronic endometrial infection occurs:

* in association with intrauterine contraceptive devices (IUD, 'coil')
* in patients with chronic PID
* in association with retained products of pregnancy
* in tuberculosis – diagnosis can be difficult as cyclical endometrial shedding prevents the formation of typical caseating granulomas
* without other associated factors (15%).

Treatment depends on the underlying cause – antibiotics, removal or replacement of the IUD or endometrial curettage to remove retained gestational tissue.

Lichen sclerosus

Lichen sclerosus a chronic inflammatory skin condition that most commonly affects the vulva. Classically, the surface keratin is thickened, the epidermis is atrophic and the dermis is abnormally fibrotic. There is an increased risk of developing squamous cell carcinoma.

Endometriosis

Endometriosis a common condition in which endometrial glands and stroma are present in organs other than the uterus (Box 28 and Figure 57). Typical sites of endometriosis include the ovaries, fallopian tubes, uterosacral ligaments, Pouch of Douglas and cervix, but it can occur throughout the peritoneum and even within distant organs such as the lung. The process is not neoplastic but the mechanism(s) by which endometrial tissue establishes itself in these extrauterine sites remains uncertain. Theories include:

* endometrial metaplasia
* retrograde flow through the fallopian tube at menstruation
* implantation after surgery
* bloodstream spread of viable endometrial fragments.

Endometriotic foci may show proliferative and secretory activity in response to oestrogen and progesterone, in the same way as normal uterine endometrium. Endometriosis in the ovary is associated with clear cell adenocarcinoma (see below). The presence of endometrial glands and stroma within the myometrium is called adenomyosis.

Polyps

Polyps are benign polypoid proliferations of glandular epithelium and stroma. They can arise in the endocervix and endometrium and may cause abnormal vaginal bleeding. Endometrial polyps occur most frequently after the menopause, and the incidence is increased in breast carcinoma patients receiving treatment with tamoxifen.

Ovarian cysts

Benign follicle ('follicular') and corpus luteum cysts are very common, but sometimes raise clinical suspicion of malignancy if seen on an ultrasound scan. Multiple bilateral follicular cysts, associated with ovarian enlargement, menstrual irregularities, hirsutism, obesity and infertility, are features of polycystic ovarian disease. The underlying cause seems to be abnormal release of pituitary hormones.

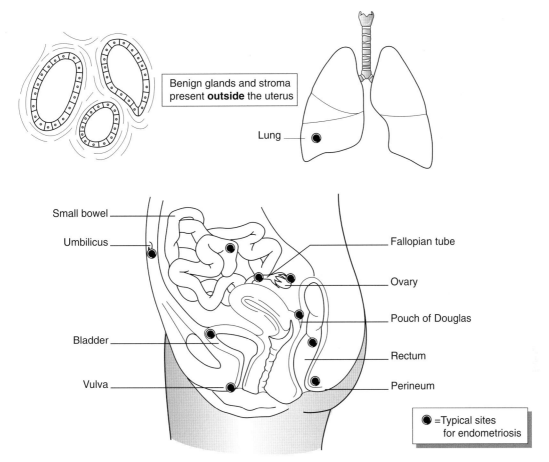

Benign glands and stroma present **outside** the uterus

Lung

Small bowel

Umbilicus

Fallopian tube

Ovary

Pouch of Douglas

Bladder

Rectum

Vulva

Perineum

● =Typical sites for endometriosis

Figure 57 Endometriosis.

21.2 Dysplasia and neoplasia

Learning objectives

You should:
- understand the concepts of dysplasia and intra-epithelial neoplasia in the female genital tract
- understand the principles and practice of the NHS Cervical Screening Programme
- have sufficient knowledge of neoplastic disease of the female genital tract to interpret histopathology reports of these tumours.

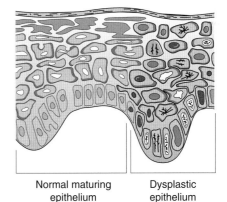

Normal maturing epithelium

Dysplastic epithelium

Figure 58 Dysplastic epithelium.

Dysplasia means abnormal growth. Dysplastic epithelium shows morphological changes of neoplastic cells but without evidence of invasion (Figure 58). Dysplastic changes include:

- increased nuclear to cytoplasmic ratio
- nuclear pleomorphism (variation in size and shape)
- nuclear hyperchromatism (increased intensity of staining)
- abnormal mitoses
- abnormal cellular crowding
- failure of epithelial maturation.

Epithelial dysplasia occurs throughout the lower female genital tract:

- vulval intra-epithelial neoplasia (VIN)
- vaginal intra-epithelial neoplasia (VAIN)
- cervical intra-epithelial neoplasia (CIN)
- cervical glandular intra-epithelial neoplasia (CGIN)
- atypical endometrial hyperplasia.

The intra-epithelial neoplasia of squamous epithelium in the vulva, vagina and cervix (VIN, VAIN and CIN) is

223

numerically graded from 1 to 3, according to the severity of dysplastic changes. Thus, CIN 1 is low-grade cervical dysplasia in which the cellular abnormalities are confined to the lower third of the squamous epithelium. In CIN 3 (high-grade dysplasia, also called carcinoma in situ), the entire thickness of the epithelium is abnormal, showing cytological features of malignant cells. However, there is no invasion of the atypical cells beyond the epithelial basement membrane and so there is no capacity for local spread or distant metastasis. CGIN describes dysplasia of endocervical glandular epithelium, and is classified as either low or high grade.

Abnormal proliferation within the endometrium is known as hyperplasia, and occurs in response to unopposed oestrogen stimulation:

- **simple hyperplasia** – diffuse proliferation of both endometrial glands and stroma
- **complex hyperplasia** – focal glandular proliferation only, no cytological atypia
- **atypical hyperplasia** – glandular proliferation and crowding (usually focal) with atypical cytological changes.

Only atypical hyperplasia is regarded as a high-risk pre-malignant change. Like other adaptive tissue changes, hyperplasia remains under the control of the eliciting stimulus. If the oestrogen excess is neutralised, for example by exogenous progesterone administration, the hyperplasia will regress. Even early stage endometrial carcinoma may be effectively treated in some cases with progestogens rather than surgery.

Cervical screening

The ability to recognise the abnormal cells from dysplastic cervical epithelium forms the basis of the NHS Cervical Screening Programme. All women between the ages of 25 and 65 are invited to have a cervical smear examination every 3–5 years. A brush is used to gently remove cells from the surface of the cervix, ensuring that the cervical os is adequately visualised and the transformation zone is sampled. The cells are examined under the microscope for nuclear changes – enlargement, chromatin abnormalities and nuclear membrane irregularities – which might indicate a dysplastic or malignant lesion. The cytological changes are called dyskaryosis and graded as mild, moderate or severe. The screening programme was originally intended to identify dyskaryosis in the squamous epithelial cells, but it is possible to detect endocervical glandular abnormalities in some cases. Smears that show changes of HPV infection in the absence of dyskaryosis are still regarded as abnormal and warrant further follow-up, in view of the association between HPV and cervical neoplasia. Cytological abnormalities that do not amount to unequivocal dyskaryosis may be described as 'borderline', and again these changes require more regular follow-up smears to exclude significant disease.

The success of the programme depends on the detection and treatment of women with asymptomatic dysplastic lesions (CIN and CGIN) before they progress to invasive carcinoma. The degree of dyskaryosis in the cervical smear

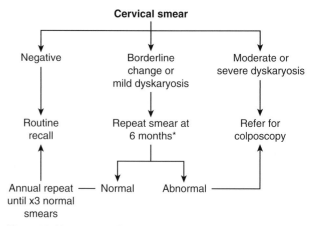

Figure 59 Management of normal and abnormal cervical smears. This is a simplified management scheme. *Mild dyskaryosis may be managed with a repeat smear a 6 months or referred directly to colposcopy.

is an indication of the likely severity of dysplasia in the epithelium. High-grade smear abnormalities or persistent low-grade changes require colposcopic examination of the cervix by a gynaecologist, with tissue biopsy for histological confirmation of dysplasia (Figure 59). Treatment by laser, cold coagulation or tissue resection is followed up with regular smears, until it is safe for the patient to return to routine recall.

As with all screening programmes, there are advantages and disadvantages in participation, with both false-positive and false-negative results possible. False positives may be caused by:

- HPV infection without dysplasia
- cervical inflammation
- degenerate cellular changes that mimic dyskaryosis.

False negatives may result from:

- failure to sample the dysplastic focus within the smear
- small numbers of dyskaryotic cells being 'missed' by the cervical screener
- dyskaryotic cells being misinterpreted by the screener or cytopathologist.

Treatment of dysplastic lesions is not without significant adverse effects, as cervical stenosis secondary to tissue resection or ablation can cause infertility. Not all women with CIN, even of high grade, will definitely progress to invasive carcinoma if left untreated. However, the risk of a CIN lesion progressing to cancer cannot be predicted for individual women.

Neoplasia

Vulva

Cancer is relatively uncommon; the majority are squamous cell carcinomas (>90%) and usually occur in elderly women, but the incidence is increasing in younger women. Prognosis is closely related to spread, especially to inguinal and pelvic lymph nodes. Vulval malignant melanoma is rare, but has a poor prognosis. Extramammary Paget's disease occurs in the vulva and anogenital region. This is an intra-epidermal proliferation of adenocarcinoma cells, which clinically manifests as a well-demarcated, crusted, red lesion. Unlike Paget's disease of the nipple, underlying invasive malignancy is uncommon.

Vagina

Malignant neoplasms are rare. In infants the vagina is a site for embryonal rhabdomyosarcoma. There is an association between clear cell adenocarcinoma of the vagina and exposure to diethylstilboestrol during intrauterine life. Squamous cell carcinoma is the most frequent tumour in adults, but is rarely seen clinically. There is an association with both vulval and cervical carcinoma.

Cervix

Up to 90% of malignancies are squamous cell carcinomas (Table 38); the role of HPV in carcinogenesis, and the role of cervical screening in prevention of cervical cancer have already been discussed. Cervical cancers arise from the junctional region between squamous ectocervical epithelium and columnar endocervix, also known as the transformation zone. Adenocarcinoma accounts for approximately 10% of cervical malignancies, but is increasing in incidence.

Staging of cervical cancer

- Stage I – confined to cervix.
- Stage II – extends beyond cervix but does not involve pelvic wall or lower third of vagina.
- Stage III – involvement of pelvic wall or lower third of vagina.
- Stage IV – extension beyond pelvis or involvement of bladder or rectal mucosa.

Endometrium

Endometrial adenocarcinoma is the commonest invasive tumour of the female genital tract (Table 39).

Myometrium

The commonest neoplasm arising in the female genital tract is the leiomyoma (benign smooth muscle tumour), also known as a 'fibroid'. Growth of leiomyomas is stimulated by oestrogen, hence these are tumours of reproductive life that can grow rapidly in pregnancy but may atrophy after the menopause. Leiomyomas are often multiple and can reach many centimetres in diameter. They can cause pelvic pain, abnormal uterine bleeding, urinary symptoms and infertility or complications of pregnancy. Malignant smooth muscle tumours (leiomyosarcomas) are rare.

Ovary

The ovary can harbour a wide variety of benign and malignant neoplasms (Table 40), the more frequent examples are listed in Box 29. Most adult tumours arise from the surface epithelium of the ovary. In children germ cell tumours predominate. Most ovarian tumours (80%) are benign.

Table 38 Cancer checklist: cervical squamous cell carcinoma

Incidence	Age >20, peak incidence around 40
Risk factors	HPV infection with specific subtypes – multiple sexual partners, male partner with multiple previous partners, early age of first intercourse, smoking, HIV, herpes simplex type 2
Protective factors	Celibacy, barrier contraception
Associated lesions	High grade CIN
Clinical presentation	Abnormal vaginal bleeding, pain/bleeding after sexual intercourse
Location	Initially arises in transformation zone
Macroscopic appearance	Exophytic, ulcerating or infiltrative mass
Histological features	Squamous cells +/– keratinisation
Pattern of spread	Local spread to uterine body, vagina, pelvic wall, bladder, ureters and rectum
	Local and distant lymph nodes
	Distant metastases in liver and lung
Prognosis (per cent 5-year survival)	Stage I 80–90%
	Stage IV 10–15%
	Advanced tumours often cause death through renal tract obstruction

Table 39 Cancer checklist: endometrial carcinoma

Incidence	Age >40, usually post-menopausal
Risk factors	Excessive oestrogen exposure – early menarche and late menopause, nulliparity, obesity (increased oestrogen production in peripheral fat), family history, diabetes, hypertension, oestrogen-producing tumours
Protective factors	Ovarian agenesis or removal
Associated lesions	Atypical endometrial hyperplasia
Clinical presentation	Abnormal vaginal bleeding (often post-menopausal)
Location	Anywhere in endometrium
Macroscopic appearance	Polypoid or diffuse growth pattern
Histological features	Mild, moderately or poorly differentiated according to the extent of glandular and solid growth pattern
	Aggressive subtypes: clear cell carcinoma; serous papillary carcinoma
Pattern of spread	Myometrium, cervix and pelvic organs
	Lymph nodes
Prognosis (per cent 5-year survival)	Most cases are Stage I (confined to uterus) and well or moderately differentiated, with 90% survival
	Extrauterine spread, poor differentiation or aggressive histological subtypes have worse prognosis (20–50% survival)

Twenty one

Table 40 Cancer checklist: ovarian malignancy

Incidence	Carcinoma >40 years
	Malignant germ cell tumours <30 years
Risk factors	Abnormal gonadal development
	Nulliparity
	Family history
	BRCA1 gene
Protective factors	Oral contraceptive use
Associated lesions	Breast cancer in *BRCA1*-related cases
Clinical presentation	Abdominal mass/pain, hormonal symptoms
Location	20–65% of carcinomas are bilateral, germ cell malignancies usually unilateral
Macroscopic appearance	Partly cystic or solid masses, papillary areas, necrosis and haemorrhage
Histological features	Very variable, according to tumour type
Pattern of spread	Into peritoneal cavity – ascites
	Contralateral ovary, omentum, local lymph nodes, lung, liver
Prognosis	Carcinomas dependent on stage – spread beyond ovary usually means poor outcome
	Some germ cell tumours respond well to chemoradiotherapy

However, ovarian malignancies cause more deaths than all other female genital-tract cancers combined. See Box 30 for clinical features.

Surface epithelial tumours

Surface epithelial tumours are the most frequent. Histologically, they show serous, mucinous, transitional or endometrial differentiation. Benign tumours are often cystic. Malignant tumours may be partly cystic and partly solid. Tumours may affect both ovaries, especially with serous neoplasms. Prognosis of carcinomas largely depends on stage. Clinical presentation in the majority of cases is late, and many carcinomas have reached an advanced stage at diagnosis. There is also a group of 'borderline' tumours – these show cytological features of carcinoma (loss of cell polarity, hyperchromatic nuclei, abnormal mitoses) but without evidence of stromal invasion. Borderline tumours usually behave in a benign fashion or show low malignant potential.

Germ cell tumours

Germ cell tumours are a diverse group of lesions, the commonest of which is the benign dermoid cyst (mature cystic teratoma). The tumour consists of differentiated somatic tissues, and may include skin, with sebaceous glands and hair, teeth, fat, bone, cartilage, nervous tissue, respiratory epithelium and thyroid epithelium. Malignant germ cell tumours include yolk sac tumour, dysgerminoma (the

---

Box 29 Ovarian tumours

Surface epithelial tumours (70%)
Benign:

- serous cystadenoma
- mucinous cystadenoma
- Brenner (transitional cell) tumour

Borderline (low malignant potential):

- serous borderline tumour
- mucinous borderline tumour
- serous cystadenocarcinoma

Malignant:

- serous adenocarcinoma
- mucinous adenocarcinoma
- endometrioid adenocarcinoma
- clear cell carcinoma

Germ cell tumours (20%)
Benign:

- cystic teratoma ('dermoid cyst')

Malignant:

- yolk sac tumour
- dysgerminoma
- choriocarcinoma (non-gestational)

Stromal tumours (10%):*

- fibroma, thecoma
- granulosa cell tumour
- Sertoli–Leydig cell tumours

*Also called sex cord–stromal tumours; most cases are benign but a small proportion of each of these lesions will show malignant behaviour.

Box 30 Clinical notes: presentation of ovarian tumours

- Abdominal mass (tumour itself ± ascitic fluid)
- Pain/discomfort
- Symptoms related to hormone production (abnormal vaginal bleeding in oestrogen-producing tumours; masculinisation if excess androgens are produced)
- Raised serum CA125 or ovarian mass on pelvic ultrasound in women at risk of carcinoma (e.g. families with known *BRCA1* gene)

---

female equivalent of seminoma) and choriocarcinoma (trophoblastic differentiation).

Stromal tumours

Stromal tumours are less common. Most are benign, but they may cause symptoms due to hormone production. Granulosa cell tumours, thecomas and fibromas can secrete oestrogens, and they may be associated with endometrial hyperplasia or carcinoma. Some stromal tumours can produce androgens and clinically present with masculinisation. These include Sertoli–Leydig cell tumours and hilus cell tumours.

Metastatic tumours

Metastatic tumours form a small proportion of ovarian tumours. They may arise from primaries elsewhere in the female genital tract. The most frequent distant primary source of ovarian metastases is the breast. Bilateral ovarian enlargement due to metastatic adenocarcinoma from the gastrointestinal tract (particularly stomach) is known as Krukenberg's tumour.

21.3 Pathology related to pregnancy

Learning objectives

You should:
- understand the terms pre-eclampsia, gestational trophoblastic disease and hydatidiform mole
- know the possible causes of spontaneous abortion.

Ectopic pregnancy

Extrauterine implantation of the fetus occurs in approximately 1 in 150 pregnancies. The fallopian tube is by far the commonest site; predisposing factors include pelvic inflammatory disease and previous tubal surgery. Tubal pregnancy frequently ruptures within the first trimester, with serious intraperitoneal haemorrhage. Ectopic pregnancy is also associated with a greater risk of hydatidiform mole (see below).

Spontaneous abortion

Early pregnancy loss (before the fetus is viable) can result from:

- chromosomal abnormalities
- congenital abnormalities
- uterine or placental malformations and abnormalities, including fibroids and cervical incompetence
- infections, including toxoplasmosis, listeriosis, mycoplasmosis and viral diseases.

Pre-eclampsia

Pre-eclampsia is the development of proteinuria, hypertension and oedema in late pregnancy. It is associated with young maternal age, twin pregnancy, diabetes, chronic hypertension and a history of pre-eclampsia in previous gestations. Central to the pathogenesis is defective uteroplacental blood circulation. This probably arises from failure of trophoblastic tissue to adequately invade the maternal spiral arterioles, resulting in placental ischaemia. Imbalance of arachidonic acid metabolites (prostacyclin and thromboxane) have also been identified and immune-related mechanisms may be important in some cases. Management includes monitoring, bed rest and antihypertensive medication. Delivery is curative, and may be expedited by caesarean section. Some cases may progress to eclampsia, a serious condition characterised by fits and disseminated intravascular coagulation.

Gestational trophoblastic disease

Gestational trophoblastic disease is a group of conditions characterised by abnormal proliferation of trophoblastic tissue.

Hydatidiform mole

Hydatidiform mole is composed of abnormal chorionic villi, which are enlarged and oedematous with excess cytotrophoblast and syncytiotrophoblast. There are partial and complete forms of mole. Both contain an abnormal karyotype. In complete mole, all of the genetic material is derived from paternal chromosomes (46 XX). Partial moles have triploidy with an extra set of paternal chromosomes (69 XXY). There is a marked geographical variation in incidence, with much higher rates in Asian than European or North American populations. Women over the age of 50 also have a greatly increased risk.

Molar pregnancy clinically presents in the mid-trimester of pregnancy with abnormal uterine bleeding, but earlier detection is possible with routine antenatal ultrasound. A fetus may be present in partial moles but not in complete moles. The uterus is often large for dates, and the swollen villi may be detected on scanning or on naked eye examination of aborted tissue passed vaginally. Serum levels of β-human chorionic gonadotrophin are markedly elevated. Serial measurement of this hormone is used in follow-up of treated patients to detect any recurrence or malignant transformation. Occasionally the molar tissue extends deeply into the myometrium and causes uterine rupture. Although hydatidiform mole is the commonest predisposing factor to gestational choriocarcinoma, progression to this neoplasm is rare (2%).

Gestational choriocarcinoma

Gestational choriocarcinoma is a malignant tumour of trophoblast, which develops following hydatidiform mole, abortion, normal pregnancy or ectopic gestation. The malignant trophoblast does not form chorionic villus structures. Gestational choriocarcinoma metastasises widely but is responsive to chemotherapy.

Placental site trophoblastic tumour

Placental site trophoblastic tumour is a rare neoplasm derived from intermediate trophoblast. No chorionic villi structures are formed.

Twenty one

Self-assessment: questions

One best answer questions

1. A 43-year-old woman presents with post-coital bleeding. She had a mildly abnormal cervical smear 8 years earlier, but had not attended for further follow-up smears. At colposcopy, an ulcerated mass is seen at the cervical os. The likely diagnosis is:
   a. squamous cell carcinoma
   b. CIN
   c. CGIN
   d. adenocarcinoma
   e. HSV type 2

True-false questions

1. The following statements are correct:
   a. simple hyperplasia of the endometrium is usually a premalignant lesion
   b. CIN inevitably progresses to invasive carcinoma if left untreated
   c. the incidence of hydatidiform mole shows marked geographical variation
   d. endometriosis frequently involves the ovaries
   e. polypoid growths in the endometrium are always benign

2. HPV infection is associated with the following diseases:
   a. squamous cell carcinoma of the vulva
   b. adenocarcinoma of the cervix
   c. serous cystadenocarcinoma of the ovary
   d. condylomata lata
   e. endometrial hyperplasia

3. Chronic endometritis:
   a. is diagnosed histologically by the presence of lymphocytes in the endometrium
   b. is associated with intrauterine contraceptive devices
   c. can be part of pelvic inflammatory disease
   d. can follow a normal pregnancy
   e. is associated with endometrial carcinoma

4. The following primary malignant tumours commonly arise in the ovary:
   a. cystic teratoma ('dermoid cyst')
   b. Krukenberg's tumour
   c. leiomyoma
   d. choriocarcinoma
   e. embryonal rhabdomyosarcoma

5. Concerning pre-eclampsia:
   a. symptoms begin in early pregnancy
   b. it occurs most commonly in the first pregnancy
   c. it is characterised by hypertension and haematuria
   d. the fetus may be small for dates
   e. the underlying pathology is defective uteroplacental circulation

6. The following are correctly paired:
   a. intrauterine contraceptive devices – *Actinomyces* infection
   b. toxic shock syndrome – *Neisseria gonorrhoeae*
   c. infertility – endometriosis
   d. nulliparity – ovarian carcinoma
   e. smoking – squamous cell carcinoma of the cervix

Case history questions

Case history 1

A 68-year-old woman presents to her general practitioner with post-menopausal bleeding. She is mildly obese and diabetic. Her previous cervical smear tests have been normal. She was diagnosed with breast cancer 3 years ago and has been taking tamoxifen.

1. What is the likely diagnosis?
2. What diagnostic procedure should be performed?

Case history 2

A 26-year-old woman attends the casualty department with acute abdominal pain. On questioning she describes her menstrual cycle as irregular. She has a previous history of pelvic inflammatory disease.

1. What differential diagnoses should you consider?
2. What immediate investigations are appropriate?

Viva questions

1. Discuss the advantages and disadvantages of a population-screening programme for cervical carcinoma.
2. How does pathological examination contribute to the management of patients with ovarian cancer?

Self-assessment: answers

One best answer

1. a. Over 90% of invasive cancers in the cervix are squamous cell carcinomas; most of the remainder are adenocarcinomas. CIN and CGIN are dysplastic lesions (intra-epithelial neoplasia); they do not present as mass lesions.

True-false answers

1. a. **False.** Simple hyperplasia without atypia is rarely associated with subsequent endometrial carcinoma. There is a much greater risk of atypical hyperplasia progressing to invasive malignancy.
   b. **False.** The natural history of CIN is not fully known. Some, but not all, cases of high-grade CIN will progress to invasive carcinoma over a variable period of time. Lower-grade CIN may progress, remain stable, or regress. It is not possible to predict the risk of progression for an individual patient.
   c. **True.**
   d. **True.**
   e. **False.** Most polyps in the endometrium are benign growths of endometrial glands and stroma. Submucosal leiomyomas (fibroids) can also project into the uterine cavity. However, endometrial carcinoma frequently has a partly exophytic polypoid growth pattern.

2. a. **True.** HPV is associated with squamous cell carcinoma of the vulva, vagina, cervix, anus and non-genital skin.
   b. **True.** HPV DNA can be detected with similar high frequency in both squamous and glandular carcinomas of the cervix.
   c. **False.**
   d. **False.** Condylomata lata are genital lesions seen in secondary syphilis. Condylomata acuminata are HPV-related genital warts.
   e. **False.**

3. a. **False.** Lymphocytes can be seen in normal endometrium. Plasma cells are required for the diagnosis of chronic endometritis.
   b. **True.**
   c. **True.**
   d. **True.** Retained placental material following normal vaginal delivery can become chronically inflamed.
   e. **False.**

4. a. **False.** Cystic teratomas do occur in the ovary, but these are benign germ cell neoplasms.
   b. **False.** Krukenberg's tumours are bilateral ovarian metastases, usually from gastric adenocarcinomas. The most common ovarian metastases, however, arise from primary malignancies elsewhere in the female genital tract or from the pelvic peritoneum.
   c. **False.** Leiomyomas are benign smooth muscle neoplasms, which are very common in the myometrium.
   d. **True.** Choriocarcinoma can arise as a non-gestational germ cell tumour in the ovary, or as a pregnancy-related uterine malignancy.
   e. **False.** This rare malignant skeletal muscle tumour occurs in the vagina in young girls.

5. a. **False.** Symptoms begin in the third trimester.
   b. **True.**
   c. **False.** Hypertension, proteinuria and oedema are characteristic.
   d. **True.**
   e. **True.**

6. a. **True.**
   b. **False.** The causative agent is *Staphylococcus aureus*.
   c. **True.**
   d. **True.**
   e. **True.**

Case history answers

Case history 1

1. Abnormal vaginal bleeding may be:
   - intermenstrual
   - post-coital
   - due to irregular menstrual cycles, often peri-menarchal and perimenopausal
   - due to menorrhagia (heavy prolonged periods)
   - post-menopausal.

There are many potential causes, including benign and malignant tumours and pregnancy-related bleeding. Abnormal bleeding during the reproductive years is most frequently related to altered oestrogen and progesterone balance (dysfunctional uterine bleeding), including anovulatory cycles and inadequate corpus luteum function. Post-coital bleeding is a classic symptom of cervical carcinoma, although benign causes are more commonly responsible. Post-menopausal bleeding – other than that related to hormone replacement therapy – suggests the presence of an endometrial polyp, endometrial hyperplasia or endometrial carcinoma.

Relevant risk factors for carcinoma include diabetes and obesity. Tamoxifen is a drug used successfully in breast cancer; it blocks oestrogen receptors on breast tumour cells. However, tamoxifen has a stimulatory effect on the endometrium, promoting growth. An increased incidence of both endometrial hyperplasia and carcinoma has been attributed to tamoxifen use, and this may limit the length of time that the drug is given to women who have not had a hysterectomy.

2. The nature of any endometrial pathology must be established. Ultrasound scan may demonstrate increased endometrial thickness or a mass lesion. Histological sampling is necessary for definitive diagnosis. Suction biopsy may be performed by the general practitioner or in an out-patient clinic, but the tissue yield can be very low. More extensive material can be obtained by dilatation and curettage under general anaesthesia.

Case history 2

1. Potential serious causes of acute abdominal pain in a woman of this age include appendicitis, cholecystitis and ruptured ectopic pregnancy. Other possible gynaecological causes include endometriosis, an exacerbation of pelvic inflammatory disease, ovarian torsion and 'mittelschmerz' (cramping pain experienced in the middle of the menstrual cycle, due to ovulation).

2. It is vital to ascertain whether there is any chance of pregnancy and perform a pregnancy test. Ruptured tubal ectopic pregnancy occurs in the first trimester. It is a surgical emergency, and can cause shock with life-threatening intraperitoneal haemorrhage. The woman may be unaware of her pregnancy. Ultrasound scan helps confirm the diagnosis, as no gestational sac is identified within the uterus. The tubal abnormality might also be visualised. Often there is a little vaginal bleeding, which adds to the initial clinical suspicion of a ruptured ectopic gestation.

Viva answers

1. *Comment*: Be prepared to describe the pathological basis for cervical screening and to outline the management of a patient with an abnormal smear (Figure 59). You should know potential causes for false-positive and false-negative results and ways of minimising these – such as proper training of smear takers, cytoscreeners and pathologists, and regular audit.

2. Pathological examination is necessary for accurate initial diagnosis of ovarian carcinoma, either through ovarian histology or cytology of ascitic fluid. Histological examination of cancer resection specimens provides prognostic information, particularly related to tumour stage – spread to other organs and lymph nodes – and histological tumour type. Cytological examination of peritoneal washings obtained at operation forms part of the staging investigation. Serum tumour markers are specific proteins elaborated by the neoplasm, which can be helpful in initial diagnosis and during follow-up of treated patients to detect recurrent disease. Markers include CA125 in surface epithelial carcinomas, α-fetoprotein in yolk sac tumour and β-hCG in choriocarcinoma.

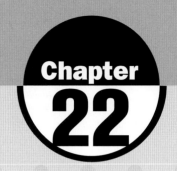

Male genital tract

Chapter overview

The male genital tract consists principally of the penis, foreskin, testes, epididymes and prostate gland. A large range of disease processes affect the male genital tract, but inflammation and tumours are probably the most important clinically. Malignancies of the testis and prostate are particularly common tumours and it is important that you have a working knowledge of these. Sexually transmitted diseases (STDs) are also seen and may affect a variety of organs in the male genital tract. Congenital diseases are also common and vary from the relatively insignificant (overly long foreskin) to the very significant (e.g. the maldescended testis with the associated increased risk of malignancy).

22.1 The penis and scrotum

Learning objectives

You should:
- know the basic anatomy of the penis
- have a working understanding of the common congenital and acquired disorders, in particular inflammatory and malignant diseases.

The penis is a skin-covered organ (as is the scrotum) and can therefore exhibit many of the common skin disorders (e.g. eczema/dermatitis). In addition, the penile urethra may be susceptible to tumours of the urothelium (proximally) and squamous epithelium (distally).

Congenital disorders

Abnormalities include an excessively small penis (micropenis) or a urethra that opens either on the ventral (under) surface (hypospadias) or dorsal surface (epispadias) of the penis rather than at the tip.

Acquired disorders

Inflammatory disorders

Many inflammatory skin conditions can occur in the penis, foreskin and scrotum, such as eczema, psoriasis and lichen planus. In addition, more specific inflammatory diseases may cause penile (skin) inflammation.

Granuloma inguinale

Granuloma inguinale is caused by the Gram-negative bacillus *Calymmatobacterium granulomatis*. This is an STD and causes an ulcer on the glans.

Lymphogranuloma venereum

Lymphogranuloma venereum is an STD caused by *Chlamydia trachomatis* (which also causes non-specific urethritis). Males may be asymptomatic carriers of the organism. The infection causes a spontaneously healing red papule on the penis. Enlarged lymph nodes in the groin then develop, which then become soft and attach to the overlying skin. Sinus formation occurs.

Syphilis (caused by the spirochaete, *Treponema pallidum*), herpes simplex and human papilloma virus (HPV) are all important causes of penile infection (see Table 41).

Peyronie's disease is a penile disease of unknown cause in which the penis becomes excessively curved or bowed due to accumulation of scar tissue (the curvature may make sexual intercourse impossible).

Tumours

The penis can be affected by both in situ and invasive (squamous) malignancies. Benign tumours of the penis are rare.

Intra-epithelial neoplasia

Unfortunately, there are three very confusing historical names for intra-epithelial dysplasia in the region of the penis and scrotum (see Table 42).

Squamous cell carcinoma

This is a relatively rare tumour in Western countries (and very rare in circumcised males), but occur more frequently in parts of Asia and Africa. A poorly retracting infected foreskin and infected glans are probably risk factors. There is an association between HPV 16 and 18 infection and

Table 41 Penile infections

Infection	Organism	Clinical features
Syphilis	*Treponema pallidum* (bacterium, spirochaete)	Rare Penis usually involved in primary syphilis ('chancre' seen – nodule on penis). Heals after about 1 month Penis can be involved in secondary syphilis (papular rash)
Herpes simplex	Herpes simplex virus (herpes virus)	Common Painful recurrent blisters/ulcers on penile skin May last 2–3 weeks then resolve Virus can remain latent in sacral sensory ganglia and reactivate/recur
Human papilloma virus	Human papilloma virus (HPV; papillomavirus)	Causes condylomata acuminata ('venereal warts') Especially types 6 and 11 Types 16 and 18 can cause premalignant and malignant conditions
Chancroid	*Haemophilus ducreyi*	Rare Penile ulceration and inguinal lymphadenopathy

Table 42 Carcinoma in situ of the penis

On glans	On shaft	Glans + shaft
Erythroplasia of Queyrat	Bowen's disease	Bowenoid papulosis
Red patches	Pale, thickened areas	Velvety papules (younger men)
		HPV-associated in most cases

squamous cell carcinoma. The tumour may vary from a papillary and well-differentiated malignancy with abundant keratin formation to a solid, ulcerated, widely invasive, poorly differentiated lesion (which spreads via lymphatics to local lymph nodes).

Verrucous carcinoma

Verrucous carcinoma is the name given to a (very) well-differentiated, squamous cell carcinoma with surface papillae and a deep, rounded, bulbous growth pattern. It is believed to be caused by HPV.

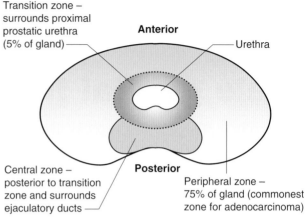

Figure 60 The zones of the prostate gland.

22.2 The prostate

> **Learning objectives**
>
> You should:
> * understand the basic anatomical relations and zones of the prostate
> * understand benign prostatic hyperplasia and carcinoma of the prostate.

The prostate is a 20 g, walnut-shaped gland located in the male perineum. The exact function of the gland is still unclear. The gland lies subjacent to the bladder and is traversed by the urethra. Any enlargement of the prostate gland, particularly that part surrounding the urethra (see Figure 60 for zones of the prostate), can lead to reduction/obstruction of flow of urine –dribbling, hesitancy, poor stream or complete blockage (retention). The prostate is composed of glandular and fibromuscular components, and it is hyperplasia/hypertrophy of both of these elements and malignancy of the glandular elements that commonly lead to urinary symptoms.

Hyperplasia of the prostate

This is such a common finding in adult men that it is often considered to be a normal part of ageing (probably about 80% of 80-year-olds will have evidence of prostatic hyperplasia). The prostate has a nodular, whorled appearance to the naked eye (nodular hyperplasia). It is mainly the periurethral and transition zones that are affected. Down the microscope, the glandular and/or stromal components may be affected. The glands may become papillary in form, or cystically dilated. However, hyperplastic glands have two cell layers – an inner clear cell layer and an outer, more darkly staining, basal cell layer. Hyperplasia of the prostate is often accompanied by areas of infarction, chronic inflammation and glandular atrophy.

Acute and chronic prostatitis can also occur in the setting of urinary tract infection (UTI) with organisms such as *Escherichia coli*, *Pseudomonas* and *Klebsiella*.

Table 43 Cancer checklist: Prostatic adenocarcinoma

Incidence	Age >50 years (very common in >80-year-olds)
Risk factors	Black men > white men > Asians + family history
	?fats in diet
	?androgen-driven
Associated lesions	High-grade PIN (particularly multifocal)
Clinical presentation	Incidental finding
	Urinary symptoms
Diagnosis	Per rectal examination, ultrasound scan and biopsy
	Blood levels of prostatic-specific antigen (PSA)
Macroscopic	Usually invisible to the naked eye
Microscopic	Gleason scoring system (see Table 44)
Pattern of spread	Local versus lymphatic versus blood
Treatment	Carefully supervised 'watch and wait' (small intraprostatic lesions)
	Surgery
	Radiotherapy

Table 44 The Gleason grading system

Gleason grade (or pattern)	Characteristics
1	**Uncommon**
	Very round, regular, monotonous, closely packed glands
	Well circumscribed
2	Similar to 1, *but* less circumscribed, some variation in gland size and shape
3	**Commonest grade**
	May be small or large glands or cribriform (sieve-like) pattern
	May be marked variation in size/shape of glands
	Ragged edges and infiltrates widely
4	Glands now fused together
	Nests and streams of cells seen
5	Large sheets of malignant cells
	Necrosis may be seen
	May be very undifferentiated

Chronic granulomatous prostatitis can be due to tuberculosis but is often idiopathic and possibly due to an inflammatory response to ruptured ducts.

Carcinoma of the prostate

Carcinoma of the prostate is a very common malignancy. The biological behaviour of this tumour is poorly understood – a significant number of latent and incidental cancers are found at autopsy or in tissue removed at operation on an apparently benign prostate (e.g. transurethral resection of the prostate, TURP). Thus, it is likely that some prostatic cancers either never progress or only do so very slowly. The disease is more common in older men (particularly those aged over 60) and is seen more often in black men than in white men or Asian men. A small number of prostatic cancers appear familial. Most cases (about 70%) arise in the peripheral zone of the prostate.

Macroscopically, it is usually difficult to see prostatic cancer (it may or may not cause gland enlargement). On microscopy, prostatic cancer is usually an adenocarcinoma (although leiomyosarcoma and lymphoma occur, and rhabdomyosarcoma may be seen in children; Table 43). The Gleason grading system is now widely used for prostatic adenocarcinoma. This system depends on the glandular differentiation and pattern of infiltration of the tumour (see Table 44).

The higher the Gleason score (achieved by adding together the commonest two patterns or doubling a single pattern tumour) the more poorly differentiated the tumour. There is a correlation between the score of the tumour and its biological behaviour (the higher the score, the higher the cancer mortality rate). The tumour may be associated with high-grade prostatic intra-epithelial neoplasia (PIN; thought to be a likely precursor lesion). Adenocarcinoma of the prostate typically invades locally through the gland and into surrounding pelvic tissues and then by lymphatics to local/regional lymph nodes. Prostatic cancer has a propensity to metastasise via the bloodstream to bones (particularly the spine).

22.3 The testis and epididymis

Learning objectives
You should:
- have a working knowledge of the histology of the testis
- be familiar with the basic classification of testicular tumours.

The testis

Each testis is composed of densely packed, coiled seminiferous tubules, which are lined by Sertoli cells (regulatory cells) and germ cells (which mature into spermatozoa). In the normal adult testis, luminal spermatozoa are seen. Between the tubules lies the interstitium, which has the Leydig cells. These cells secrete testosterone under the influence of luteinising hormone from the anterior pituitary gland.

Congenital abnormalities of the testis

The immature (prepubertal) testis has small seminiferous tubules, which contain mainly Sertoli cells and only a very small number of germ cells.

Cryptorchidism

In this condition, the testis (most cases are unilateral) stops somewhere along the normal pathway of descent and fails to reach the scrotum. The testis may be found in the inguinal canal or abdomen. The most serious consequence of this is the increased risk of development of testicular cancer (about 10 times that of a normal, scrotum-sited testis). Even when surgical correction is done there is still a small increased risk of malignancy.

Torsion

Torsion of the testis, i.e. twisting of the spermatic cord, leading to vascular (most often venous) obstruction of the testis, is usually caused by a congenital, structural abnormality of the testis and may lead to haemorrhagic necrosis.

Inflammatory conditions

Inflammation of the epididymis is more common than the testis. There may be severe pain in the scrotal area. Non-specific epididymitis and orchitis are usually associated with UTIs. Causative bacteria include *E. coli* in older men and *Neisseria gonorrhoeae* in young adults.

Histologically, non-specific acute/acute-on-chronic inflammation may be seen, together with abscess formation and, eventually, scarring.

Table 45 Classification of germ cell tumours of the testis

British Testicular Tumour Panel	WHO
Seminoma	Seminoma
Classical	Typical
Spermatocytic	Spermatocytic
Malignant teratoma	
Undifferentiated (MTU)	Embryonal carcinoma and teratoma
Intermediate (MTI)	Teratoma, mature/immature/with malignant transformation
Differentiated (MTD)	Choriocarcinoma
Trophoblastic (MTT)	Yolk sac tumour

Table 46 Germ cell tumours of the testis

	Seminoma	Embryonal carcinoma	Yolk sac tumour	Choriocarcinoma	Teratoma
Behaviour	Low-grade malignancy	Aggressive	Variable	Very aggressive	Variable
Frequency	Commonest type of germ cell tumour		Commonest testicular tumour in infants (pure form). Usually mixed with embryonal carcinoma in adults	Rare	Common in infants to adults but pure forms common in infants. Adults – usually mixed
Naked eye appearance	Large, white mass	Variegated appearance with haemorrhage and necrosis	Yellowish, mucinous appearance	Small haemorrhagic nodule	Large, cystic solid masses
Microscopy	Large cells with large nuclei and clear cytoplasm. Well-demarcated cell membranes. Fibrous septae with chronic inflammatory cells	Large, pleomorphic overlapping cells with numerous mitoses	Lacy lines of tumour cells. Pink globules (containing α-fetoprotein and α_1-antitrypsin, seen in and outside cells	Cytotrophoblastic and syncytiotrophoblastic cells seen (latter contain human chorionic gonadotrophin)	Haphazard arrangement of often mature tissues such as cartilage, muscle, neural tissue, fat, etc. Rarely a focus of squamous cell carcinoma or adenocarcinoma may be seen (malignant transformation)

NB: Testicular germ cell tumours secrete hormones/enzymes/proteins into the patient's blood and these can be used as a 'marker' for progression/response to treatment/relapse of the tumour. Examples include α-fetoprotein, human chorionic gonadotrophin and lactate dehydrogenase. Treatment/prognosis of these tumours depends on histology and extent of spread. Options include surgery alone, or with chemoradiotherapy.

Granulomatous orchitis is thought to be an autoimmune reaction. The testis may be tender and granulomas are seen in and around the seminiferous tubules. Tuberculosis (also causing a granulomatous orchitis), mumps virus and syphilis can all affect the testis.

Testicular tumours

Testicular tumours are an important cause of morbidity and mortality in young and middle-aged men. There is a wide range of tumours of the testis and the nomenclature can be confusing and, unfortunately, different systems are used in different parts of the world. Most testicular tumours present as painless enlargement of the testis.

Broadly speaking, tumours of the testis can be divided into two groups:

- germ cell tumours (about 90%)
- non-germ cell tumours.

Germ cell tumours

These can be:

- seminomas
- non-seminomatous tumours
- combined seminomas and non-seminomatous tumours.

Classification of germ cell tumours of the testis

The two main classification systems are the World Health Organization (WHO) system and the British system (Table 45).

Both systems are based on recognition of the wide spectrum of morphological patterns seen in germ cell tumours (Table 46). It is believed that the precursor lesion for most germ cell tumours is intratubular germ cell neoplasia. In this condition, large, pleomorphic, vacuolated malignant cells are seen in atrophic (non-spermatozoa-producing) seminiferous tubules (often seen around invasive germ cell tumours).

Germ cell tumours tend to spread initially by lymphatics to the iliac and retroperitoneal (para-aortic) lymph nodes. Bloodstream spread occurs to the lungs, liver, bones and brain. Clinical staging of germ cell tumour is shown in Table 47.

Table 47 Staging of germ cell tumours

Stage	Definition
PT0	Histological scar in testis
PTis	Intratubular germ cell neoplasia
T1	Tumour confined to testis/epididymis No lymphatic/vascular invasion Tunica albuginea may be invaded
T2	As for T1, *but* lymphatic/vascular invasion seen or tumour extends through tunica albuginea and invades tunica vaginalis
T3	Tumour invades spermatic cord ± lymphatic or vascular invasion
T4	Tumour invades scrotum ± lymphatic or vascular invasion
N0	No regional lymph node metastasis
N1	Metastasis with a lymph node mass ≤2 cm and up to five positive nodes (≤2 cm)
N2	Lymph node mass >2 cm but ≤5 cm, or more than five positive nodes (≤5 cm), or extranodal tumour spread
N3	Lymph node mass >5 cm
M0	No distant metastases
M1	Distant metastases
M1a	Non-regional lymph nodes or lung
M1b	Other sites

Other testicular tumours

Other testicular tumours include sex cord stromal tumours, Sertoli cell tumours and lymphomas.

Epididymis

The epididymis is posterolateral to the testis and functions to store, concentrate and transport spermatozoa. The epididymis is most often affected by inflammatory conditions (epididymitis). This may then affect the testis (epididymoorchitis). The inflammation is often bacterial in origin (*E. coli*, *Gonococcus* or *Chlamydia*).

Twenty two

Self-assessment: questions

One best answer questions

1. Which of the following statements regarding the prostate gland is correct?
   a. prostatic carcinoma is usually apparent on macroscopic examination of the gland
   b. prostatic carcinoma is most common in Asian men
   c. prostatic hyperplasia is evident in 30% of men by the age of 80
   d. malignant prostatic glands are composed of two cell layers
   e. prostatic hyperplasia mainly affects the central region of the gland

True-false questions

1. Germ cell tumours of the testis:
   a. are most common in the over 70s
   b. may be associated with in situ malignancy
   c. can produce human chorionic gonadotrophin (hCG)
   d. are of uniformly poor prognosis
   e. commonly spread by the lymphatics

2. Prostatic adenocarcinoma:
   a. may be incidental
   b. is the only cause of a raised serum prostatic-specific antigen (PSA)
   c. is usually centrally located in the prostate gland
   d. has a predilection for metastasising to bone
   e. is staged using the Gleason system

3. The following statements are correctly paired:
   a. maldescent of the testis – increased risk of testicular lymphoma
   b. squamous cell carcinoma of the foreskin – circumcised men
   c. epididymitis – E. coli urinary tract infection
   d. spermatocytic seminoma – widespread metastases
   e. yolk sac tumour – α-fetoprotein (AFP) production

4. The following statements are correct:
   a. testicular torsion is usually painless
   b. balanitis xerotica obliterans is similar to lichen sclerosus
   c. epispadias is a condition of the epididymis
   d. cancer of the glans penis is usually a squamous cell carcinoma
   e. a poorly differentiated prostatic adenocarcinoma would have a Gleason score of about 8–10

Case history questions

Case history 1

A 30-year-old man noticed a steadily enlarging, painless lump in his right testis. He had no significant medical or surgical history. His general practitioner refers him for an urgent ultrasound examination. This showed a cystic and solid tumour mass. Special blood tests were performed. The following day his right testis was removed.

1. What are the likely differential diagnoses?
2. What is the most likely diagnosis now and what 'special blood tests' would have been done?

Histology showed a malignant teratoma and areas of classical seminoma.

3. What does the term teratoma mean?

Case history 2

A 93-year-old man presented to his general practitioner having noticed a hard, painless lump under his foreskin. He did not know how long the lump had been there. On examination, he had a craggy 15 mm mass under the foreskin.

1. What is the likely diagnosis? What are the risk factors for this?

He was referred to a urologist who did a biopsy. The report read: 'This is an ulcerated, invasive, moderately differentiated squamous cell carcinoma. Tumour is seen in lymphatic channels . . .'.

2. Where is the tumour likely to spread?

Short note questions

Write short notes on:

1. Testicular swellings/tumours.
2. Prostatic adenocarcinoma.
3. Penile cancer.
4. Principles of grading and staging – use the male genital tract to illustrate your answer.

Viva questions

1. What are the risk factors for prostatic/testicular cancer?
2. What is the definition of teratoma (versus hamartoma)?
3. What are the methods of monitoring effects of treatment in prostatic and testicular cancer?

Self-assessment: answers

One best answer

1. e. Prostatic hyperplasia mainly affects the central region of the gland, in contrast with carcinoma, which usually arises in the gland periphery. As hyperplasia affects the central periurethral region, it often presents with symptoms of urinary obstruction. Hyperplasia affects the majority of older men (probably 80% by 80 years of age). Benign prostate glands (normal or hyperplastic) have two layers – a basal outer layer and an inner luminal cell layer. Malignant prostatic glands are composed of only one layer. Prostatic carcinoma is commoner in black and white men than in Asian men. It often cannot be seen on naked-eye examination of the gland.

True-false answers

1. a. **False.** Germ cell tumours of the testis are commonest in the 15–40-year-old age group. In fact, testicular tumours in men over the age of 70 are quite unusual – many turn out to be lymphomas.

   b. **True.** In many cases, in situ germ cell tumour (germ cell tumour confined inside the seminiferous tubules) will be seen around the periphery of the frankly invasive tumour. The tubules containing the tumour cells are usually atrophic (showing no spermatogenesis).

   c. **True.** Testicular seminomas may contain giant cells and syncytial-like cells (i.e. resembling normal human placental tissues) and human chorionic gonadotrophin is contained in, and secreted by, these cells. This can lead to a modestly elevated level of hCG in the blood of these patients. In addition, choriocarcinoma, a highly malignant tumour made up of cytotrophoblast and syncytiotrophoblast (again tissue seen in the normal human placenta), can cause a massive outpouring of hCG into the bloodstream (since urinary hCG is the basis of the pregnancy test, it is therefore possible for a man to have a positive pregnancy test). Markers like hCG can be used to monitor the success of treatment (has all the hCG-producing tumour been removed and the level therefore fallen to baseline?) and relapse (the level did fall to baseline but now it has risen again – is there a new tumour somewhere in the body?).

   d. **False.** The prognosis for many of the testicular germ cell tumours is excellent. For instance the survival for a stage I (testis-confined) seminoma is almost 100%.

   e. **True.** Germ cell tumours spread by the lymphatics and bloodstream. The common lymph node groups involved are the retroperitoneal para-aortic lymph nodes (further spread to the mediastinal and supraclavicular lymph nodes then occurs). Blood spread is to lungs, liver, central nervous system and bones.

2. a. **True.** Carcinoma of the prostate is a very common malignancy. A small, but significant, number of tumours are found incidentally (e.g. when prostatectomy tissue is examined under a microscope during life or after autopsy).

   b. **False.** An elevated PSA in the blood is not only malignancy related. Prostatitis, and digital examination/instrumentation of the prostate are among other causes of a raised blood PSA (there is still much controversy whether PSA should be used as a screening test for prostatic cancer).

   c. **False.** About 70% of cases of prostatic cancer are found in the peripheral part of the gland (usually posteriorly, hence the importance of good digital rectal examination of the prostate).

   d. **True.** Prostate cancer tends to spread initially locally through the capsule into surrounding nearby structures such as the seminal vesicles and bladder. Lymphatic spread may occur to the obturator, perivesical, iliac and para-aortic lymph node groups and by the bloodstream to bone (remember that cancers of the breast, kidney, thyroid, lung and prostate have a tendency to metastasise to bone). Prostatic metastases tend to induce new bone formation (i.e. they are osteoblastic).

   e. **False.** Gleason is a grading system *not* a staging system.

3. a. **False.** Abnormalities of the descent of the testis are associated with an increased risk of germ cell tumours, not lymphomas.

   b. **False.** Uncircumcised men have an increased risk of carcinoma of the foreskin/glans.

   c. **True.**

   d. **False.** Spermatocytic seminomas are a special category of seminoma. They are often found in older men and are composed of a mixed population of cells, which look like various sperm precursors. In situ germ cell tumour is not associated with these tumours, which do not metastasise.

   e. **True.** This pattern of differentiation resembles adenocarcinoma but the cells form tubules or papillae. It reflects an extraembryonic differentiation pattern. The normal human yolk sac produces AFP in the embryo and usually does so when malignant yolk sac tissue is produced in the testis. Again this protein will be found in the blood and can be used to monitor treatment/relapse of the tumour.

4. a. **False.** Testicular torsion is usually very painful.
   b. **True.** Balanitis xerotica obliterans is, in fact, the male analogue of lichen sclerosus of the vulva. Neither condition is well understood. Both present as thickened, white patches and, on microscope examination, show reactive/atrophic epithelial changes with a subjacent zone of hyalinised connective tissue, below which chronic inflammation is seen. It may be a premalignant condition.
   c. **False.** Epispadias and hypospadias are both conditions relating to the position of the urethral opening on the penis.
   d. **True.**
   e. **True.** The higher the Gleason score of a prostatic cancer, the poorer the degree of differentiation (i.e., roughly speaking, a score of 2–4 = well differentiated; 5, 6 = moderate; and 7–10 = poorly differentiated).

Case history answers

Case history 1

1. Obviously, a full history with clinical examination is required. Often, the fact that the lump is growing and is painless is actually more worrying (and more strongly suggests cancer) than if the lump was painful (which may suggest inflammation/infection). It is probably better to assume the lump is malignant and send the patient for urgent ultrasound. This type of investigation is often conclusive as to whether the lump is benign or malignant (or inflammatory, etc.).

2. With the ultrasound results strongly suggesting this is tumour, preoperative blood tests should be done, including the 'markers' of hCG and AFP (looking for choriocarcinoma and yolk sac tumour elements in the tumour). After the operation, further imaging (of abdominal lymph node groups for instance) may be required.

3. Teratomas are tumours that show endodermal, mesodermal and ectodermal elements of differentiation. In essence, they may be *mature* (showing fully differentiated elements such as intestinal epithelium, muscle and skin), *immature* (incomplete differentiation of any of the elements of the tumour seen) or show *malignant transformation* (cancer, e.g. adenocarcinoma, seen developing in a mature teratoma). Some germ cell tumours contain both seminoma and teratoma.

Case history 2

1. This is very likely to be a squamous cell carcinoma of the glans penis. The risk factors for this tumour include:

- uncircumcised penis
- poor penile hygiene, with carcinogen accumulation in smegma
- infection with HPV types 16 and 18.

2. Squamous cell carcinoma of the glans penis is usually a slow growing tumour of older men and spreads to the inguinal and iliac lymph node groups (the 5-year survival rate is about 30% for tumours that have metastasised to regional lymph nodes).

Short note answers

1. With all these types of questions, it is important to set out the response in a logical fashion.
   Comment: Remember, common things are common. Congenital as well as acquired things should be on your list (consult surgical textbooks for comprehensive guides for examining the testis and its lumps/bumps!).

2 and 3. *Comment*: In these sorts of questions you need to go through your 'memory jogger list' again (e.g. definition, age, sex, incidence, geography, aetiopathogenesis, macro-, micro-, spread, management) to try to shape your answer into a well-drilled, succinct response. It is worth having a set of hand-written or typed revision sheets/cards for important tumours (set out with these similar headings).

4. *Comment*: Applications of grading and staging is a very common question in undergraduate (and, for that matter, postgraduate) exams.

Viva answers

1. *Comment*: See Tables 43 and 48.

2. A hamartoma is a mass made up of haphazardly arranged, but differentiated, tissues normally found in the area in which the mass is found. Thus, a lung hamartoma may contain a jumble of cartilage and glandular epithelium. Although it may be rapidly growing, it is not malignant.

3. Blood markers can be used (PSA in prostate cancer and AFP/hCG in testicular cancer).

Table 48 Risk factors for testicular germ cell tumours

Risk factor	Comments
Age	Peak age for germ cell tumours is 25–45 years
	Only yolk sac tumour is common in children
Cryptorchidism	A non-descended testis has an increased risk of developing a tumour
Genetics	Some testicular tumours are familial
Abnormally formed gonad	Testicular dysgenesis predisposes to malignancy

Urinary tract

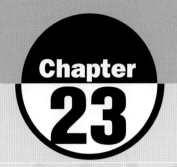
Chapter overview

The urinary tract comprises the kidneys, ureters, bladder and urethra. In males, the prostate gland surrounds a small proportion of the mid-to-lower urethra. This chapter will discuss the pathology of the kidney, ureter, bladder and urethra. Chapter 22 deals with the pathology of the prostate, testis, penis, foreskin and scrotum (i.e. the male genital tract). Some of the pathological processes of the urinary tract are very common (e.g. urinary tract infection), but some are rare (e.g. glomerulonephritis). Urine, the modified ultrafiltrate of blood produced by the kidneys, is often used to assess the general health of a person. There are many simple, colour-based 'stick tests' that enable patients and doctors to monitor substances that may leak into the urine (e.g. glucose, blood, protein).

23.1 The kidneys

Learning objectives

You should:
- understand that many of the broader subsets of kidney disease do not fit conveniently into simple classification systems (e.g. 'inflammatory disease'). This is because diseases like glomerulonephritis and tubulointerstitial disease often have a complex aetiopathogenesis and histological appearance, which may involve two or more pathological processes, e.g. local inflammation and immunological reactions
- know that renal diseases can be simply classified as medical (e.g. glomerulonephritis, where therapy usually relies on pharmacological treatments) or surgical (e.g. tumours or large urinary tract stones, where an operation is often involved in the management of the patient)
- be aware that medical diseases of the kidney (and particularly the glomerulus) are often complex with a

confusing nomenclature. It is more important that you have a working understanding of the underlying basic pathological processes, rather than trying to memorise the classification systems involved.

Structure and function

Each kidney lies in the upper retroperitoneum and has a large number of complex functions including salt and water balance and pH homeostasis. The kidneys receive about 25% of the cardiac output. With the naked eye, the kidney is seen to have a tough external capsule covering an outer 'rind' of cortex, which itself covers the inner medulla (see Figure 61). Histologically, the kidney is made up of four discrete, but interdependent, compartments:

- glomeruli
- tubules
- interstitium
- vessels.

It is probably easiest to tackle each compartment in turn.

Glomeruli

Despite the confusing nomenclature surrounding the pathologies that affect the glomerulus, it is a relatively simple structure. The glomerulus is essentially a highly specialised, incredibly leaky, sieve under high hydrostatic pressure. It is composed of tiny, anastomosing capillaries held together by a specialised matrix and covered by two layers of epithelium (Figure 62). The glomerular capillary wall is the main filtration barrier of the glomerulus and has a unique structure, directly related to its function.

There are some general 'rules' that apply to many of the diseases that affect the glomerulus:

- most primary glomerular diseases are mediated by the immune system (and involve the deposition of immunoglobulins and/or complement in some part of the glomerular structure)
- often, glomerular diseases will present with proteinuria (if heavy, the nephrotic syndrome) or haematuria
- some diseases that affect the glomerulus are relatively acute/sudden in onset and are entirely reversible (clinically and histologically). However, chronic glomerular diseases can lead to scarring of the

glomeruli, death of nephrons and eventually renal failure.

Tubules

The kidney is made up of about a million nephrons, each of which is composed, simplistically, of a glomerulus and its attached tubule (into which the filtrate from the glomerular sieve percolates). This tubule is hollow and is lined, along its complex, writhing course, by epithelial cells. Essentially, the structure of the tubular epithelial cell varies with its function (usually related to its position along the course of the tubule). The proximal tubular cells reabsorb much of the sodium, water, glucose and protein

that filters through the glomerulus. It is not surprising, therefore, that their structure (microvilli projecting into the tubular lumen to increase surface area and plentiful mitochondria providing energy for absorption pumps) is much more complex than many distal tubular cells (flat, nondescript cells that may function only to 'line' the tubule and make it watertight). The specialised function and microanatomy of the proximal tubular cells make them more susceptible to certain cellular insults such as ischaemia/poisons.

Interstitium

Previously thought to be an inert, fibrous compartment of the kidney that binds the glomeruli, tubules and vessels together, we now realise that the interstitium is very important in renal function. Indeed, scarring of the interstitium is important in the degree of impairment of renal function and progression of renal disease (see below). The cortical interstitium is inconspicuous in the normal kidney (the tubules are virtually back to back), but contains peritubular capillaries and fibroblast-like cells (these latter cells communicate with each other and with their neighbouring tubular epithelial cells by means of growth factors and other molecules). In the medulla, however, the amount of interstitium increases and the tubules are more separated from each other (Figure 63).

There are some general 'rules' that apply to many of the diseases affecting the tubules and interstitium:

- most diseases that affect the tubules and/or interstitium are mediated by ischaemia, toxins or infection
- many diseases of the tubules and/or interstitium present as acute renal failure or abnormalities of urine volume/concentration/electrolytic composition
- diseases of the tubules are potentially entirely reversible. The tubular epithelial cells are stable cells and surviving cells can therefore undergo mitosis,

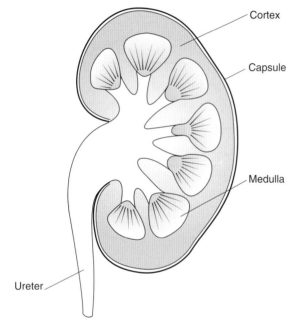

Figure 61 Structure of the kidney.

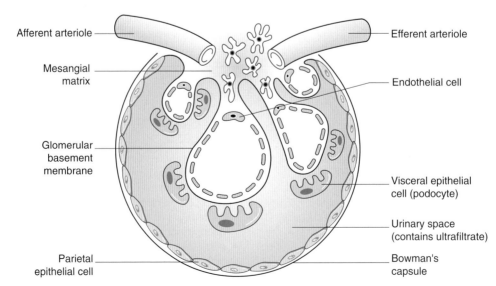

Figure 62 Ultrastructure of the glomerulus.

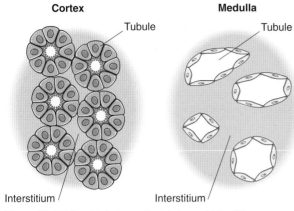

Figure 63 Relationship between the tubules and interstitium.

and regenerate and replenish their numbers/make up new tubules. However, diseases targeting the interstitium may lead to scarring and loss of renal function.

Vessels

Combined, the kidneys weigh only a fraction of the total body weight, yet they receive 25% of the cardiac output (the cortex is much more vascular than the medulla). The kidney receives its blood supply from the main renal artery, which subdivides into anterior and posterior branches at the hilum of the kidney. There is then progressive subdivision of the arterial supply until small afferent arterioles enter the glomerulus. Efferent arterioles are formed by merging of the glomerular capillaries. These efferent arterioles form tiny calibre plexuses of vessels, which surround cortical tubules (peritubular capillaries) and are found in the medulla (these arterial 'vasa recta' ultimately become the venous vasa recta and drain into the systemic venous system via the intrarenal veins/main renal vein).

Remember that the glomerulus is a leash of capillary-sized vessels, therefore diseases that affect capillaries (e.g. vasculitis) are likely to affect the glomerulus.

The compartments of the kidney, although structurally separate, are intimately interrelated and interdependent. This means that chronic (scarring) pathology in one compartment will almost inevitably lead to scarring/loss of function in the other compartments. For example, chronic glomerular disease, which leads to scarring of the glomerulus, will cause atrophy of the attached tubule, scarring in the interstitium (mediated by the fibroblast-like cells) and loss of the specialised capillary plexuses. This is one of the reasons that nephrologists try to do a biopsy in patients early in the course of their renal disease. If the disease is a chronic (potentially scarring-type) process, eventually, as nephrons are lost and the interstitium fibroses, the kidney will become a shrivelled, scarred structure and the compartment of origin of the disease will not be evident (and the initial compartment target of the disease process may be important in the treatment/prognosis of the disease).

23.2 Congenital renal disease

Learning objectives

You should:
- have a working knowledge of the embryology of the kidney and urinary tract
- be able to apply this to the more common abnormalities.

There are numerous possible congenital abnormalities of the kidneys from non-formation of one kidney (unilateral agenesis), which is compatible with a normal life (and may only be discovered incidentally at autopsy), to congenital absence of both kidneys, which usually leads to death in utero. Sometimes the upper or lower poles of the kidneys are fused (forming a so-called 'horseshoe kidney'). This type of kidney malformation may be found in fetuses/children who have chromosomal abnormalities such as Turner's syndrome (45XO). Congenital cystic disease of the kidney is clinically important (Table 49).

23.3 Acquired renal disease

Learning objectives

You should:
- understand the four compartments of the kidney
- realise their interdependence and understand the basic principles of the diseases targeting each of them.

Glomerular disease

Glomerular diseases (glomerulonephritis/glomerulonephritides; glomerulopathy/glomerulopathies) are often caused by the immune system. Chronic glomerular disease is an important cause of chronic renal failure (CRF) worldwide. Severe chronic renal failure is associated with high morbidity and mortality, and renal function often needs to be maintained by artificial means, either haemodialysis or peritoneal dialysis, or by kidney transplantation from a living or dead person (living-related or cadaveric transplantation). There are numerous glomerulonephritides and their nomenclature is confusing (Table 50).

Primary glomerulonephritis

This is essentially a disease process in which the glomerulus is mainly or exclusively affected (i.e. no non-renal organs are involved), e.g. membranous glomerulonephritis.

Secondary glomerulonephritis

This by contrast, involves the glomerulus being affected as part of a widespread, multisystem disease, e.g. diabetes mellitus, amyloidosis and systemic lupus erythematosus (SLE), all of which can affect many organs including the lung, liver, kidney, etc.).

Table 49 Renal cystic disease

Cystic renal dysplasia	Autosomal dominant polycystic kidney disease	Autosomal recessive polycystic kidney disease	Medullary sponge kidney
• Commonest cystic renal disease in children • Caused by disorganised renal development • Can be unilateral or bilateral • Often associated with poorly formed ureter • Rarely part of a syndrome	• Progressive distension of kidney by enlarging cysts • 1–2 cases per 1000 live births • Usually present in adults • Caused by mutation in two genes PKD1 (85% of cases; chromosome 16) and PKD2 (15% of cases; chromosome 4) (? also PKD3 in rare cases) • 10% new mutations • Maybe associated with cysts in liver, pancreas, spleen and cerebral/coronary artery and aneurysms • About 10% require dialysis/transplantation	• Rare, 1 case per 20 000 live births • Gene on chromosome 6 • Liver also always affected • Larger kidneys at birth (may cause death soon after birth due to renal failure)	• Dilated collecting ducts giving 'spongy' appearance • ? 1 case per 5000 population • May present with renal infections in adult life • No obvious genetic link

Table 50 Glomerular disease

Non-proliferative	Proliferative
(no increase in glomerular cells) • Minimal change disease • Focal segmental glomerulosclerosis • Membranous GN • Focal segmental necrotising/crescentic GN	(increase in one or more cell type in glomerulus) • Mesangial proliferative GN • Membrano-proliferative/mesangio-capillary GN • Diffuse/post-infectious proliferative GN • Focal segmental GN • Crescentic GN

Focal – some glomeruli (often quoted as about ≤20% involved)
Diffuse – majority of glomeruli (≥80% involved)
Segmental – part of a glomerulus
Global – whole glomerulus

Aetiopathogenesis of primary glomerulonephritis

Most forms of primary glomerular disease appear to be mediated, in some way, by the immune system. Unfortunately, in most cases, we do not know what causes the immune 'attack'. However, a number of 'tests' are performed on renal biopsies and this has helped in our understanding of glomerular disease. The biopsy is stained with a number of 'routine' stains (e.g. haematoxylin and eosin; H&E) and 'special stains', e.g. Congo red for amyloid and Martius yellow-scarlet-blue (MSB) for fibrin, which allow recognition of the nucleus and cytoplasm of cells, as well as the deposition of matrix and the presence of necrosis when looking at the biopsy under the light microscope. In addition, and importantly in defining the aetiopathogenesis of glomerular disease, highly specialised immunohistological techniques (e.g. immunoperoxidase or immunofluorescence) are used, which allow human immunoglobulin and complement components to be visualised in the biopsy. Electron microscopy (EM) is also performed, and gives very high magnification of the renal structures (and particularly the glomerulus), allowing accurate assessment of the pathological processes, including the site of deposition of any immune complexes.

Using these immunological and ultrastructural techniques (and a wealth of information from experimental models of glomerular disease), it is apparent that there are several possible mechanisms by which immune-mediated glomerular disease occurs.

Pre-formed circulating immune complexes

Pre-formed circulating immune complexes (made up of antibody and antigen) may lodge in any part of the glomerulus and set up a chain of reactions leading to a change in the fine structure/charge of the glomerulus, with altered function. This type of scenario probably occurs in SLE (in which the antigen that sets up this reaction is likely to be normal nuclear-associated protein) and some glomerular diseases associated with infections (e.g. hepatitis B; here the foreign antigen is part of the virus).

Immune complexes may be formed in the glomerulus

(i.e. in situ immune complex formation rather than circulating immune complexes). In this case, antibodies against certain components of the glomerulus are found in the circulation and these attack normal constituents of the glomerulus (e.g. antiglomerular basement membrane disease; in this disease, antibodies attack part of the type IV collagen molecule in the glomerular basement membrane). Alternatively, the antibodies may 'home in' on proteins that have become stuck in the glomerulus because of their physicochemical properties (e.g. certain parts of bacterial cell walls may have a positive charge, bind to negative charges in the glomerulus and then be attacked by antibodies).

No immune complexes

It is now well established that certain glomerular diseases (e.g. minimal change disease) show no evidence of immune complex deposition (using the immunohistological/ultrastructural techniques described above). It is postulated that these diseases may be mediated by T cells or macrophages (or, more specifically, signalling molecules produced by these cells).

Types of glomerulonephritis

As can be seen from Table 50, there are numerous forms of glomerular disease, and it is beyond the scope of this book to detail them all. However, four types of glomerulonephritis will be discussed in an attempt to illustrate important aspects of glomerular pathology:

- post-infectious glomerulonephritis
- minimal change disease
- membranous glomerulonephritis
- IgA disease.

Post-infectious glomerulonephritis

Often considered to be the prototypic glomerular disease, post-infectious glomerulonephritis can occur after a large number of infections (mainly bacterial). Classically, the disease occurs in children/young adults and follows a sore throat caused by group A β-haemolytic streptococci. There is a time lag of about 1–2 weeks between the sore throat (often a very bad one) and a feeling of being unwell with the appearance of red- or cola-coloured urine (macroscopic haematuria), poor urine output (oliguria) and a mild-to-moderate elevation of protein excretion (proteinuria). Some patients have high blood pressure (the combination of haematuria, oliguria and hypertension is known as the nephritic syndrome).

Renal biopsy will usually show enlarged, hypercellular glomeruli, which contain numerous neutrophils and increased numbers of swollen endothelial cells with proliferating mesangial cells. Immunohistological stains reveal IgG, IgM and C3 in glomerular capillary walls and mesangial regions, and electron microscopy (EM) will show these immune deposits as electron dense (black) humps on the epithelial side of the glomerular basement membrane (GBM) as well as deposits in the subendothelial and mesangial regions.

Interestingly, the vast majority of patients will get entirely better – the hypercellular glomeruli will return to normal (cell death by apoptosis) and the deposits will be cleared by phagocytosis (mesangial cells are phagocytic). A few (often older) patients may develop very profound renal failure and go on to have chronic renal failure with the need for dialysis/transplantation.

Minimal change disease

Minimal change disease is the commonest cause of the nephrotic syndrome in children (especially in children aged 2–5 years). Nephrotic syndrome is defined as heavy protein loss in the urine with low levels of albumin in the blood and peripheral oedema as a consequence of the reduced colloid osmotic pressure. Microscopically, this disease is characterised by normal-looking glomeruli (the tubules, interstitium and vessels are also usually normal). Classically, immunohistological stains are negative (i.e. there are no immune complexes in the glomeruli). The only significant finding is foot process fusion (spreading of the feet of the podocyte, leading to apparent loss of the 'feet' on which the podocyte stands on the glomerular basement membrane), seen on electron microscopy (this is actually a non-specific finding as foot process fusion is seen in most glomerular diseases where there is heavy proteinuria). Most patients respond well to oral corticosteroid administration (although the disease may recur when the steroids are reduced/withdrawn).

Membranous glomerulonephritis

Membranous glomerulonephritis is the commonest cause of the nephrotic syndrome in adults. In established membranous glomerulonephritis, light microscopy classically shows glomeruli with thick capillary walls. The glomerulus is otherwise normal. A special silver deposition stain will show epithelial-directed 'spikes' poking out from the glomerular basement membrane. Immunohistologically, there is immunoglobulin (often IgG) and complement (C3) deposition along/in the capillary walls. Electron microscopy reveals variably sized subepithelial or intramembranous electron-dense deposits (see Figure 64). The 'spikes' seen on light microscopy represent 'fingers' and 'tongues' of glomerular basement membrane insinuating up between the deposits. The disease is idiopathic in about 85% of patients, but can be associated with drugs (e.g. penicillamine), tumours (e.g. lung cancer), infections (e.g. human immunodeficiency virus (HIV) and hepatitis B) and SLE. Prognosis depends, at least in part, on the underlying disease, but at least a third of idiopathic patients will eventually require dialysis or transplantation.

IgA disease

IgA disease is thought to be the most common glomerulonephritis in the world. It tends to affect young men and may present as macroscopic haematuria, which comes on at almost the same time as an upper respiratory tract infection (compare post-infectious glomerulonephritis). By

Twenty three

243

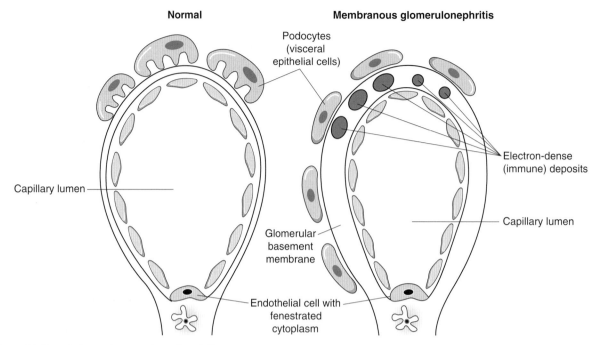

Normal

Membranous glomerulonephritis

Podocytes
(visceral
epithelial cells)

Electron-dense
(immune) deposits

Capillary lumen

Capillary lumen

Glomerular
basement
membrane

Endothelial cell with
fenestrated
cytoplasm

Figure 64 Deposits in membranous glomerulonephritis.

light microscopy, the glomeruli show a variable increase in mesangial cells (this may affect only part of some glomeruli, i.e. be a focal and segmental process). By immunohistological techniques the expanded, hypercellular mesangial regions are seen to be full of granules of IgA (often accompanied by C3) and electron microscopy confirms mesangial electron-dense deposits. The cause of the IgA deposition is still uncertain (but it is likely to be related to increased mucosal IgA production/decreased hepatic metabolism). Initially, it was thought that IgA disease was a recurrent, but benign, process. However, it is now known that a significant number of patients will ultimately require long-term dialysis or transplantation.

Tubular disease

Probably the most important tubular disease in clinical practice is acute tubular necrosis (ATN). ATN is the commonest cause of acute renal failure (ARF). As the name suggests, there is death of tubular epithelial cells. However, tubular epithelial cells are stable cells. These cells are normally in the G0 phase of the cell cycle and will only become actively mitotic if stimulated to do so. ATN is such a stimulus, causing preserved epithelial cells (probably stem cells) to undergo mitosis. There are two main categories of ATN:

- nephrotoxic
- ischaemic.

Nephrotoxic ATN

Nephrotoxic ATN can be caused by a very wide range of drugs, chemicals and poisons. Examples include: gentamicin, an antibiotic used widely in hospitals; contrast media used for radiological investigations such as an intravenous pyelogram (IVP) used for examining renal and urinary

tract structures; toxins such as ethylene glycol, used in antifreeze solutions; and substances found in some types of mushroom.

Ischaemic ATN

Ischaemic ATN is most often associated with 'shock' (particularly related to burns, sepsis or haemorrhage). The actual pathogenesis of the ARF in ATN is still uncertain; theories range from physical obstruction of tubular lumina (by shedding of dead cells/debris) to alterations in intrarenal vascular tone and glomerular ultrafiltration (see physiology textbooks for details).

Interstitial disease

It is important to recognise the close relationship between the interstitium and the tubules. The intimacy of the relationship is shown by the fact that even in ATN, a tubulecentred disease process, there may be (reactive) oedema and mild inflammation in the interstitium. It is no surprise, therefore, that in disease processes which target the interstitium, some form of tubular damage can often be seen. Interstitial diseases (interstitial nephritis or tubulointerstitial disease) are usually subdivided into acute and chronic processes.

Acute interstitial nephritis

The patient may present with ARF. There is expansion of the interstitium by oedema and inflammatory cells. Often neutrophils (acute inflammatory cells) are quite sparse and the dominant cells are actually lymphocytes, plasma cells and eosinophils. There is acute damage to tubules. The causes of acute interstitial nephritis (AIN) include:

- drugs, e.g. non-steroidal anti-inflammatory drugs (NSAIDs) and antibiotics, especially penicillins (in drug-induced AIN eosinophils are often very conspicuous)

- infections (acute pyelonephritis should be excluded, see below), e.g. leptospirosis.

A significant number of cases will be idiopathic.

Chronic interstitial nephritis

The patient is likely to have chronic renal failure (CRF). Rather non-specific features are seen histologically with small, shrunken (atrophic) tubules, interstitial chronic inflammation and scarring. Causes include:

- progression of AIN
- toxic damage, e.g. by mercury, lead or lithium
- chronic pyelonephritis (see below)
- tuberculosis.

Vascular disease

The kidney is not protected from systemic vascular diseases (it is important to remember that the kidney contains a wide range of vessels from large renal arteries to the tiny glomerular and peritubular capillaries). Hypertension, vasculitis, emboli and diabetes mellitus all affect the kidney.

Thrombotic microangiopathies (e.g. haemolytic uraemic syndrome and thrombotic thrombocytopenic purpura) are so-called because these diseases affect small vessels and lead to thrombus formation. The 'trigger factor' may be an infection or an inborn abnormality in the clotting/anti-clotting cascades leading to endothelial cell injury with subsequent platelet aggregation.

Pyelonephritis

Pyelonephritis literally means inflammation of the renal pelvis and kidney and is best considered as a separate entity (rather than being classified as a specific tubular, interstitial or tubulointerstitial disease). Classically, it is subdivided into acute and chronic forms.

Acute pyelonephritis

Acute pus-forming inflammation of the renal pelvis and kidney. This occurs in the context of urinary tract infection (UTI, see Table 51). The diagnosis of acute pyelonephritis is made by clinico-pathological-radiological methods (the renal pelvis may appear thickened and distorted).

Most commonly, bacterial colonisation of the distal urinary tract (urethra and bladder in women, bladder in men) can lead to ascending infection with infected urine refluxing up the ureters into the kidney itself (particularly to the poles of the kidney). The common organisms are *Escherichia coli*, *Proteus* species and *Enterobacter*. Patients often present with loin pain, fevers, rigors and pain on micturition (dysuria).

Rarely, haematogenous spread of organisms can lead to them settling in the renal pelvis/kidney and setting up an inflammatory response. This most often occurs in septicaemia or infective endocarditis, when infected emboli from the heart valves may lodge in small-calibre renal vessels.

Table 51 Urinary tract infections (UTIs)

Definition	Infection of any part of the urinary tract; commonly bladder (cystitis) and kidney (pyelonephritis)
Types	UTIs may be asymptomatic or, more usually, symptomatic (pain, frequency of micturition, fevers)
Sex predilection	Females (rarely male infants/older males)
Organisms	Most often bacteria, commonly gut/perineal organisms (*E. coli*, *Proteus*, *Klebsiella*)
Predisposing factors	Urological procedures/operations (e.g. catheterisation of bladder)
	Obstruction to outflow
	Pregnancy
	Congenital abnormalities of the genital tract (posterior urethral valves in young boys)
	Vesicoureteric reflux (pyelonephritis)
	Diabetes mellitus
	Immunosuppression
Pathology	Congestion/granularity of bladder/kidney
	Pus formation
	Neutrophils in urine/tissues
Sequelae	May lead to chronic cystitis or pyelonephritis

On microscopy, pus may be seen in the renal tubules with oedema and (acute) inflammation of the interstitium. Tubular necrosis may be seen, but the glomeruli are usually normal. Severe, untreated disease may lead to abscess formation in the renal pelvis/kidney (pyonephrosis), death of the renal papillae (papillary necrosis) and even perinephric abscess formation. The inflammation in acute pyelonephritis usually responds to the appropriate antibiotic, but repeated (untreated) attacks can lead to renal scarring and chronic pyelonephritis (see below).

Chronic pyelonephritis

This diagnosis is made by patho-radiological means. Classically, the radiological appearances are of deformed, scarred kidneys/kidneys with blunted calyces and histologically there is tubular atrophy or dilatation (with large hyaline casts) and chronic interstitial inflammation/scarring. Chronic pyelonephritis is an important cause of CRF. Some authorities subdivide chronic pyelonephritis into obstructive and reflux associated (see Figure 65 and Section 23.5).

Renal stones

Stones (calculi) are a relatively common problem in the urinary tract and occur most commonly in the kidneys, ureters or bladder. They can cause problems such as pain, bleeding and obstruction. Most stones (75%) contain calcium and are associated with hypercalcaemia/hypercalciuria. A minority (about 15%) are composed of magnesium ammonium phosphate, urate or cystine.

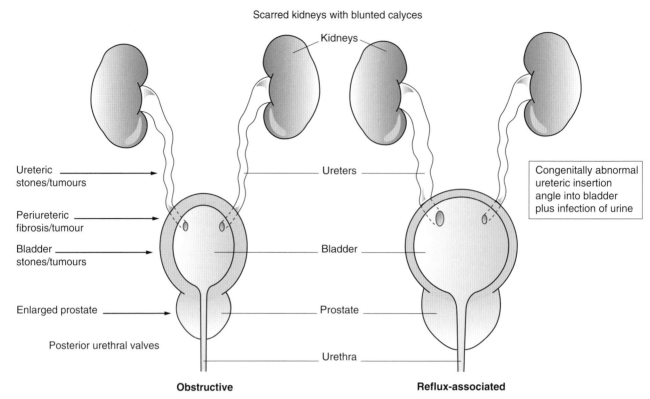

Scarred kidneys with blunted calyces

Kidneys

Ureteric stones/tumours

Periureteric fibrosis/tumour

Bladder stones/tumours

Ureters

Enlarged prostate

Bladder

Prostate

Posterior urethral valves

Urethra

Congenitally abnormal ureteric insertion angle into bladder plus infection of urine

Obstructive

Reflux-associated

Figure 65 Chronic pyelonephritis.

Table 52 Benign tumours of the kidney*

Structure	Possible benign tumours
Renal capsule/perinephric fat	Fibroma, leiomyoma, lipoma
Renal parenchyma	Adenoma (often defined as a very small renal cell carcinoma <0.5 cm in diameter; these tiny lesions rarely metastasise)
	Oncocytoma (some authorities believe that these tumours virtually never metastasise)
	Angiomyolipoma (may be seen in tuberose sclerosis; considered by some authorities to be a hamartoma)
Renal vessels	Haemangioma

*As in all organs, benign tumours can arise from any of the anatomical structures of the kidney.

Tumours of the kidney

Benign tumours

See Table 52.

Malignant tumours

The two most important malignant tumours of the kidney are renal cell carcinoma and transitional cell carcinoma.

Renal cell carcinoma

Renal cell carcinoma is the commonest renal malignancy (85% of all renal cancers) and may occur in young patients in the setting of genetic syndromes such as von Hippel–Lindau syndrome (when the tumour may be multiple and bilateral and the patients are usually carefully screened). In sporadic (i.e. non-familial) cases, the tumour may be picked up during investigation for other diseases (e.g. abdominal ultrasound scan done for abdominal pain). The tumour may cause haematuria or paraneoplastic symptoms such as fever and polycythaemia or hypercalcaemia. The tumour is more common in men and the peak incidence is in the fifth and sixth decades. Macroscopically, the tumour is most often well circumscribed, yellow, with areas of haemorrhage, necrosis and cyst formation. Histologically, there are several subtypes, but the commonest is the clear cell (conventional) renal cell carcinoma. Renal cell carcinomas tend to spread by the bloodstream and may spread up the inferior vena cava as far as the right atrium.

The prognosis depends on factors such as the size, nuclear grade and local/distant spread of the tumour.

Transitional cell carcinoma

Transitional cell carcinoma arises in the renal pelvis from the urothelium, and makes up about 10% of all renal cancers. The tumour may present with haematuria or obstruction of the kidney, and is mainly found in older patients. Histologically, tumours may vary from well differentiated, non-invasive papillary tumours to poorly differentiated solid lesions, which widely invade the wall of the renal pelvis and/or the kidney.

The prognosis will depend particularly on the stage of the tumour (see also bladder tumours in Section 23.5).

Wilms' tumour (nephroblastoma)

In children this is the commonest malignant tumour of the kidney. The tumour is derived from the embryonic components of the kidney and occurs mainly in young children (less than 5 years of age). Mutations in the tumour suppressor gene *WT1* (found on chromosome 11) are thought to be important in tumorigenesis. Prognosis (and treatment) depends on the degree of spread (stage) of the tumour and whether or not it contains high-grade areas ('anaplasia').

23.4 The ureters

Learning objectives

You should:
- know the normal histology and function of the ureters
- have a basic knowledge of congenital and acquired abnormalities of the ureter.

These epithelium-lined, muscular tubes convey the urine from the kidney to the bladder.

Congenital abnormalities

There are many congenital abnormalities of the ureters from duplication to stenosis and atresia. Congenital pelvi-ureteric junction obstruction may be picked up in utero as hydronephrosis.

Acquired abnormalities

Many of the acquired abnormalities of the ureters lead to obstruction (Table 53).

23.5 The bladder

Learning objectives

You should:
- have a sound knowledge of the normal anatomical relations and histology of the bladder
- have a working knowledge of the important congenital abnormalities of the bladder
- be acquainted with the important acquired bladder diseases (particularly inflammation-related and tumours).

The mature urinary bladder is essentially a distensible, muscular bag found in the pelvis. Urine is conveyed to the bladder by the ureters. The lining of the urinary bladder (and that of the ureters, renal pelvis and proximal urethra) is transitional cell epithelium (urothelium). Irrespective of its site, the urothelium is a watertight, multilayered epithelium covered by large specialised cells called 'umbrella cells'. The urothelium rests on a basal lamina and subjacent to this is the lamina propria (in which is found loose connective tissue, thin-walled blood vessels, twigs of smooth muscle and scattered inflammatory cells). There is a thick muscular coat to the human bladder (detrusor muscle), which consists of interwoven bundles. This allows complete emptying of the bladder. The bladder is innervated by both sympathetic and parasympathetic fibres originating from T11 to S4.

Congenital abnormalities

There are numerous congenital abnormalities of the bladder, including diverticula and fistulas (an important example is a fistula between the bladder and umbilicus, persistent urachus). Exstrophy is a rare, but important, abnormality in which there is absence of part of the anterior abdominal wall and anterior (ventral) bladder wall with eversion and exteriorisation of the rest of the urinary bladder. Other urinary tract and non-urinary tract abnormalities are often associated with exstrophy.

Vesicoureteric reflux (VUR) is also an important congenital abnormality. This may be caused by abnormal positioning (altered angle of entry) of one or both ureters as they course into the bladder wall (to open into the trigone of the bladder). Severe VUR can lead to UTI, reflux-type chronic pyelonephritis and advanced renal scarring in children (see pyelonephritis, Section 23.3).

Acquired abnormalities

The most important acquired pathologies of the bladder are inflammation (cystitis) and neoplasms (transitional cell carcinoma, TCC). As in other sites along the urinary tract, stones can also cause problems.

Cystitis

Inflammation of the bladder is common. Usually it is bacterial in origin. Bacterial colonisation of the urine may be asymptomatic (e.g. as has been found when screening the urine of normal schoolgirls) or symptomatic (features

Table 53 Abnormalities of the ureters

Congenital		Acquired	
Mega ureter	Large, dilated ureters	Ureteric obstruction due to abnormalities:	
Ureteral stricture or valves	Congenital narrowing of the ureter or 'flaps' obstructing lumen	in lumen of ureter	Stones, fragments of renal papillae (sickle cell disease)
Diverticula	Outpouchings made up of all layers of the ureteric wall	of ureteric wall	Inflammation/scarring tumours (benign or malignant)
Duplication	Double ureters on either one or both sides	from outside ureter	Inflammation/scarring/tumour (can cause dilatation above blockage)

include pain on micturition and increased frequency of passing urine). The diagnosis is, not surprisingly, made on examination of a urine sample, which will show large numbers of bacteria. These bacteria are usually intestinal in origin with *E. coli* being the commonest. Cystitis/UTI is more common in women (presumed to be because of the shorter female urethra), but becomes more frequent in older men (presumed to be secondary to bladder outflow obstruction, which occurs with an enlarging prostate). Any trauma to, or congenital/acquired abnormalities of, the bladder often increases the risk of cystitis/UTI. Bladder biopsies during an 'attack' of cystitis often show rather non-specific features such as congestion or acute or chronic inflammation.

Infection/inflammation of the bladder can also be caused by *Mycobacterium tuberculosis* (usually by way of infected urine from a tuberculous kidney), *Candida* species (especially in neonates and the immunosuppressed) and schistosomes (in particular, *Schistosoma haematobium* causing bilharzia). Adenovirus infection can also cause cystitis.

Cystitis may also be caused by non-infective agents such as radiation and drugs (e.g. cyclophosphamide causing haemorrhagic cystitis).

Two 'special' forms of cystitis are important to know:

- **Interstitial cystitis (sometimes called Hunner's ulcer)** – usually occurs in middle-aged women and often causes pain. Histologically there may be ulceration of the urothelium and mast cells are very numerous, particularly in the muscular layer.
- **Malacoplakia** – this appears to be a reaction to bacterial infection. The bladder shows yellow patches on the urothelium and down the microscope numerous foamy and granular macrophages are seen containing intracellular structures (partially digested bacterial debris) called Michaelis–Guttmann bodies. Malacoplakia is not confined to the kidney, but may be found widely in the urinary tract, lungs or bones.

Tumours of the bladder

Benign tumours of the bladder

These are rare, but include haemangiomas, neurofibromas and paragangliomas.

Malignant tumours of the bladder

By far the commonest malignant tumour of the bladder in adults is the urothelial-derived transitional cell carcinoma (TCC). However, in the paediatric age group a common malignant tumour of the bladder is the rhabdomyosarcoma (Table 54).

Transitional cell carcinoma in situ (TCCis)

Believed by many authorities to precede the development of TCC in some patients (as evidenced by the presence of TCCis in the majority of cases of TCC), TCCis is characterised by flat and thickened or gently undulating full-thickness dysplastic urothelium (nuclear pleomorphism, abnormal mitoses and apoptotic figures are seen). Often

Table 54 Bladder rhabdomyosarcoma

Definition	Malignant mesenchymal tumour, showing evidence of skeletal muscle differentiation
Age group	Usually ≤5 years old
	Male > female
Naked-eye appearance	May look like a 'polyp' or 'bunch of grapes' protruding into the bladder lumen
Microscopic appearance	May have very cellular areas and acellular areas
	Malignant cells may be small and nondescript or 'strap-like', or even look like mature skeletal muscle
Prognosis	Generally good but depends on subtype and stage

Table 55 Confirmed or suspected risk factors for transitional cell carcinoma of the bladder

Smoking	Increases risk up to five times
Analgesics	Mainly associated with renal pelvis transitional cell carcinoma, but also bladder tumours
Occupation	Workers in aniline dye, rubber and chemical industries due to exposure to β-naphthylamine (which in the liver is converted to a carcinogen that must be activated in the bladder). These workers need regular bladder checks
Cyclophosphamide	Can cause bladder cancer in the long term (although used for cancer treatment)
Schistosomiasis	Causes chronic inflammation and metaplasia (squamous) of the bladder mucosa (leading to squamous cell carcinoma)
Chronic infections/ inflammation	Some authorities believe that any chronic inflammatory process may predispose to cancer

appearing as a red patch, the disease may be multifocal within the bladder.

Transitional cell carcinoma

Overall, TCC accounts for about 5% of all malignancies in adults in the UK. Most patients are over 50 years of age and there are definite risk factors for development of TCC, the most important of which are shown in Table 55. The tumour may present with haematuria, frequency or urgency. TCC may be multifocal either within the bladder or the urinary tract.

As in other parts of the urothelium-lined urinary tract, the tumour can have a very varied appearance, both macroscopically (fronded and seaweed-like to solid) and microscopically (well differentiated and papillary to poorly differentiated and widely muscle invasive). The

Table 56 Grading and staging of bladder transitional cell carcinoma (TNM)

Grade	Definition
G1	Well differentiated
G2	Moderately differentiated
G3	Poorly differentiated/undifferentiated
Stage	**Definition**
Tis	In situ carcinoma
Ta	Non-invasive, papillary tumour
T1	Tumour invades subepithelial connective tissue
T2	Tumour invades detrusor muscle
T3	Tumour invades beyond detrusor muscle
T4	Tumour invades prostate, uterus, vagina or pelvic wall/abdominal wall
N1	Single lymph node metastasis (≤2 cm)
N2	Single metastasis (>2 cm) or multiple metastases (≤5 cm)
N3	Multiple metastases (>5 cm)

Prognosis
• About half (or more) of all newly diagnosed bladder TCCs are G1 or G2, Ta or T1 (good prognosis)
• Most patients who have had a G1/G2 Ta/T1 tumour and have a recurrence will have another similar tumour
• 10% of patients with these tumours eventually develop invasive or metastatic tumours (poor prognosis)
• About 25% of newly diagnosed bladder TCCs will be muscle invasive (and G2/G3), and about half will have metastases
• Most patients with metastatic bladder TCC die within 5 years

grading and staging system for bladder TCC is shown in Table 56, together with prognosis.

Numerous cytogenetic and molecular alterations have been found in TCC, including monosomy or deletions of the short (p) or long (q) arm of chromosome 9 and deletions of 17p (which involves the *p53* gene).

Squamous metaplasia of the urothelium can occur in a variety of circumstances, for example as a response to bladder stones, indwelling catheters and infection by *Schistosoma* (schistosomiasis is endemic in countries such as Egypt). Under these circumstances, squamous cell carcinoma of the bladder can develop. Often this tumour has invaded the bladder wall at presentation.

23.6 The urethra

Learning objectives

You should:
• know the normal anatomy and histology of the urethra
• know the principal diseases that affect this structure.

The mature male urethra is lined predominantly by transitional epithelium and has a spindle-shaped expansion in its prostatic portion (the verumontanum) into which the ejaculatory ducts drain. The distal end of the penile urethra is lined by squamous epithelium. The female urethra is much shorter than in the male and is lined mainly by squamous epithelium.

Inflammation of the urethra is relatively common (but rarely biopsied) and is caused by gonococci (gonorrhoea, *Neisseria*) and non-gonococcal organisms (such as *E. coli*, *Chlamydia* and *Mycoplasma*).

A urethral caruncle is essentially a painful, red, polypoid nodule found in females at the urethral meatus (it may represent inflamed, prolapsed tissue). The lesion is usually about 1 cm in diameter and excision is curative.

Urethral malignancies are rare. Squamous cell carcinoma of the distal urethra is the commonest.

Self-assessment: questions

One best answer questions

1. A 3-year-old boy is found to have a polypoid tumour in his bladder. The most likely diagnosis is:
   a. transitional cell carcinoma
   b. squamous cell carcinoma
   c. neurofibroma
   d. rhabdomyosarcoma
   e. Wilms' tumour

2. Which of the following laboratory investigative techniques is not routinely used when examining renal biopsy sample from patients with suspected glomerulonephritis?
   a. Congo red staining
   b. polymerase chain reaction
   c. immunohistology
   d. electron microscopy
   e. haematoxylin and eosin staining

True-false questions

1. Concerning the kidney:
   a. there are approximately 1000 nephrons in each kidney
   b. the glomerular basement membrane is a positively charged filtration unit
   c. the tubular compartment is the largest, by volume, in the kidney
   d. acute renal failure may be caused by drugs
   e. chronic renal failure inevitably leads to dialysis or transplantation

2. The following statements are correct:
   a. membranous glomerulonephritis is the commonest cause of the adult nephrotic syndrome
   b. minimal change disease is mediated by immune complexes
   c. the glomerular basement membrane is full of cationic macromolecules
   d. post-infectious glomerulonephritis is usually triggered by viruses
   e. IgA disease is a rare form of glomerulonephritis

3. Acute pyelonephritis:
   a. is commonly due to blood spread of organisms to the kidney
   b. is commoner in men than women
   c. is often caused by *E. coli*
   d. even if promptly treated results in scarring of the kidney

   e. classically results in two small, but symmetrical, kidneys

4. Concerning the renal tubules and interstitium:
   a. tubular diseases are usually mediated by immune complexes
   b. interstitial nephritis may be caused by non-steroidal anti-inflammatory drugs (NSAIDs)
   c. the amount of inflammation and scarring in the interstitium is important in the progression of renal disease
   d. acute tubular necrosis is usually irreversible and leads to permanent kidney damage
   e. granulomas may be seen in the interstitium in renal sarcoidosis

5. The following are correctly paired:
   a. renal cell carcinoma – schistosomal infestation
   b. renal angiomyolipoma – massive haemorrhage
   c. transitional cell carcinoma of the bladder – cigarette smoking
   d. Wilms' tumour – nephroblastoma
   e. Malacoplakia – malignant tumour of B lymphocytes

6. The following statements are correct:
   a. diabetes mellitus is a cause of hyaline arteriolosclerosis
   b. haemodialysis is the only method of long-term renal replacement therapy
   c. renal amyloidosis is seen in patients with multiple myeloma
   d. vesicoureteric reflux may lead to kidney scarring in children
   e. acute renal failure is commonly caused by IgA disease

Case history questions

Case history 1

A 75-year-old man presented to his general practitioner with a 3-month history of feeling generally unwell. He has noted that both his legs are puffy and he thought his urine seemed rather frothy. Blood tests show that his albumin is 9 g/L (normal about 40) and his urine contains about 10 g/L of protein.

1. What is the syndrome that this patient has?

His renal function (i.e. creatinine clearance) is normal and he undergoes a renal biopsy.

2. What is the likeliest cause of his syndrome?

He is treated appropriately, but 3 months later is found to have lung cancer.

3. What is the relationship between the tumour and his renal disease?

Case history 2

Whilst having a routine life assurance medical, a 52-year-old man is found to present with haematuria.

1. List the common causes of haematuria in a 52-year-old man.

Further tests show that he has a 10 cm mass that has replaced one pole of his right kidney.

2. What could this mass be?

A biopsy of the mass is performed, and it is found to be a renal cell carcinoma. At operation, it appears to have invaded into the right renal vein.

3. How do renal cell carcinomas spread?

4. What is understood by the 'stage' of a tumour?

Short note questions

1. Briefly describe the possible mechanisms of pathogenesis of immune-mediated glomerulonephritis.

2. Write short notes an pyelonephritis.

3. Write short notes an bladder cancer.

Viva questions

Discuss:

1. Grading and staging of urinary tract tumours.

2. UTIs and common organisms/complications.

3. The immune system and glomerular disease.

Self-assessment: answers

One best answer

1. d. The patient's age is an important consideration. Transitional cell carcinoma is the commonest bladder tumour in adults. Wilms' tumour also affects children but is a neoplasm of the kidney.

2. b. Many primary glomerular diseases are immune-mediated, and the pattern of deposition of immune complexes within the glomerulus contributes considerably to the diagnostic pathological features of these diseases. Such deposits can be demonstrated using electron microscopy and by applying specific antibodies to tissue sections (immunohistology). Congo red staining is a method for demonstrating amyloid on light microscopy (the stained tissue appears bright green when viewed with polarised light); as amyloid is a relatively common cause of glomerular disease, this stain is often routinely performed on diagnostic renal biopsy samples. Haematoxylin and eosin remains the standard initial light microscopy stain used for all histopathology specimens, including renal biopsy specimens.

True-false answers

1. a. **False.** The quoted figure is 1 000 000.
   b. **False.** The glomerular basement membrane is certainly a charge-selective filtration barrier. However, it is full of *negatively* charged macromolecules such as collagen and heparan sulphate.
   c. **True.**
   d. **True.** Drugs (often widely used drugs such as non-steroidal anti-inflammatories, NSAIDs) can cause acute renal failure (often by provoking an interstitial nephritis). Remember that acute renal failure can be classified as:

   - pre-renal, i.e. caused by poor perfusion of the kidney as seen in severe heart failure or patients with extensive burns
   - renal, i.e. the abnormality causing renal dysfunction is in the kidney itself, e.g. glomerulonephritis
   - post-renal, i.e. usually caused by relatively sudden blockage to urine flow, e.g. prostatic enlargement with urine retention.

   In any of these instances, there may be dramatic, life-threatening alterations in electrolyte, water and acid–base balance. Acute renal failure is a medical emergency.

   e. **False.** There are many patients with renal disease who have impaired renal function, but it is not severe enough to require dialysis or transplantation. Chronic renal failure will often be characterised by a slow, predictable decline in renal function, which can be monitored by urea and creatinine levels in the blood. There will be wide-ranging changes in salt and water, acid–base and calcium and phosphate homeostasis (to name but a few). Chronic renal failure is also a cause of (normocytic normochromic) anaemia.

2. a. **True.** The nephrotic syndrome is defined as heavy proteinuria (the cut-off point is often quoted as 3.5 g/day) combined with hypoalbuminaemia and peripheral oedema. In addition, nephrotic patients often have hypercholesterolaemia and a tendency to thrombosis.
   b. **False.** No immune complexes can be demonstrated.
   c. **False.** Cationic molecules are *positively* charged.
   d. **False.** Post-infectious glomerulonephritis is usually triggered by bacteria (especially group A β-haemolytic streptococci).
   e. **False.** Many authorities believe it is the commonest glomerulopathy in the world.

3. a. **False.** Ascending infection is far more common.
   b. **False.** Females are far more likely to have urinary tract infections (UTIs) than men and acute pyelonephritis is a sequel to this. This is probably due, at least in part, to the shorter urethra in females.
   c. **True.**
   d. **False.** Early treatment should lead to complete resolution of the inflammatory process.
   e. **False.** Interestingly, recurrent attacks of acute pyelonephritis may lead to chronic pyelonephritis and scarred kidneys, but there is usually asymmetrical, coarse scarring. Thus, one kidney may be very shrivelled and shrunken (perhaps because there was severe bladder-to-ureter-to-kidney reflux on this side) while the other is relatively normal or shows only one or two small scars. In chronic glomerular diseases and hypertension the kidneys become symmetrically reduced in size with a finely granular surface (due to loss of nephrons).

4. a. **False.** They are usually caused by ischaemia, toxins and infections.
   b. **True.**
   c. **True.**

d. **False.** Many cases of acute renal failure due to acute tubular necrosis will, with supportive measures, completely resolve.

e. **True.** Sarcoidosis is a multisystem granulomatous disease of unknown aetiology that usually targets lymph nodes, the lung and liver. The kidney can be involved. The two 'oids', amyloid and sarcoid, often crop up in multiple choice or short answer questions and it is worth knowing a few facts about each.

5. a. **False.** Schistosomiasis is endemic in countries such as Egypt and causes squamous metaplasia of the bladder urothelium. Thus, there is an unusually high number of cases of squamous cell carcinoma of the bladder in these countries.

b. **True.** Angiomyolipoma is a rare (benign) kidney tumour (some authorities think that it is a hamartoma rather than a tumour, i.e. a haphazard collection of tissue normally found in and around the kidney). The 'tumour' is made up of adipose tissue with thick-walled blood vessels. This tumour has an association with tuberous sclerosis, an autosomal dominant disease in which patients can also have rhabdomyomas of the heart and skin lesions (called adenoma sebaceum). Angiomyolipomas can be very vascular and may present as a massive bleed into the retroperitoneum.

c. **True.** Cigarette smokers have a significantly increased risk of bladder transitional cell carcinoma. Other 'smoking-related' tumours are found in the mouth, oesophagus, lung and cervix.

d. **True.** Wilms' tumour is also known as nephroblastoma. There are several important childhood 'solid tumours' that you should be aware of (remember that haematological malignancy is common in children, e.g. acute leukaemia). Many of the childhood solid malignancies look similar down the microscope and are often called 'small blue cell tumours'. Among these are neuroblastomas, rhabdomyosarcomas, nephroblastomas, and some lymphomas. Many of these tumours contain primitive or precursor cells normally found in the developing tissue/organ. Deciding which tumour is which can be difficult, but is helped by immunocytochemistry and molecular biology.

e. **False.** Malacoplakia is a rare inflammatory disease. In the bladder (it can also occur in the bowel and respiratory tract), yellow mucosal plaques are seen and histologically these are collections of macrophages with cytoplasmic and extruded, dark-coloured, Michaelis–Guttmann bodies (which are probably bacterial-derived).

6. a. **True.** Hyaline arteriolosclerosis – thick, bright pink arteriolar walls on staining with haematoxylin and eosin – is seen in conditions such as diabetes, amyloidosis and hypertension.

b. **False.** Peritoneal dialysis and transplantation are two others.

c. **True.** In multiple myeloma, the amyloid is light chain derived (AL amyloid).

d. **True.** See 3e above.

e. **False.** IgA disease could theoretically cause acute renal failure, but usually presents as haematuria with or without proteinuria.

Case history answers

Case history 1

1. This man has the nephrotic syndrome.

2. The commonest cause of the nephrotic syndrome in adults is membranous glomerulopathy.

3. Interestingly, although in the vast majority of cases membranous nephropathy is idiopathic it can be rarely associated with/caused by tumours (possibly by tumour-containing immune complexes becoming lodged in the glomerulus). There have been cases where removal of the tumour has led to resolution of the glomerular disease.

Case history 2

Comment: This is quite a common exam question. Essentially, whether in an essay, short answer or viva format, this type of question tests how well you can logically approach a clinical problem (and mimics how, for instance, casualty officers or general practitioners have to think with the patient in front of them). The best way to tackle this type of question is to mentally (or physically, on a piece of exam paper) jot down the components of the urinary tract (kidney-to-ureter-to-bladder, etc.) and then use a set of general headings to describe the possible pathologies (usable for any organ), e.g. congenital vs. acquired, inflammatory (bacterial, viral, etc.), neoplastic (benign vs. malignant, primary vs. secondary), metabolic, etc. The list you make should, of course, be modified to the age of the patient (it is less likely that a congenital abnormality will present in a man of 52 than an acquired, inflammatory or neoplastic condition).

1. The commoner causes of haematuria in a 52-year-old man are as follows.

Kidney:

- tumours (renal cell carcinoma, transitional cell carcinoma)
- stones with inflammation/ulceration
- trauma.

Ureter:

- tumours (transitional cell carcinoma)
- stones ± inflammation.

Bladder

- tumours (transitional cell carcinoma)
- acquired diverticula with inflammation/stones
- infection (less likely than in females but instrumentation, diabetes, etc.).

Prostate

- benign prostatic enlargement/tumours.

2. The mass is a renal cell carcinoma.

3. Renal cell carcinomas may spread locally or to distant sites. Classically, the tumour may permeate the renal vein and may grow up this structure as far as the right atrium. Distant metastases can occur in any organ but particularly the bones.

4. Remember that *stage* is a reflection of the degree of spread of a tumour (*grade* is how malignant the tumour looks down the microscope).

Short note answers

1. *Comment*: Include circulating and in situ immune complex formation and the possibility of T cell/macrophage products as a cause of glomerular dysfunction.

2. *Comment*: Set out your answer logically. Tackle acute and chronic pyelonephritis (have your memory-jogger headings ready: definition; incidence; age of patient; sex distribution; aetiology/pathogenesis; naked eye, i.e. macroscopic, appearances; microscopic appearances; spread; complications; treatment; etc.).

3. *Comment*: Set out your response in a logical fashion (remember bladder cancer implies a malignant process, so spend most of your time on transitional cell carcinoma).

Viva answers

Comment: All three questions should be approached logically; remember to define the terms you use, this shows the examiner that you understand the nomenclature that you are using.

Lymphoreticular system

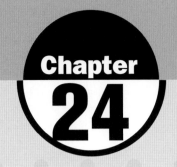

Chapter overview

The lymphoreticular system consists of organs (lymph nodes, spleen, thymus) and ill-defined tissues (mucosa-associated lymphoid tissue) that are concerned with the growth, development and deployment of white blood cells. White blood cells are crucial for immune responses. The lymph nodes lie along the course of the lymphatics, receiving lymph from the tissues and destroying or mounting immune responses to foreign agents before they reach the bloodstream. Both benign and malignant disorders of the lymph nodes often manifest as lymph node enlargement (lymphadenopathy), and lymph node biopsy is sometimes necessary to determine the diagnosis and indicate further management. The spleen receives blood from the arterial system. It functions as a filter by removing obsolescent red blood cells and particulate matter from the blood, and mounts immunological responses against foreign agents. Most benign and malignant disorders of the spleen manifest as splenic enlargement (splenomegaly). Rupture of the spleen is a potentially life-threatening condition that requires prompt management. The thymus is an important component of the lymphoreticular system in fetal life, but probably has no significant role in adults. Failure of normal development of the thymus causes deficient immune responses and, in adults, thymic hyperplasia and thymic tumours may develop.

Basic principles

The cells which circulate in the peripheral blood can be classified simply into those that are non-nucleated (erythrocytes and platelets) and those that are nucleated (leucocytes or white blood cells). White blood cells can be further subclassified into three main cell types:

- granulocytes
- monocytes
- lymphocytes.

The main function of these cells is to protect against infection. Lymphocytes and monocytes circulate around the body in blood vessels and lymphatic vessels, but they also accumulate in organised masses called lymphoid tissues. These organised masses together are known as the lymphoreticular system and the main components of this system are the lymph nodes, thymus, spleen, tonsils, adenoids, and the Peyer patches. The latter three tissues are known as mucosa-associated lymphoid tissue (MALT).

24.1 Lymph nodes

Learning objectives

You should:
- understand the structure and function of lymph nodes
- know the causes of lymphadenopathy
- have a basic understanding of the lymphoid neoplasms.

Structure and function

Lymph nodes are ovoid, encapsulated structures, which range in size from a few millimetres to a few centimetres. They are situated along the course of lymphatic vessels and tend to occur in groups where these vessels converge (e.g. the axilla, groin, neck and mediastinum). Lymph is essentially interstitial fluid containing proteins that need to return to the bloodstream, but which are prevented from doing so within the tissues because of overwhelming hydrostatic pressure. Lymph is therefore carried away from the tissues in small peripheral lymphatic vessels, which converge to form larger vessels, until eventually a single large lymphatic vessel called the thoracic duct ultimately drains the lymph into the bloodstream at the root of the neck. Before the lymph enters the bloodstream, it must pass through one or more lymph nodes. Within the lymph nodes, foreign agents and unwanted materials, which have gained access to the tissues, are entrapped and an immune response is mounted.

Each lymph node is divided into three main regions: the cortex, the paracortex and the medulla (Figure 66).

The cortex

The cortex is the area just beneath the capsule, and it contains spherical aggregations of B lymphocytes (B cells). These aggregations are called primary follicles. B cells are involved in humoral immunity and the primary follicle is the principal site of B cell activation in response to anti-

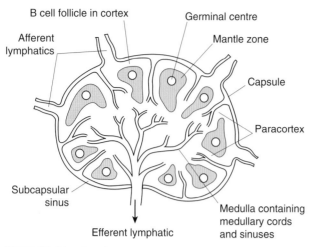

B cell follicle in cortex

Germinal centre

Afferent lymphatics

Mantle zone

Capsule

Paracortex

Subcapsular sinus

Efferent lymphatic

Medulla containing medullary cords and sinuses

Figure 66 A lymph node.

genic stimulation. Antigens that enter the lymph node are presented to the B cells in the primary follicle. Activated B cells enlarge and undergo a series of changes, resulting ultimately in the production of immunoglobulin-secreting plasma cells. Hence, after antigenic stimulation, the primary follicle enlarges and develops a pale-staining germinal centre that contains large, activated B cells. The germinal centre is surrounded by a rim of small unchallenged B cells called the mantle zone.

The paracortex

The paracortex is the area between the follicles and is rich in T lymphocytes (T cells). T cells are involved in cell-mediated immunity. Scattered histiocytic cells are also present.

The medulla

The medulla contains the medullary cords and sinuses. The sinuses are lined by macrophages, which phagocytose particulate material within the lymph. The medullary cords contain numerous plasma cells, which secrete immunoglobulins (antibodies).

Lymph enters the lymph node via multiple afferent lymphatic vessels, which perforate the fibrous capsule and empty into a slit-like space just beneath the capsule called the subcapsular sinus. From there, the lymph enters the cortex via multiple, small cortical sinuses, which penetrate into the node. In the medulla, these sinuses begin to converge into larger sinuses (the medullary sinuses) and, in turn, the medullary sinuses join to form a single efferent lymphatic vessel.

Lymphadenopathy

When there is a pathological process affecting a lymph node, it usually becomes enlarged. Lymphadenopathy is a term used to denote lymph node enlargement. Lymphadenopathy may be localised or widespread. There are two main causes:

- non-neoplastic (reactive) lymphadenopathy
- neoplastic lymphadenopathy.

Neoplasms of the lymph nodes can be divided into primary (lymphoma) or secondary (metastases).

Non-neoplastic (reactive) lymphadenopathy

Lymph node enlargement is a common response to antigenic stimuli. These may be:

- infecting organisms
- non-infectious agents such as foreign material, cell debris, metabolites or drugs
- unknown agents.

Reactive lymph nodes enlarge because there is proliferation of one or more cell types within them. The various antigenic stimuli evoke the reactive proliferation of particular cell types within the lymph node, and may induce other changes. In many cases, the morphological changes induced by these aetiological agents are non-specific, such that precise diagnosis of the causal agent is not possible on histological grounds alone (blood tests may be needed). In other cases, the reactive changes are entity specific, such that the pathologist is able to make an exact diagnosis.

Non-specific reactive changes

Lymph nodes may react in one of five different ways to antigenic stimulation. Often, a combination of one or more of these patterns is seen.

Acute non-specific lymphadenitis This occurs when there is direct drainage of pyogenic infectious microbes into a lymph node, causing a localised acute inflammatory response. Affected lymph nodes become enlarged and tender. Microscopically, there is lymph node oedema and hyperaemia, and neutrophil polymorphs migrate from the vasculature into the nodal parenchyma. There may be progression to abscess formation.

Follicular hyperplasia This occurs when there is a B cell response, and is characterised by marked enlargement and prominence of the germinal centres.

Paracortical hyperplasia This is the result of a T cell response. The paracortex expands and encroaches on the follicles. This pattern is often encountered in reactions induced by drugs and acute viral infections.

Sinus histiocytosis This is seen if there is a marked proliferation of histiocytic cells, which normally occupy the sinuses. The sinuses become dilated and engorged with numerous histiocytes.

Granulomatous lymphadenitis This term refers to the formation of granulomas within a lymph node. A granuloma is a collection of macrophages. Causes include:

- tuberculosis
- sarcoidosis
- cat scratch disease
- Crohn's disease
- toxoplasmosis
- reaction to foreign material.

Entity-specific reactive changes

A number of reactive conditions affecting lymph nodes induce morphological appearances which, although often complex, may be distinctive enough to enable the pathologist to make an exact diagnosis. Such conditions include certain infections (e.g. toxoplasmosis, human immunodeficiency virus (HIV) infection, Epstein–Barr virus infection), some connective tissue diseases (e.g. systemic lupus erythematosus), reactions to types of foreign material (e.g. silicone), certain drug reactions (e.g. some anticonvulsants) and conditions of uncertain aetiology (e.g. Castleman disease).

Neoplastic lymphadenopathy

Lymphoma

Lymphomas are primary neoplasms of the cells native to the lymphoid tissues. The term 'lymphoma' is a misnomer, because all lymphomas are potentially malignant.

Lymphomas are classified into subtypes according to histological appearance and immunophenotype (i.e. the staining patterns on immunohistochemistry). Different subtypes behave differently, have different prognoses, and require different treatments. Hence, classification of lymphoma is the means by which pathologists convey meaningful information to the clinicians. There have been a number of classification systems in the past (e.g. Kiel classification, Working Formulation for Clinical Usage), all of which have had their merits. However, many entities went by different names in the different classification systems, and this was a source of confusion for both pathologists and clinicians. In addition, there have been major advances in our knowledge and understanding of lymphoid neoplasms since the 1980s, and many new entities have now been recognised. To overcome these problems, a new unifying lymphoma classification system was devised and published by the International Lymphoma Study Group in 1994, and it was called the 'Revised European-American Classification of Lymphoid Neoplasms' (REAL). A few years later, when the World Health Organization (WHO) was developing a new classification system for neoplastic diseases of the haematopoietic and lymphoid tissues, it adopted the REAL classification, making only a few modifications. It is the 2001 WHO Lymphoma Classification System that is currently used in clinical practice.

There are two main types of lymphoma – Hodgkin's lymphoma and non-Hodgkin's lymphoma. They are considered separate for two main reasons:

- Hodgkin's lymphoma is characterised morphologically by the presence of unique neoplastic cells called Reed–Sternberg cells
- Hodgkin's lymphoma may be associated with certain clinical symptoms.

Hodgkin's lymphoma

Hodgkin's lymphoma is differentiated from the other types of lymphoma by the presence of distinctive and diagnostic tumour cells called Reed–Sternberg cells (RS cells), although for the diagnosis of Hodgkin's lymphoma to be made, the RS cells must be associated with the appropriate cellular background. Classically, the RS cell is large with a pale, bilobed nucleus and large, prominent, eosinophilic nucleoli. The nucleoli are bounded by a clear zone, giving the cell a characteristic 'owl-eye' appearance. The various subtypes of Hodgkin's lymphoma are shown in Table 57.

Clinical features Typical patients are young adults, the peak incidence being in the third and fourth decades of life. Patients usually present with painless lymphadenopathy, which typically affects the upper half of the body. The enlarged lymph nodes are discrete, mobile, and rubbery in consistency. Patients may also present with systemic symptoms (unexplained pyrexia, drenching night sweats, unexplained weight loss).

Staging Staging is an important determinant of treatment and prognosis. The staging system used is the Ann Arbor system:

- **Stage I** – involvement of a single lymph node region (I) or single extranodal organ or site (Ie).
- **Stage II** – involvement of two or more lymph node regions on the same side of the diaphragm (II), or one extranodal organ plus one or more lymph node regions on the same side of the diaphragm (IIe).
- **Stage III** – involvement of lymph regions on both sides of the diaphragm (III), which may be associated with splenic involvement (IIIs), or localised involvement of an extranodal site (IIIe), or both (IIIse).
- **Stage IV** – diffuse or disseminated involvement of one or more extralymphatic sites, such as the liver, lung, or bone marrow, with or without lymph node involvement.

Any of these stages may be followed by the suffix A or B, depending on whether the systemic symptoms are absent (A) or present (B). The presence of systemic symptoms is associated with a poorer prognosis.

Treatment and prognosis Factors associated with a poorer prognosis are:

- advancing age
- systemic symptoms
- advanced stage
- aggressive histological subtype (e.g. lymphocyte-depleted Hodgkin's lymphoma)
- abnormal blood markers.

With advances in treatment during the late 1990s, the prognosis of Hodgkin's lymphoma has generally improved, so that even with advanced disease, the 5-year disease-free survival is 60–70%.

Non-Hodgkin's lymphoma

Within this category, there is a much wider spectrum of lymphoid neoplasms, showing a marked diversity in their histological appearance, immunophenotype, biological behaviour, response to therapy, prognosis, and clinical settings, including typical age at onset. Because of the extremely complex nature of this group of lymphoid neoplasms, only a framework for the basic understanding of non-Hodgkin's lymphoma will be presented here as detailed descriptions of the various subtypes are not necessary in this text. The most frequently encountered subtypes are shown in Table 57. In basic terms, non-Hodgkin's lymphoma can be subdivided according to the type of lymphoid cell of origin into B cell non-Hodgkin's lymphoma and T cell/natural killer (NK) cell non-Hodgkin's lymphoma. These B and T cell neoplasms can be further subdivided into precursor (lymphoblastic) neoplasms or

Table 57 The WHO lymphoma classification system

Hodgkin's lymphoma	• Nodular lymphocyte-predominant Hodgkin's lymphoma		
	• Classical Hodgkin's lymphoma	• Nodular sclerosing Hodgkin's lymphoma	
		• Lymphocyte-rich classical Hodgkin's lymphoma	
		• Mixed-cellularity Hodgkin's lymphoma	
		• Lymphocyte-depleted Hodgkin's lymphoma	
Non-Hodgkin's lymphoma*	• B cell neoplasms	• Precursor B cell neoplasms	• Precursor B lymphocytic leukaemia/lymphoma§
		• Mature B cell neoplasms	• B cell chronic lymphocytic leukaemia/small lymphocytic lymphoma†
			• Plasma cell myeloma†
			• Extranodal marginal zone B cell lymphoma of MALT type
			• Follicular lymphoma†
			• Mantle cell lymphoma
			• Diffuse large B cell lymphoma†
			• Burkitt's lymphoma§
	• T/NK cell neoplasms	• Precursor T cell neoplasms	• Precursor T lymphoblastic lymphoma§
		• Mature T cell neoplasms	• Mycosis fungoides/Sézary syndrome
			• Peripheral T cell lymphoma
			• Angioimmunoblastic T cell lymphoma
			• Anaplastic large-cell lymphoma

*Within the non-Hodgkin's group, only the most common subtypes are shown.
†The subtypes which constitute the majority of lymphoid neoplasms in adults.
§The subtypes most common in children.

mature (peripheral) neoplasms. Within these categories, the various distinct entities are then listed.

In the past, grading of lymphomas has sometimes been used, but the current convention is to grade only follicular lymphomas, because only for this particular lymphoma subtype does grading add any further information. Low-grade follicular lymphomas have an indolent clinical course but respond poorly to therapy, and high-grade follicular lymphomas behave more aggressively but respond well to therapy. With all other subtypes of lymphoma, the behaviour and expected response to therapy is implied by the diagnosis. For example, Burkitt's lymphoma is always a high-grade tumour, and therefore behaves aggressively but responds quite well to very aggressive therapy.

Diagnosis of lymphoma

In order to make a definitive diagnosis of lymphoma, a lymph node biopsy is often performed and the node examined histologically. In some cases, cytogenetic analysis is used in conjunction with histological assessment in order to make the correct diagnosis. Lymph node biopsy may be preceded by fine-needle aspiration cytology.

Secondary tumours

The tumours most often encountered in the lymph nodes are metastatic rather than primary. Most carcinomas, mel-anomas, and some sarcomas have the capacity to metasta-sise via the lymphatic system.

24.2 The thymus

> **Learning objectives**
>
> You should:
> • understand the structure and function of the thymus
> • know the common disorders of the thymus.

Structure and function

The thymus is an encapsulated bilobed structure, which is situated in the anterior superior mediastinum.

It is embryologically derived from the third and, occasionally, fourth pharyngeal pouches. The gland grows in size until puberty (weighing up to 50 g), thereafter undergoing progressive atrophy and gradual replacement by fibrofatty tissue.

The thymus has a central role in cell-mediated immunity. During fetal development, stem cells derived from the bone marrow migrate to the thymus where they differentiate and mature into T cells. A small population of B cells is also present. The thymus has a lymphoid component and an epithelial component.

Disorders of the thymus

Agenesis and aplasia

These conditions are the result of failure of development of either the epithelial or lymphoid component of the thymus. In DiGeorge syndrome, there is failure of development of the third and fourth pharyngeal pouches that normally give rise to the thymus and parathyroid glands. Affected infants have grossly reduced cell-mediated immunity due to absence of the thymus, and hypocalcaemia leading to tetany due to absence of the parathyroids. Cardiac defects and abnormal facies may also be a feature. In Nezelof syndrome, which is an inherited condition, only the thymus is affected.

Thymic hyperplasia (thymic follicular hyperplasia)

This condition is characterised by the presence of lymphoid follicles with germinal centres within the thymus. Thymic hyperplasia is seen in ~70% of patients with the autoimmune condition myasthenia gravis. In these patients, the thymus appears to be the main source of the autoantibody, and thymectomy may therefore be of benefit. A degree of thymic hyperplasia may also be seen in other autoimmune disorders such as Graves' disease, systemic lupus erythematosus, systemic sclerosis and rheumatoid arthritis.

Neoplasms of the thymus

The main types of neoplasms that can arise within the thymus are:

- thymoma
- thymic carcinoma
- lymphoma
- germ cell tumours (rare)
- neuroendocrine tumours (rare).

Thymomas

Thymomas are tumours of thymic epithelial cells. Many are asymptomatic and are only detected on chest X-ray performed for other reasons. Others become manifest clinically through local pressure symptoms, e.g. stridor, cough or dyspnoea, or through their association with myasthenia gravis. The majority of thymomas are completely benign.

Thymic carcinomas

They are usually highly aggressive.

Lymphoma

Can occur in the thymus. The thymus is not an uncommon site for Hodgkin's lymphoma and thymic involvement by non-Hodgkin's lymphoma, mostly T cell neoplasms or large B cell lymphomas, is frequently encountered.

Germ cell tumours

Tumours such as seminomas and teratomas may be encountered. They are derived from germ cells that have failed to migrate to the gonads during fetal life.

Neuroendocrine tumours

Thymic carcinoids may arise from neuroendocrine cells that are scattered throughout the gland.

24.3 The spleen

Learning objectives

You should:
- understand the structure and function of the spleen
- know the major causes of splenomegaly
- understand the importance of splenic rupture.

Structure and function

The spleen is an encapsulated organ, which is situated in the left upper quadrant of the abdomen. The spleen receives blood from the splenic artery and, in general, it is to the circulatory system what the lymph nodes are to the lymphatic system. The adult organ has two main functions:

- filtration and phagocytosis of obsolescent red blood cells and bacteria
- mounting immunological responses.

Reflecting these functions, the spleen has two main components: the white pulp, which is lymphoid tissue and is where immunological responses are mounted, and the red pulp, which is the site of blood filtration and phagocytosis.

The white pulp

The splenic artery enters the spleen at the hilum and then divides to give rise to numerous central arteries, which ramify through the organ. Each central artery becomes ensheathed in lymphoid cells, which constitute the white pulp. The white pulp consists of periarteriolar lymphoid sheaths (PALS) of T cells, which are intermittently expanded by B cell follicles. The unstimulated B cell follicle consists of a nodule of small B lymphocytes surrounded by a rim of larger, marginal zone B cells. If the B cell follicle is stimulated, a germinal centre forms in the centre, surrounded by a mantle zone of small unchallenged B cells, which are surrounded by the marginal zone (Figure 67).

The red pulp

The red pulp consists of sinusoids separated by splenic cords (Figure 68). The splenic cords contain numerous macrophages. Once blood has left the central artery of the white pulp, it passes into capillaries. Blood within the capillaries can either drain directly into the sinusoids and then into the splenic veins ('closed' circulation), or it can first enter the splenic cords and then pass into the sinu-

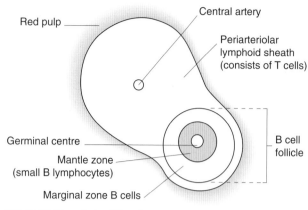

Figure 67 The splenic white pulp.

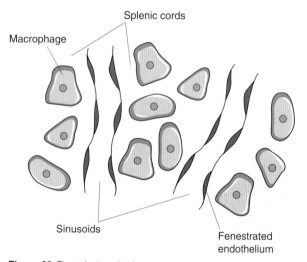

Figure 68 The splenic red pulp.

soids through fenestrations in the sinusoid epithelium ('open' circulation). In the open circulation, red blood cells must undergo extreme deformation to pass from the cords into the sinusoids. Obsolescent, damaged or abnormal red blood cells have reduced deformability and, therefore, become trapped within the splenic cords where they are phagocytosed.

Macroscopically, the cut surface of the spleen is red (red pulp) dotted with grey specks (white pulp).

Disorders of the spleen

Congenital abnormalities

An accessory (supernumerary) spleen is not uncommon, the most usual location being the hilum of the spleen. Congenital absence of the spleen (asplenia) and polysplenia are rare and are often associated with other congenital defects.

Splenomegaly

This term refers to enlargement of the spleen. With very few exceptions, pathological states in the spleen are manifest as splenomegaly, and there are numerous causes. However, apart from being an indicator of an underlying disorder, splenomegaly may itself cause problems by inducing portal hypertension (because of increased blood flow though the organ) and hypersplenism. Hypersplenism is characterised by splenomegaly, a deficiency in one or more of the cellular elements in the blood, and correction of the cytopenia(s) by splenectomy.

Causes of splenomegaly include:

- infections (e.g. acute non-specific splenitis, infectious mononucleosis, malaria, miliary tuberculosis)
- congestion (e.g. cardiac failure, cirrhosis, portal hypertension)
- lymphohaematogenous disorders and neoplasms (e.g. lymphoma, leukaemia, haemolytic anaemia)
- immune inflammatory disorders (e.g. rheumatoid arthritis, systemic lupus erythematosus)
- storage diseases (e.g. Gaucher's disease)
- amyloidosis and sarcoidosis.

Infection

The morphological changes which occur in the spleen during infection often vary depending on the particular infecting organism. In acute non-specific splenitis due to sepsis, the spleen becomes very soft and, when sliced, the substance of the spleen typically flows out from the cut surface. In infectious mononucleosis the splenic capsule is particularly vulnerable to rupture. In malaria, the spleen can reach a massive size and is markedly congested.

Congestive splenomegaly

Persistent elevation of the splenic or portal venous blood pressure can cause splenomegaly. The pressure may be raised due to prehepatic, hepatic or post-hepatic causes. Prehepatic causes include thrombosis of the splenic or portal veins. The most important hepatic cause is cirrhosis. Post-hepatic causes include thrombosis of the hepatic veins (Budd–Chiari syndrome), and raised inferior vena cava pressure associated with right heart failure.

The spleen may be considerably enlarged and the capsule is often thickened and fibrotic. The cut surface is dark red with inconspicuous white pulp. Microscopically, the increased venous pressure is reflected by distension of the sinusoids by red blood cells. Collagen may be laid down in the basement membranes of distended sinusoids, resulting in impairment of blood flow from the cords to the sinusoids. The red blood cells are therefore exposed to the cord macrophages for much longer, and hypersplenism may result. The elevated venous pressure can lead to sinusoid rupture and intraparenchymal haemorrhage. Organisation of these areas gives rise to small brown nodules called Gamna–Gandy bodies, which are visible with the naked eye.

Lymphohaematogenous neoplasms

The spleen is not infrequently involved in a number of lymphoid and haematological neoplasms. Each type of neoplasm is associated with a different pattern of splenic involvement. For example, in chronic myeloid leukaemia, the red pulp is filled with mature myeloid precursors, and in Hodgkin's lymphoma, the white pulp is preferentially involved with the formation of expansile nodules.

Non-lymphohaematogenous tumours of the spleen are rare, but include hamartomas, lymphangiomas and haemangiomas.

Splenic infarction

Splenic infarcts are due to occlusion of the splenic artery or one of its branches, and are usually secondary to emboli that arise in the heart. Occasionally, infarction is due to localised thrombosis (e.g. in sickle cell disease). Infarcts are characteristically pale and wedge shaped. They may be single or multiple, and healing leads to the formation of scars, which depress the surface.

Splenic rupture

Rupture of the spleen is most commonly the result of blunt trauma, such as can occur during a car accident when the steering wheel may inflict a severe blow to the upper abdomen. Spontaneous splenic rupture may occur if the organ is enlarged and abnormally soft, as in infectious mononucleosis. Rupture is followed by extensive intra-peritoneal haemorrhage. Prompt splenectomy is necessary to prevent death from hypovolaemic shock.

Twenty four

Self-assessment: questions

One best answer question

1. A 25-year-old woman presents to her general practitioner with a lump in the right side of the neck. She also states that she has lost weight recently and has been experiencing night sweats. On examination, the lump measures about 3 cm across, is painless, discrete and mobile, but does not move on swallowing. An excisional biopsy was performed and this showed an abnormal lymph node with a completely effaced architecture and scattered single atypical cells with bilobed nuclei and large eosinophilic nucleoli. The most likely diagnosis is:
   a. non-specific reactive lymphadenopathy
   b. lymphoma
   c. metastatic carcinoma
   d. tuberculosis
   e. thyroid neoplasm

2. A 60-year old man died at home. He had a history of increasing shortness of breath. A coroner's post mortem was carried out to determine the cause of death. The main findings were a fish-mouth deformity of the mitral valve, left atrial dilatation and right ventricular hypertrophy, markedly congested and oedematous lungs, a 'nutmeg liver' and a mildly enlarged spleen containing small, firm, brown nodules. The most likely diagnosis is:
   a. carcinomatosis
   b. infective endocarditis
   c. sarcoidosis
   d. pulmonary thromboembolism
   e. congestive cardiac failure

True-false questions

1. The following statements are correct:
   a. lymph nodes are only found in the neck
   b. after passing through lymph nodes, lymph enters the bloodstream via the thoracic duct
   c. lymph node enlargement always indicates a malignant process
   d. acute viral infections cause paracortical expansion
   e. the primary follicles within a lymph node are composed of T cells

2. The following statements are correct:
   a. lymphomas may affect the gastrointestinal tract
   b. Hodgkin's lymphoma is one of the most common forms of malignancy in young adults

   c. lymph nodes involved by Hodgkin's lymphoma may become painful on consumption of alcohol
   d. non-Hodgkin's lymphomas are characterised by the presence of Reed–Sternberg cells
   e. the definitive diagnosis of lymphoma requires histological assessment of a lymph node biopsy specimen

3. The following statements regarding the thymus are correct:
   a. the thymus is situated in the anterior superior mediastinum
   b. thymomas are tumours of thymic T cells
   c. thymic hyperplasia may be associated with myasthenia gravis
   d. DiGeorge syndrome is associated with thymic enlargement
   e. the thymus is most active in late adult life

4. The following statements regarding the spleen are correct:
   a. the spleen is composed of white pulp and red pulp
   b. malaria is associated with development of massive splenomegaly
   c. splenomegaly may be associated with leucopenia
   d. spontaneous rupture of the spleen refers to splenic rupture when there is no underlying pathology
   e. splenectomy should be supplemented by vaccination against *Pneumococcus*

5. The following statements are true:
   a. reactive lymphadenopathy is usually self-limiting
   b. lymph node enlargement associated with pyrexia and night sweats is always due to infection
   c. lymphoma hardly ever occurs in young people
   d. the diagnosis of lymphoma is made on clinical grounds alone
   e. high-grade lymphomas always respond poorly to treatment

Case history questions

Case history 1

A 32-year-old woman presented to her general practitioner with unexplained weight loss and drenching night sweats for the last 6 months. On examination she has right-sided cervical lymphadenopathy.

1. What diagnoses would you consider?
2. What further information would you seek from the history and examination to help determine the diagnosis?
3. What tests might you perform to establish the diagnosis?

Viva questions

1. How are lymphomas classified?
2. How might thymic tumours present clinically?
3. What are the main causes of congestive splenomegaly?

Self-assessment: answers

One best answer

1. b. Lymphoma. The atypical cells described in the lymph node biopsy are consistent with Reed–Sternberg cells seen in Hodgkin's lymphoma. The combination of young age, painless lymphadenopathy, systemic symptoms and Reed–Sternberg cells in the lymph node biopsy all point to this diagnosis. However, remember that a lump in the neck could represent any number of pathological processes – an enlarged lymph node, a thyroid mass, a salivary gland mass (the parotid gland also extends into the neck in many people), a branchial cyst or a soft tissue lesion. An adequate history and examination together with imaging studies and fine-needle aspiration cytology (FNAC) usually indicates the tissue involved and possibly the nature of the lump, but if lymphoma is suspected, excision biopsy is mandatory for confirmation of the diagnosis and accurate subtyping. Thyroid lumps usually move on swallowing, so a thyroid neoplasm is unlikely, and metastatic carcinoma would be unusual in a patient of this age. Tuberculosis may present with lymphadenopathy, weight loss and night sweats, but a history of recent travel abroad may be given and the lymph node biopsy would typically show numerous caseating granulomas. With non-specific reactive lymphadenopathy, the lymph node is typically painful on palpation and there is usually a history of recent illness (e.g. tonsillitis). Weight loss and night sweats would be unusual. However, imaging studies, FNAC and/or excision biopsy would be required to confirm the diagnosis.

2. e. Congestive cardiac failure. The fish-mouth deformity to the mitral valve denotes mitral stenosis. This leads to increased pressure in the left atrium (causing left atrial dilatation) and pulmonary veins (causing raised pulmonary venous pressure, pulmonary oedema and right ventricular hypertrophy). The 'nutmeg liver' represents chronic passive venous congestion of the liver and the small, firm, brown nodules in the spleen are most likely to be Gamna–Gandy bodies seen in longstanding severe congestive splenomegaly. All of the changes in the cardiac chambers, lungs, liver and spleen can be explained by the haemodynamic disturbances caused by severe mitral stenosis. The history of shortness of breath is consistent with cardiac failure. Carcinomatosis would appear as multiple tumour nodules at many sites. The characteristic vegetations observed on cardiac valves complicated by infective endocarditis were not seen in this case. Sarcoidosis can cause hepatosplenomegaly, but the changes described in the heart do not fit with this diagnosis. Thromboembolism can be seen in patients with mitral stenosis through the increased risk of atrial fibrillation (leading to thrombus formation), but since the thrombus would form in the left atrium it would enter the systemic circulation, not the pulmonary circulation. Systemic thromboembolism could lead to infarction of the spleen, but splenic infarcts usually appear pale and wedge shaped.

True-false answers

1. a. **False.**
   b. **True.**
   c. **False.**
   d. **True.**
   e. **False.** Primary follicles are composed predominantly of B cells.

2. a. **True.** The gastrointestinal tract contains mucosa-associated lymphoid tissue within its wall, which may be involved by lymphoma.
   b. **True.**
   c. **True.**
   d. **False.** Reed–Sternberg cells are seen in Hodgkin's lymphoma.
   e. **True.**

3. a. **True.**
   b. **False.** Thymomas are tumours of thymic epithelial cells.
   c. **True.**
   d. **False.**
   e. **False.** The thymus undergoes progressive atrophy after puberty.

4. a. **True.**
   b. **True.**
   c. **True.** Splenomegaly may induce hypersplenism.
   d. **False.** Spontaneous splenic rupture refers to non-traumatic rupture. If rupture is spontaneous, an underlying pathology predisposing to rupture must be considered.
   e. **True.** Patients who have had a splenectomy have a life-long increased risk of infection with *Pneumococcus* and other encapsulated bacteria. Hence they should be considered for vaccination.

5. a. **True.**
   b. **False.** Hodgkin's disease can present in a similar way.

c. **False.**

d. **False.** Clinical and radiological findings may suggest lymphoma, but histological examination (± cytogenetic analysis) is required for definitive diagnosis in all cases.

e. **False.**

Case history answers

Case history 1

1. There are two main causes of lymph node enlargement – a reactive process and a neoplastic process. In this case the lymphadenopathy is associated with a 6-month history of unexplained weight loss and drenching night sweats. This should raise the possibility of Hodgkin's lymphoma, and the age of the patient and apparent involvement of only one group of nodes in the upper part of the body is supportive of this diagnosis. However, this combination of symptoms and findings is also seen during the course of some infections. Although an acute infection is unlikely with this long history, a chronic infection should be considered. For example, tuberculosis could cause pyrexia with night sweats, weight loss and cervical lymphadenopathy. Secondary involvement of the lymph nodes by a malignant tumour is unlikely in this age group.

2. *Comment*: Ask questions to determine if an infective process could be causing the symptoms, e.g. chronic cough, pharyngitis, laryngitis, etc. You should also ask if there has been any recent travel abroad where an unusual infection, such as tuberculosis, could have been contracted. Remember that lymph nodes affected by Hodgkin's lymphoma may be painful on consumption of alcohol, so you should enquire about this. All systems should be examined in the physical examination to exclude an infective aetiology. Remember that a low-grade pyrexia may be present in Hodgkin's lymphoma. Lymph nodes involved by an infective process may be tender on palpation. Lymph nodes affected by Hodgkin's lymphoma are said to be discrete, mobile, and rubbery in consistency. You would also need to examine for lymphadenopathy elsewhere on the body, and see if there is any associated splenomegaly or hepatomegaly. Remember that the spleen may be enlarged in some infective processes, most notably infectious mononucleosis.

3. If the possibility of lymphoma is not excluded on history or examination, the next step is either to remove part, or all, of an affected lymph node for formal histological assessment or to perform a fine-needle aspiration (FNA) and examine the extracted cells for any signs of a neoplastic process. If signs of neoplasia are present on FNA, the lymph node must then be removed for formal histological assessment and diagnosis. Other tests may aid the diagnosis of infections. To diagnose tuberculosis, a chest X-ray should be the performed but ultimately the bacillus must be isolated in a tissue specimen, usually either sputum or a biopsy. Serology may be helpful in the diagnosis of some infections, e.g. infectious mononucleosis.

Viva answers

1. The classification of lymphoma has been a hot topic lately. The classification system now used by most clinicians is the WHO classification, which is based on the REAL classification. Lymphomas are divided into two main types – Hodgkin's lymphoma and non-Hodgkin's lymphoma. Within these two groups there are a number of separate entities that differ in their histological appearance, immunophenotype, clinical behaviour and prognosis (see Table 57).

2. Many thymic tumours are discovered incidentally during the course of thoracic surgery or imaging studies. Thymic abnormalities are actively sought in patients with myasthenia gravis. When they reach a certain size they produce local pressure symptoms relating to their location in the anterior mediastinum, e.g. stridor, cough or dyspnoea.

3. Congestive splenomegaly arises when there is persistent or chronic venous congestion. The venous congestion may be systemic (such as in right-sided cardiac failure) or localised, but traditionally the causes of congestive splenomegaly are divided into three categories:

- prehepatic causes
- hepatic causes
- post-hepatic causes.

Prehepatic causes include obstruction of the extra-hepatic portal vein or splenic vein by thrombus or an inflammatory process. By far the most common hepatic cause is cirrhosis. Post-hepatic causes include right-sided cardiac failure and thrombosis of the hepatic veins (Budd–Chiari syndrome).

Bones and soft tissue

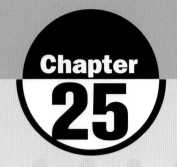

Chapter overview

Within the osteoarticular system, the bones provide structural support for the body and have an important role in mineral homeostasis and haematopoiesis, and the joints permit movement. Disorders of the osteoarticular system can, therefore, cause significant disability and deformity. Most of the more common disorders such as osteoarthritis, osteoporosis and rheumatoid arthritis are chronic and progressive, causing significant morbidity among the general population, especially the elderly. Bone tumours affect all age groups, show marked diversity in their behaviour and different types target particular age groups and anatomic sites. Connective tissue diseases form an important group of multisystem disorders, and they are presented here because a feature common to most of them is their propensity to involve the joints and soft tissues. 'Soft tissue tumours' form a highly heterogeneous group of neoplasms that are important because benign tumours are relatively frequent and sarcomas are often highly aggressive.

25.1 Bone

Learning objectives

You should:
- know the structure and function of bones
- know the major bone diseases, their pathogenesis and clinicopathological features
- know the major types of bone tumour.

Structure and function

The skeletal system is composed of 206 bones, and has a number of functions:

- Structural support.
- Protective. The skull and the vertebral column protect the brain and spinal cord respectively. The ribs protect the thoracic and upper abdominal organs to a lesser degree.
- Mineral homeostasis. Bone is a reservoir for the body's calcium, phosphorus and magnesium.
- Haematopoiesis. Under normal conditions in the adult, bone is the sole site of haematopoietic marrow.

Bone is a special type of connective tissue, which is mineralised, and therefore has an organic and inorganic component. The organic component is the connective tissue matrix composed predominantly of type I collagen. The organic matrix undergoes mineralisation by the deposition of the mineral calcium hydroxyapatite. This mineral is the inorganic component of bone. Mineralisation gives bone its strength and hardness. Unmineralised bone is called osteoid. Bone formation, maintenance and remodelling is performed by the bone cells, of which there are three main types:

- **Osteoblasts** – these cells are responsible for bone formation. They synthesise the type I collagen that forms osteoid, and also initiate the process of mineralisation.
- **Osteoclasts** – these are multinucleate cells responsible for bone resorption.
- **Osteocytes** – evidence suggests that these cells have an important role in the control of the daily fluctuations in serum calcium and phosphorus levels and the maintenance of bone.

Bone can be formed quickly or slowly. When bone is formed quickly, such as in fracture repair or fetal development, the osteoblasts deposit the collagen in a random weave arrangement. This type of bone is called woven bone. Woven bone is replaced by lamellar bone, which is formed much more slowly.

In lamellar bone, the collagen is arranged in parallel sheets. Lamellar bone can also form without a woven bone framework. There are two types of mature lamellar bone:

- **Cortical (compact) bone** – this is composed of numerous units called haversian systems. In each haversian system the lamellar bone is arranged concentrically around a central canal called the haversian canal, through which arteries and veins run.
- **Cancellous (spongy) bone** – this consists of lamellar bone arranged in a meshwork of bone trabeculae.

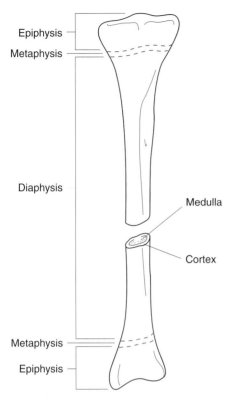

Epiphysis
Metaphysis
Diaphysis
Medulla
Cortex
Metaphysis
Epiphysis

Figure 69 Parts of a bone.

Most bones are tubular, hollow structures that consist of a shaft, called the diaphysis, expanded end regions, called the epiphyses, and a region between the diaphysis and each epiphysis, called the metaphysis (Figure 69). The sleeve-like tube (or cortex) of each bone is composed of compact sheets of cortical bone. The inner portion of bone is not quite hollow and is called the medulla. The medulla contains cancellous bone, connective tissue, nerves, blood vessels, fat, and haematopoietic tissue. All bones are covered by a periosteum composed of connective tissue.

Development and growth of the skeleton

During fetal development, bone can be formed either directly in mesenchyme, as in the case of the skull and clavicles (intramembranous ossification), or on pre-existing cartilage (endochondral ossification). In intramembranous ossification, bone is laid down as woven bone that eventually matures into lamellar bone. In endochondral ossification, the cartilaginous template undergoes ossification at particular sites along the bone known as ossification centres. In long bones, the cartilage at the epiphysis persists until after puberty, allowing growth. This area of persisting cartilage is called the growth plate.

Once the bones are fully formed, further growth occurs by the laying down of further bone onto the pre-existing bone. The coordinated actions of the osteoblasts and osteoclasts are paramount in bone development and maintenance. In bone development, the action of osteoblasts predominates. When the skeleton has reached maturity, the bones are continually renewed and remodelled, which requires the actions of the osteoblasts and osteoclasts to be in equilibrium. By the third decade, osteoclastic resorption begins to predominate, with a resultant steady decrease in skeletal mass.

Developmental disorders

Achondroplasia

Achondroplasia is a major cause of dwarfism, and is due to mutation of a single gene. The condition can be familial, with autosomal dominant inheritance, or sporadic. The defective gene leads to abnormal ossification at the growth plates of bones formed by endochondral ossification. Intramembranous ossification is unaffected. Affected individuals have a characteristic appearance, with shortening of the proximal extremities, a relatively normal-sized trunk, and a disproportionately large head with typical bulging of the forehead and depression of the nasal bridge.

Osteogenesis imperfecta ('brittle bone' disease)

This is a rare group of genetic disorders that have in common the abnormal synthesis of type I collagen. In addition to bone, the other tissues rich in type I collagen are tendons, ligaments, skin, dentine and sclera. Affected individuals have brittle bones and spontaneous fractures may occur. The sclera appears blue because it is so thin that the underlying uveal pigment becomes visible. Some variants of osteogenesis imperfecta are fatal early in life while others are associated with survival.

Acquired disorders

Osteoporosis

Osteoporosis is characterised by reduced bone mass, making bone vulnerable to fracture. Trabecular bone is affected before cortical bone. Trabecular bone is found in the greatest amounts in the vertebral bodies and pelvis, and cortical bone is found in the greatest amounts in the long bones.

Aetiology and pathogenesis

Osteoporosis may be primary or secondary. Primary osteoporosis refers to senile osteoporosis and post-menopausal osteoporosis. Secondary osteoporosis is due to conditions other than age or menopause, such as reduced mobility (e.g. after fracture or associated with rheumatoid arthritis), smoking and alcohol consumption, endocrine disorders (e.g. Cushing's syndrome, hyperthyroidism, diabetes) and corticosteroid therapy. Obesity and exercise appear to be protective against osteoporosis.

Senile osteoporosis There is a normal progressive loss of bone mass after around the age of 30 years, and so all elderly people will have some degree of osteoporosis. Bone loss rarely exceeds 1% per year. The higher the initial bone density, the lower the risk of significant osteoporosis. Women are at higher risk than men, and white people are at higher risk than black people.

Post-menopausal osteoporosis Post-menopausal osteoporosis is characterised by hormone-dependent acceleration of bone loss. Post-menopausal women may lose up to 2% of cortical bone per year and up to 9% of trabecular bone per year for 8–10 years, declining to the normal rate of bone loss after that. Oestrogen deficiency is thought to have a major role, and oestrogen replacement at the beginning of the menopause reduces the rate of bone loss.

Clinical features

The major complication of osteoporosis is bone fracture. The sites most commonly affected are the vertebral bodies, the distal radius (Colles' fracture) and the hips. Fractures of the vertebral bodies can be of the 'crush' variety leading to progressive loss of height and considerable pain, or of the 'wedge' variety causing deformity of the spine (kyphosis). Hip fractures are important because they cause major disability and lead to hospital admission. Secondary complications such as pneumonia and pulmonary thromboembolism are common with hip fractures, and account for the high mortality rate associated with hip fractures.

Treatment

Women who take hormone replacement therapy have a reduced risk of developing post-menopausal osteoporosis. Also, oral bisphosphonates and vitamin D may be effective.

Metabolic bone disease

Rickets and osteomalacia

Osteomalacia is characterised by defective mineralisation of the osteoid matrix, and is associated with lack of vitamin D. When the condition occurs in the growing skeleton (children) it is called rickets. Vitamin D is important in the maintenance of adequate serum calcium and phosphorus levels, and deficiency impairs normal mineralisation of osteoid laid down in the remodelling of bone. The result is osteomalacia. In children, lack of vitamin D leads to inadequate mineralisation of the epiphyseal cartilage as well as the osteoid, resulting in rickets.

Aetiology

There are two main sources of vitamin D – dietary and endogenous. Consequently, there are four main causes of osteomalacia:

- **Dietary deficiency of vitamin D** – this used to be a common cause of rickets and osteomalacia. Improvements in diet and the addition of vitamin D to foodstuffs has drastically reduced the incidence of osteomalacia due to nutritional deficiency.
- **Intestinal malabsorption** – this is now the commonest cause of osteomalacia. Vitamin D is fat soluble. Any condition that causes malabsorption or poor absorption of fat (steatorrhoea) can cause osteomalacia. Causes include coeliac disease and Crohn's disease.
- **Deficiency of endogenous vitamin D due to defective synthesis in the skin** – more than 90% of circulating vitamin D is photochemically synthesised in the skin. A steroid molecule precursor found in the epidermis is converted to vitamin D by UV light from the sun. Decreased exposure to sunlight or increased skin pigmentation hinders synthesis of vitamin D.

- **Renal or liver disease** – newly synthesised vitamin D is biologically inactive. A number of metabolic steps are required to convert vitamin D into its active form. The first of these steps is carried out by hepatocytes. The resulting compound is converted to the active form of vitamin D (1,25-dihydroxycalciferol) in the kidney. Hence, renal disease and, to a lesser extent, liver disease can lead to a deficiency in the active form of vitamin D.

Clinicopathological features

The basic abnormality is deficient mineralisation of the organic matrix of the skeleton. In children, the skeleton becomes deformed because there is reduced structural rigidity and inadequate ossification at the growth plates. In pre-ambulatory infants, there is flattening of the occipital bones, and in ambulatory children, bowing of the legs and lumbar lordosis are characteristic. A pigeon breast deformity may develop due to the forces incurred on the weakened bones of the chest during normal respiration. Excess osteoid may cause frontal bossing of the head. Inadequate calcification of the epiphyseal cartilage in long bones leads to cartilaginous overgrowth at the growth plates, resulting in localised enlargement, which is seen especially at the wrists, knees and ankles. Overgrowth of the cartilage at the costochondral junctions of the chest results in an appearance that is referred to as a 'rachitic rosary'.

In adults, the osteoid that is laid down in the remodelling of bone is inadequately mineralised. The shape of the bone is usually not affected, but the bone becomes vulnerable to spontaneous fractures. Looser zones (pseudofractures) are the hallmark of osteomalacia, and they appear on X-rays as transverse linear lucencies perpendicular to the bone surface. Persistent inadequate mineralisation may eventually lead to generalised osteopenia.

Hyperparathyroidism and renal osteodystrophy

These are discussed in Chapter 19.

Paget's disease (osteitis deformans)

The aetiology of Paget's disease is uncertain. There is an initial phase of osteoclastic resorption of bone followed by a 'reparative phase' in which there is intense osteoblastic activity and overproduction of disordered and architecturally abnormal bone. Bones may become larger than normal, and are composed of structurally unsound cortical bone and thickened trabeculae with numerous prominent cement lines, which give the bone its characteristic 'mosaic pattern' on microscopy. Later, bone may become ivory hard ('sclerosis'). The abnormal bone is vulnerable to fracture.

Clinical features and complications

The clinical features and complications of Paget's disease are:

- bone pain
- fractures
- neuropathies

- deformities
- deafness
- high-output heart failure
- osteosarcoma and other bone tumours.

The usual presenting features are bone pain, deformities and fractures. The axial skeleton, skull and proximal femur are involved in the vast majority of cases. Pain is a common problem, and is localised to the affected bone. Deformities are most common when the skull is involved, resulting in enlargement of the head with protuberance of the frontal lobes and lion-like (leonine) facies. When the long bones of the lower extremities are involved, weight-bearing leads to anterior bowing of the legs. Fractures occur most commonly in the long bones of the legs, and 'crush' fractures of the spine may lead to spinal cord injury and kyphosis.

The spinal cord and nerve roots are also at risk of compression due to enlargement of the vertebral bodies. Distortion of the middle ear cavity and VIIIth nerve compression may lead to deafness. Other cranial nerves may be affected by compression. The bones in Paget's disease are extremely vascular, and the subsequent increased blood flow can (rarely) lead to high-output heart failure. Paget's disease may be complicated by the development of bone tumours, the most sinister being osteosarcoma.

Diagnosis and treatment

Paget's disease may be detected incidentally on X-ray or become manifest through the development of typical clinical features. Intense osteoblastic activity means that affected individuals have raised serum alkaline phosphatase levels. Treatment is with calcitonin and bisphosphonates.

Osteomyelitis

Osteomyelitis refers to inflammation of the bone and marrow, and is usually the result of infection.

Aetiology

Organisms may gain access to the bone by bloodstream spread from a distant infected site, by contiguous spread from neighbouring tissues, or by direct access via a penetrating injury. Almost any organism can cause osteomyelitis, but those most frequently implicated are bacteria. *Staphylococcus aureus* is responsible for many cases. Patients with sickle cell disease are predisposed to *Salmonella* osteomyelitis. *Mycobacterium tuberculosis* is sometimes implicated.

Pathogenesis

The location of the lesions within a particular bone depends on the intraosseous vascular circulation, which varies with age. In infants less than a year old, the epiphysis is usually affected. In children the metaphysis is usually affected, and in adults the diaphysis is most commonly affected.

In acute osteomyelitis, once the infection has become localised in bone, an intense acute inflammatory process begins. The release of numerous mediators into the haver-

sian canals leads to compression of the arteries and veins, resulting in localised bone death (osteonecrosis). The bacteria and inflammation spread via the haversian systems to reach the periosteum. Subperiosteal abscess formation and lifting of the periosteum further impairs the blood supply to the bone, resulting in further necrosis. The dead piece of bone is called the sequestrum. Rupture of the periosteum leads to formation of drainage sinuses, which drain pus onto the skin. If osteomyelitis becomes chronic, a rind of viable new bone is formed around the sequestrum and below the periosteum. This new bone is called an involucrum. An intraosseous abscess, called a Brodie abscess, may form.

Clinical features and treatment

Acute osteomyelitis presents with localised bone pain and soft tissue swelling. If there is systemic infection, patients may present with an acute systemic illness. Presentation may be extremely subtle in children and infants, who may present only with pyrexia (pyrexia of unknown origin, PUO). Characteristic X-ray changes consist of a lytic focus of bone surrounded by a zone of sclerosis. Treatment requires aggressive antibiotic therapy. Inadequate treatment of acute osteomyelitis may lead to chronic osteomyelitis, which is notoriously difficult to manage. Surgical removal of bony tissue may be required.

Avascular necrosis

This is necrosis of bone due to ischaemia. Ischaemia may result if the blood supply to a bone is interrupted, which may occur if there is a fracture particularly in areas where blood supply is suboptimal (e.g. the scaphoid and the femoral neck). Most other cases of avascular necrosis are either idiopathic or follow corticosteroid administration.

Bone tumours

Primary bone tumours are uncommon. They can generally be classified according to whether they are cartilage-forming or bone-forming.

Benign cartilage-forming tumours

Osteochondroma (exostosis)

Osteochondromas are cartilage-capped bony outgrowths, which most frequently occur near the metaphysis of long bones. Affected individuals are usually less than 20 years of age. Exostoses are usually solitary. Malignant change is very rare.

Chondroma (enchondroma)

Chondromas are cartilaginous tumours that usually arise within the medullary cavity of the bones of the hands and feet. They occur most frequently in the third to fifth decades of life. The lesions can sometimes cause localised pain, swelling, tenderness or pathological fracture. X-rays show the characteristic 'O-ring' sign – oval-shaped radiolucent cartilage surrounded by a dense rim of bone. Most chondromas are solitary. Malignant change is extremely rare.

Other rare benign cartilage-forming tumours are chondroblastomas and chondromyxoid fibromas.

Malignant cartilage-forming tumours

Chondrosarcoma

Chondrosarcoma is the second most common primary tumour of bone, being half as frequent as osteosarcoma. Chondrosarcomas occur most frequently in the trunk bones (ribs, spine and pelvis). A few develop within pre-existing osteochondromas, chondroblastomas, or bones affected by Paget's disease. They present as painful enlarging masses, and their nodular growth pattern gives them a scalloped appearance on X-ray. Most chondrosarcomas are low grade, and therefore pursue a relatively indolent course. However, high-grade tumours metastasise in 70% of cases, usually to other parts of the skeleton or the lungs.

Benign bone-forming tumours

Osteoma

These are bosselated tumours of bone, which most frequently occur in the skull and facial bones. Symptoms depend on the site at which they occur, e.g. symptoms due to obstruction of paranasal sinuses, symptoms related to impingement on the brain.

Osteoid osteoma

These round tumours consist of a small central area (called the 'nidus') surrounded by dense sclerotic bone. Affected individuals are usually less than 25 years old. The lesions are characteristically painful.

Malignant bone-forming tumours

Osteosarcomas

These are the commonest primary malignant tumour of bone, and they usually affect young adults. The metaphysis of long bones are the most frequently affected sites, particularly the distal femur. They present as painful enlarging masses. The tumours usually penetrate the bone cortex, causing elevation of the periosteum. This produces the characteristic triangular shadow (Codman triangle) seen on X-ray, formed by the bone cortex and the elevated ends of the periosteum. Patients with hereditary retinoblastoma are at significantly increased risk of developing osteosarcomas. Mutations in the *p53* gene have also been implicated in some cases. A few cases are secondary to Paget's disease or previous radiation. These aggressive tumours can metastasise widely, especially to the lungs, but due to advances in treatment, the 5-year survival has improved to around 50%.

Miscellaneous bone tumours

Ewing's sarcoma

This tumour is composed of small, round, darkly staining cells, which are now believed to be neuroectodermal in origin. The tumour affects children and adolescents, the average age at presentation being 10–15 years. The pelvis and the diaphysis of long bones are the most frequently affected sites. The tumour presents as a painful enlarging mass, and some patients may have systemic features such as a fever, raised white cell count, or raised erythrocyte sedimentation rate (ESR). Treatment with radiotherapy and chemotherapy has drastically improved survival rates.

Fibroblastic tumours

Although fibroblastic tumours such as malignant fibrous histiocytomas and fibrosarcomas more frequently arise within soft tissues, they can also occur in bones. A quarter of cases are secondary to pre-existing conditions such as Paget's disease, radiation, or bone infarct. The prognosis for high-grade tumours is poor.

Secondary bone tumours

The commonest malignant tumours of bone are secondary deposits from other sites. Most skeletal secondary deposits originate from malignancies at the following sites:

- lung
- breast
- thyroid
- kidney
- prostate.

These deposits cause osteolytic lesions to the bone, with the exception of secondaries originating from prostate tumours, which cause osteosclerotic lesions.

25.2 Joints

Learning objectives

You should:
- know the structure and function of joints
- know the major joint diseases, their pathogenesis and clinicopathological features.

Structure and function

Joints are of two types:

- **Solid joints** – these joints are fixed and rigid, and allow only minimal movement. Examples of solid joints include the skull sutures (where the skull bones are bridged by fibrous tissue) and the symphysis pubis (where the bones are joined by cartilage).
- **Synovial joints** – these joints have a joint space, which allows a wide range of movement. The articular cartilage in synovial joints is a specialised hyaline cartilage, which is an excellent shock absorber. The synovial membrane secretes synovial fluid into the joint space. Synovial fluid acts as a lubricant and provides nutrients for the articular hyaline cartilage (Figure 70).

Osteoarthritis (degenerative joint disease)

This is the most common type of joint disease, and is characterised by the progressive erosion of articular cartilage in weight-bearing joints. The incidence increases with age. Osteoarthritis can be primary or secondary to other bone or joint diseases, systemic diseases such as diabetes, a congenital or developmental deformity of a joint, or previous trauma including repetitive trauma.

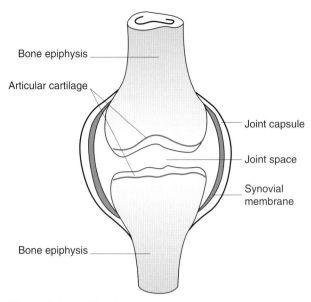

Bone epiphysis

Articular cartilage

Joint capsule

Joint space

Synovial membrane

Bone epiphysis

Figure 70 A synovial joint.

Pathology and pathogenesis

In the early stages of osteoarthritis, the articular cartilage becomes eroded and fragmented (fibrillated), and portions of the cartilage flake off. In contrast with joints affected by simple wear and tear, these changes occur well away from the articular margins, and there is eventual full thickness loss of cartilage with the underlying bone becoming exposed and developing a polished ivory appearance (eburnation). Loss of articular cartilage stimulates thickening of the subchondral plate and the adjacent cancellous bone, which impairs the ability of the joint to act as a shock absorber and results in increased damage to the residual cartilage.

Small fractures develop in the now articulating bone, allowing synovial fluid to enter the subchondral regions, with resultant formation of subchondral pseudocysts. Fragments of cartilage and bone fall into the joint space forming loose bodies (joint mice). Bony outgrowths, known as osteophytes, form at the margin of the articular cartilage. The articular surfaces become increasingly deformed.

The reason why the articular cartilage becomes predisposed to this damage appears to be related to biochemical alterations in the hyaline. In hyaline cartilage affected by osteoarthritis, the water content is increased and the proteoglycan content is decreased. The elasticity and compliance of the cartilage is, therefore, reduced. The very first change seen in osteoarthritis is proliferation of chondroblasts, and it has been proposed that these cells produce enzymes that induce these biochemical changes in the hyaline cartilage.

Clinical features

The most frequently affected joints are the hips, the knees, the cervical and lumbar vertebrae, the proximal and distal interphalangeal (PIP and DIP) joints of the hands, the first metacarpophalangeal joint and the first metatarsophalangeal joint. Osteophytes at the DIP joints produce nodular swellings called Heberden's nodes. With increasing deformity of the joint the typical symptoms develop, which are pain (which is worse with use), morning stiffness, and limitation in joint movement. With involvement of the cervical and lumbar spine, osteophytes may impinge on the nerve roots causing symptoms such as pain and pins and needles in the arms or legs. The overall result is disability. The process cannot be halted.

Rheumatoid arthritis

Rheumatoid arthritis is a chronic inflammatory multisystem disorder (hence rheumatoid 'disease'), but the joints are invariably involved. The condition can affect all age groups. When children are affected, the condition is designated Still's disease. Females are affected more often than males.

The pathogenesis is not well understood, but it is thought that an initiating agent, possibly an organism, triggers immunological dysfunction resulting in persistent chronic inflammation in genetically susceptible individuals. In the joints, the ongoing inflammation causes destruction of the articular cartilage. Circulating autoantibodies (rheumatoid factors), which are directed against autologous IgG immunoglobulins, can be detected in the serum of around 80% of affected individuals. The exact role of these autoantibodies is uncertain (see Box 9, Ch. 8).

Pathological features

Joints

The most severe morphological changes of rheumatoid arthritis are manifest in the joints. In the early stages the synovium becomes thickened, oedematous and hyperplastic. With ongoing inflammation, a pannus is formed. A pannus is a chronically inflamed fibrocellular mass of synovium and synovial stroma, which develops over the articular cartilage. As the pannus slowly spreads, it degrades the underlying cartilage, and erosions and subchondral cysts develop in the underlying bone. Small detached fragments fall into the joint space and are called rice bodies. Localised osteoporosis may also occur. The fibrous pannus eventually bridges the opposing bones causing limitation of movement, and ossification of this fibrous tissue leads to bony ankylosis. The inflammation also affects the joint capsule, tendons and ligaments causing characteristic deformities.

Skin

The most common cutaneous lesions are rheumatoid nodules, which arise in areas exposed to pressure, e.g. the extensor surfaces of the arms and the elbows. They are seen in ~30% of patients. They arise in the subcutaneous tissue and manifest as firm, non-tender skin nodules. Microscopically, they consist of a central area of fibrinoid necrosis surrounded by a palisade of histiocytes and fibroblasts.

Blood vessels

Patients with severe disease may develop a rheumatoid vasculitis. Peripheral neuropathy, skin ulceration, gangrene and nail-bed infarcts may develop. Impairment of blood supply to vital organs can be fatal.

Lungs

Parenchymal rheumatoid nodules (usually asymptomatic), chronic interstitial fibrosis and pleurisy can occur.

Eyes

Scleritis and uveitis can develop.

Heart

The development of rheumatoid nodules in the conduction system may occur, and coronary artery vasculitis may result in myocardial ischaemia. Pericarditis can also be a feature.

Bones

Patients are at increased risk of localised and generalised osteoporosis.

Lymphoreticular

Patients may develop lymphadenopathy, with or without splenomegaly. The combination of rheumatoid arthritis, splenomegaly and neutropenia is called Felty's syndrome. Approximately 50% of patients with Felty's syndrome develop secondary Sjögren's syndrome. Patients may have a normocytic normochromic anaemia.

Miscellaneous

Patients are at an increased risk of developing amyloidosis.

Clinical features

The clinical course of rheumatoid arthritis is very variable. Some patients have mild disease, whereas others have severe progressive disease quickly leading to disability. Initially patients may suffer constitutional symptoms and only after a few weeks or months do the joints become involved. Generally, the small joints (especially those in the hands) are affected before the large joints. The affected joints are swollen, painful and stiff following a period of inactivity. Symptoms may improve with the administration of anti-inflammatory drugs or immunosuppressants. As a result of the pathological processes within the articular and periarticular tissues, characteristic deformities develop. These include:

- radial deviation at the wrists
- ulnar deviation at the fingers
- flexion and hyperextension deformities of the fingers (swan neck and boutonnière deformities).

Typical X-ray changes include:

- loss of articular cartilage leading to narrowing of the joint space
- joint effusions
- localised osteoporosis
- erosions.

Fatalities are usually the result of complications such as amyloidosis, vasculitis or the iatrogenic effects of therapy (e.g. gastrointestinal bleed secondary to non-steroidal anti-inflammatory drugs (NSAIDs), infections secondary to steroids).

Seronegative spondyloarthropathies

The spondyloarthropathies are a group of disorders characterised by arthropathy associated with disease in other systems. Many are associated with human leucocyte antigen (HLA)-B27 positivity. The term 'seronegative' is used because affected individuals are seronegative for rheumatoid factors.

Ankylosing spondylitis

This condition typically affects young men and ~90% of patients are HLA-B27 positive. The changes are first seen in the sacroiliac joints and the spine. In the early stages there is inflammation of the tendo-ligamentous insertion sites, which is followed by reactive bone formation in the adjacent ligaments and tendons. This is compounded by a chronic synovitis causing destruction of the articular cartilage. With attempts at healing, the overall result is bony ankylosis and severe spinal immobility. Patients present with chronic progressive lower back pain. Further progression of the disease leads to spinal kyphosis and neck hyperextension (question mark posture). Characteristic X-ray changes include a 'bamboo spine' and squaring of the vertebral bodies. Extra-articular manifestations include:

- uveitis
- apical lung fibrosis
- aortic incompetence
- amyloidosis.

Reiter's syndrome

This condition is defined as a triad of:

- arthritis
- urethritis (non-gonococcal)
- conjunctivitis.

Typical patients are young men, and ~80% of patients are HLA-B27 positive. The condition usually follows infection of the gastrointestinal or genitourinary tract. Several weeks after the diarrhoea or urethritis, an arthritis develops, which may persist for many months. The joints of the leg are the most commonly affected sites.

Enteropathic arthropathy

Salmonella, *Shigella*, *Yersinia* and *Campylobacter* gastroenteritis may be complicated by arthritis, with HLA-B27 positive individuals being at an increased risk of developing this complication. Arthritis is also seen in 20% of patients with Crohn's disease or ulcerative colitis.

Psoriatic arthritis

An arthritis is developed by ~5% of patients with psoriasis, and these individuals are usually HLA-B27 positive.

Infective arthritis

Organisms can gain access to the joint by three main routes:

- haematogenous spread from a distant infected site (most common)

- direct access via a penetrating injury
- direct spread from a neighbouring infected site, e.g. osteomyelitis, soft-tissue abscess.

Infective arthritis, particularly bacterial and tuberculous arthritis, is potentially serious because it can cause rapid destruction of the joint.

Bacterial arthritis

Most cases of infective arthritis are caused by bacteria. The most common organisms are gonococcus (*Neisseria*), *Staphylococcus*, *Streptococcus*, *Haemophilus influenzae* and Gram-negative bacilli. In general, children are affected more commonly than adults. Gonococcal arthritis is seen mainly in late adolescence and adulthood, and patients with sickle-cell disease tend to develop *Salmonella* arthritis. Affected patients develop pain and swelling of the affected joint, and there may be systemic indicators of infection, e.g. fever. Aspiration and culture of the joint fluid gives the diagnosis. Prompt treatment with antibiotics is paramount.

Viral arthritis

Infections such as viral hepatitis, rubella and parvovirus B19 may be complicated by an arthritis. Symptoms are of a mild arthralgia (aching joints). It is not certain whether the virus directly infects the joint, or whether the arthritis is simply a reactive process due to systemic viral infection.

Rare forms of infective arthritis

Lyme disease

Lyme disease is caused by joint infection with the spirochete *Borrelia burgdorferi*, which is transmitted to humans via tick bites. Infection of the skin is followed by dissemination of the organism to many other sites, particularly the joints. The patient usually first develops a macular rash known as erythema migrans and there may be constitutional symptoms. This is followed by the development of an arthritis, which may affect more than one joint.

Tuberculous arthritis

Tuberculous arthritis is due to haematogenous spread from an established focus of infection elsewhere, usually the lungs. This condition usually presents with insidious development of joint pain associated with limitation of movement. The vertebral column is commonly involved, and when there is an associated osteomyelitis vertebral collapse may result (Pott's disease of the spine).

Crystal arthropathies

Crystal arthropathies are a group of disorders caused by the deposition of crystals within the joint resulting in an acute and chronic arthritis. Such crystals may be endogenous or exogenous. The most common crystal arthropathies, gout and calcium pyrophosphate arthropathy, are due to endogenous crystal deposition.

Gout

Gout occurs due to the crystallisation of monosodium urate within a joint, resulting in an acute (gouty) arthritis, which is characterised by extreme localised pain, erythema, and exquisite tenderness of the affected joint. The most commonly affected joint is the metatarsophalangeal joint of the great toe, followed in decreasing frequency by the ankle, and then the knee. The disorder is due primarily to raised serum uric acid levels, but only around 3% of people with hyperuricaemia will develop gout. Uric acid is the end product of purine metabolism, and is excreted by the kidneys. Purines can either be derived from the breakdown of nucleic acids or synthesised de novo. Hyperuricaemia has several causes:

- idiopathic (80% of cases)
- overproduction of uric acid due to increased purine turnover (e.g. leukaemia) or an enzyme defect
- decreased excretion of uric acid (e.g. chronic renal failure, thiazide diuretics)
- high dietary purine intake.

The events which lead to the deposition of urate crystals in the joint are uncertain, but possible triggers include alcohol, trauma, surgery and infection. The presence of urate crystals within the joint causes the accumulation of numerous inflammatory cells. The resulting arthritis remits after a few days or weeks, even without treatment. The diagnosis can be confirmed by aspirating the joint fluid and using polarising microscopy to detect the needle-shaped crystals, which exhibit negative birefringence with a red filter.

Repeated attacks of acute gouty arthritis eventually lead to chronic tophaceous gouty arthritis, where the affected joint is damaged and function is impaired. Tophi are large aggregates of urate crystals, which are visible with the naked eye. They occur in the joints and soft tissues of people with persistent hyperuricaemia. A common site for tophi is the pinna of the ear.

Urate crystals can also become deposited in the kidney, resulting in acute uric acid nephropathy, chronic renal disease, or uric acid stones causing renal colic.

Calcium pyrophosphate arthropathy (pseudogout, chondrocalcinosis)

This condition is due to the deposition of calcium pyrophosphate crystals in the synovium (pseudogout) and articular cartilage (chondrocalcinosis). It can occur in three main settings:

- sporadic (more common in the elderly)
- hereditary
- secondary to other conditions, such as previous joint damage, hyperparathyroidism, hypothyroidism, haemochromatosis and diabetes.

The crystals first develop in the articular cartilage (chondrocalcinosis), which is usually asymptomatic. From here the crystals may shed into the joint cavity resulting in an acute arthritis, which mimics gout and is therefore called pseudogout. Pseudogout can be differentiated from gout in three ways:

- the knee is most commonly involved
- X-rays show the characteristic line of calcification of the articular cartilage
- the crystals look different under polarising microscopy – they are rhomboid in shape and exhibit positive birefringence with a red filter.

25.3 Connective tissue diseases

Learning objectives

You should:
- understand the meaning of the term 'connective tissue disease'
- know the various connective tissue diseases and their clinicopathological features
- understand what is known about the pathogenesis of rheumatoid arthritis, systemic lupus erythematosus and scleroderma.

Basic principles

Connective tissue diseases is a convenient general term that covers a wide variety of disorders which have certain features in common:

- they are multisystem disorders and the joints, skin and subcutaneous tissue are often affected
- females are more commonly affected than males
- immunological abnormalities are often present
- a chronic clinical course is usual
- they usually respond to anti-inflammatory drugs.

The conditions included in this group of disorders are:

- rheumatoid arthritis (presented above)
- systemic lupus erythematosus (SLE)
- polyarteritis nodosa (PAN)
- dermatomyositis and polymyositis
- polymyalgia rheumatica
- cranial arteritis
- scleroderma (systemic sclerosis).

Systemic lupus erythematosus

SLE is a multisystem disorder of autoimmune origin. Females are affected more commonly than males (the female to male ratio is 9:1), and the disease usually arises in the second or third decade.

Aetiology and pathogenesis

The cause of SLE is unknown but most patients have circulating autoantibodies directed against nuclear antigens (antinuclear antibodies, or ANAs) and these autoantibodies are the mediators of the tissue damage. Hence B cell hyper-reactivity is implicated in the pathogenesis and evidence suggests that it is excess T cell help that drives self-reactive B cells to produce these autoantibodies. Genetic factors may also be important, since there is a strong familial tendency to develop SLE. Some cases of SLE are drug induced, hydralazine and procainamide being among the drugs implicated.

Clinicopathological features

Most visceral lesions are mediated by type III hypersensitivity (immune complex hypersensitivity reaction). The haematological effects are mediated by type II hypersensitivity. The organs and tissues affected and the various pathological manifestations are shown in Table 58.

The typical presentation of SLE is of a young woman with a butterfly rash on her face associated with a fever and arthralgia. Alternatively, fever or arthralgia may be the only symptoms, making diagnosis difficult. Some patients who have autoantibodies directed against cardiolipin develop the anti-phospholipid antibody syndrome, characterised by thrombophilia. Affected women may have recurrent miscarriages.

The clinical course of the condition is variable. That most frequently seen is a relapsing remitting course spanning years. Exacerbations are treated with steroids or other immunosuppressants. Death is usually due to renal disease, diffuse central nervous system (CNS) disease or intercurrent infection.

Polyarteritis nodosa

PAN is characterised by inflammation and fibrinoid necrosis of small or medium-sized arteries. The aetiology is unknown. Segmental artery wall damage may lead to aneurysm formation. The primary targets of PAN are the main visceral vessels, with the kidneys being affected most frequently, followed by the heart, liver and gastrointesti-

Table 58 Common clinicopathological features of SLE

Organ affected	Clinicopathological features
Skin (involved in most patients)	Symmetrical erythematous facial 'butterfly' rash, often precipitated by sun exposure
	Discoid lupus erythematosus (DLE)
Joints	Arthralgia
Kidneys	Glomerulonephritis, which may progress to renal failure
Central nervous system	Psychiatric symptoms
	Focal neurological symptoms due to non-inflammatory occlusion of small blood vessels
Cardiovascular system	Pericarditis
	Myocarditis
	Libman–Sacks endocarditis (rare)
	Necrotising vasculitis
Lungs	Pleuritis
	Pleural effusions
Lymphoreticular	Mild lymphadenopathy and splenomegaly
Haematological	Anaemia
	Leucopenia
	Thrombophilia (antiphospholipid antibody syndrome)

nal tract. Joints, muscles, nerves, the skin and the lungs may also be involved.

Clinical features

Patients usually present with non-specific features such as pyrexia and myalgia, with or without organ-specific symptoms. Renal vessel involvement may cause hypertension, haematuria or proteinuria. Involvement of the mesenteric vessels causes abdominal pain, melaena, vomiting and diarrhoea. Involvement of the arteries supplying nerves is a cause of mononeuritis multiplex. Joint involvement causes arthralgia, skin involvement causes a rash, and lung involvement causes cough and dyspnoea.

The diagnosis depends on finding a necrotising vasculitis in a biopsy specimen. The serum of affected patients often contains pANCA (perinuclear antineutrophil cytoplasmic antibody).

Therapy with corticosteroids or cyclophosphamide causes remission in most cases. If left untreated, PAN is often fatal.

Dermatomyositis and polymyositis

Both of these conditions are inflammatory disorders of muscle, and they present with gradual onset of muscular weakness. More than one muscle is usually affected and the distribution is commonly bilateral, symmetrical and proximal. The oesophagus, diaphragm and heart are not infrequently involved. In dermatomyositis, a distinctive skin rash precedes the muscular weakness. The rash is a lilac discoloration of the upper eyelids associated with periorbital oedema. A more generalised dermatitis is often present. Ten per cent of patients with dermatomyositis have an underlying malignancy, most commonly carcinoma of the lung, breast or gastrointestinal tract. Polymyositis differs from dermatomyositis because it lacks the skin changes and is seen only in adults. There is a slight increased risk of an underlying malignancy.

Diagnosis of these disorders depends on clinical symptoms, elevated muscle enzymes (e.g. creatinine phosphokinase) and muscle biopsy.

Polymyalgia rheumatica

This condition is seen in elderly individuals, and presents with pain and stiffness in the shoulder and pelvic girdles. Muscle weakness is not a feature. There may be non-specific features such as lethargy, raised ESR and mild normochromic normocytic anaemia. The condition responds well to corticosteroid therapy.

Cranial arteritis (temporal or giant cell arteritis)

Cranial arteritis is a granulomatous inflammation of small and medium-sized arteries, and is the commonest of the vasculitides. The inflammatory process principally affects the cranial vessels, especially the temporal arteries and the terminal branches of the ophthalmic artery. In such cases, prompt diagnosis is paramount because of the risk of blindness. Typical symptoms are headache, scalp tenderness in the region of the temporal artery, and jaw claudication. The condition may also be associated with polymyalgia rheumatica. A raised serum ESR should raise the possibility of cranial arteritis.

Diagnosis depends on temporal artery biopsy, which should be performed immediately if the diagnosis is suspected. Histologically, the wall of the artery is infiltrated by inflammatory cells, with or without multinucleate giant cells, and the internal elastic lamina becomes fragmented. These changes may only be focal ('skip' lesions) and may be missed on biopsy. The treatment of choice is steroids.

Scleroderma (systemic sclerosis)

This condition is characterised by excessive fibrosis of organs and tissues. The skin is almost always affected with variable involvement of the gastrointestinal tract, heart, kidneys, lungs, arteries, and musculoskeletal system. The condition is more common in women than men. In a subset of patients where the skin is the main target organ and visceral involvement is uncommon, the condition is often associated with CREST syndrome. CREST is an acronym for:

- **C**alcinosis
- **R**aynaud syndrome
- o**E**sophageal dysfunction
- **S**clerodactyly
- **T**elangiectasia

Aetiology

The principal underlying abnormality is excessive production and deposition of collagen. The mechanism by which this occurs is uncertain, but disordered immune activation appears to be involved with excess T cell help driving the production of fibrogenic mediators by inflammatory cells.

Clinicopathological features

Most patients present with Raynaud phenomenon and the characteristic skin changes, but some patients also develop symptoms related to involvement of other organs.

Skin

Becomes tight and tethered and joint mobility becomes impaired. The hands and fingers are usually affected first, the fingers become tapered and the hand takes on a claw-like configuration. Involvement of the face causes taut facial skin and the mouth appears small. At a microscopic level, there is skin oedema followed by progressive fibrosis of the dermis and epidermal atrophy. Impaired blood supply due to arterial involvement may lead to skin ulceration and autoamputation of digits.

Gastrointestinal tract

There is fibrous replacement of the muscularis. This change can affect any part of the gastrointestinal tract, but the oesophagus is frequently involved resulting in dysphagia. When other parts of the gastrointestinal tract are affected, malabsorption may result.

Kidneys

The renal abnormalities are due to changes in the vasculature. Vascular lesions are confined to the medium-sized arteries and are similar to those seen in hypertension. Ten to thirty per cent of patients with scleroderma develop hypertension, and in a proportion of these cases there is malignant hypertension, which may prove fatal.

Lungs
Patients may develop interstitial fibrosis causing dyspnoea.

Heart
Pericarditis with effusions and myocardial fibrosis are seen rarely.

Musculoskeletal
There may be polyarthritis and myositis.

Progression of the disease is usually slow, unless superseded by malignant hypertension. Death may occur from:

- renal failure secondary to malignant hypertension
- severe respiratory compromise
- cor pulmonale
- cardiac failure or arrhythmias secondary to myocardial fibrosis.

25.4 Soft tissue tumours

Learning objectives
You should:
- understand what defines soft tissue tumours
- understand the classification of soft tissue tumours
- know how benign and malignant soft tissue tumours behave
- know some common types of soft tissue tumour.

Soft tissue can be defined as non-epithelial, extraskeletal tissue of the body, exclusive of the reticuloendothelial system, glia, meninges, and the visceral parenchyma. Soft tissue tumours are a highly heterogeneous and complex

Table 59 Examples of benign and malignant soft tissue tumours

Mature tissue resembled	Benign	Malignant
Fat	Lipoma	Liposarcoma
Smooth muscle	Leiomyoma	Leiomyosarcoma
Skeletal muscle	Rhabdomyoma	Rhabdomyosarcoma
Blood vessels	Haemangioma	Angiosarcoma
Perivascular tissue	Glomus tumour	Malignant glomus tumour
Fibrous tissue	Fibroma	Fibrosarcoma
Fibrohistiocytic tumours	Fibrous histiocytoma	Malignant fibrous histiocytoma
Nerves	Schwannoma, neurofibroma	Malignant peripheral nerve sheath tumour

group of neoplasms, which are classified according to the mature tissues that they most closely resemble. For example, lipomas and liposarcomas resemble to a varying degree normal fatty tissue. Benign soft tissue tumours (particularly lipomas) are extremely common among the general population, and many never need medial attention. Malignant soft tissue tumours (sarcomas) on the other hand are relatively rare, accounting for less than 1% of all cancers. However, sarcomas often behave extremely aggressively and are capable of metastasising widely. This, together with the fact that most sarcomas tend to arise within deep soft tissues and have often grown to a large size before they become clinically apparent, means that the prognosis is generally quite poor.

Because of the complex nature of this group of tumours, we present only a framework for the basic understanding of the various types of soft tissue tumours that exist (see Table 59). For the purposes of this book, it is not necessary to detail each specific entity, but some of the more common soft tissue tumours (e.g. leiomyoma of the uterus) are presented in other chapters.

Self-assessment: questions

One best answer questions

1. Which of the following is not a primary bone tumour?
   a. Ewing's sarcoma
   b. chondrosarcoma
   c. osteoid osteoma
   d. leiomyosarcoma
   e. enchondroma

2. A 68-year-old man presents with an acutely painful, red and tender ankle. He takes diuretics for cardiac disease and regularly drinks red wine with his evening meal. What is the most likely diagnosis?
   a. tuberculous arthritis
   b. osteomyelitis
   c. Paget's disease
   d. gout
   e. osteosarcoma

True-false questions

1. The following statements are correct:
   a. osteogenesis imperfecta is caused by dietary insufficiency
   b. osteoporosis rarely occurs in men
   c. osteomalacia and rickets are caused by a lack of vitamin K
   d. bowing of the legs is a feature of osteomalacia
   e. in Paget's disease, affected bones become enlarged and are therefore not vulnerable to fracture

2. The following statements are correct:
   a. *Staphylococcus aureus* is responsible for the majority of cases of pyogenic osteomyelitis
   b. osteomyelitis may complicate compound fractures
   c. following its fracture, the scaphoid bone is particularly vulnerable to avascular necrosis
   d. osteosarcomas are the most common bone tumours
   e. bone tumours may form cartilage

3. Osteoarthritis:
   a. is caused by bacterial infection of the articular cartilage
   b. is a multisystem disorder
   c. is characterised by pannus formation
   d. usually affects the weight-bearing joints
   e. is associated with Heberden's nodes, which represent prominent osteophytes at the distal interphalangeal joints

4. The following statements are correct:
   a. rheumatoid arthritis is a multisystem disorder
   b. rheumatoid factor is an autoantibody that is directed against articular cartilage
   c. in rheumatoid arthritis, joint deformities may develop in the hands
   d. the majority of patients with ankylosing spondylitis are HLA-B27 positive
   e. in ankylosing spondylitis, the most frequently affected joints are those of the lower limbs

5. The following statements are correct:
   a. bacterial infective arthritis may cause joint destruction
   b. gout is due to deposition of calcium pyrophosphate crystals within the joint
   c. the joint most frequently affected by gout is the knee joint
   d. use of diuretics may predispose to the development of gout
   e. the crystal seen in joints affected by pseudogout are rhomboid in shape and exhibit positive birefringence on polarising microscopy

6. Systemic lupus erythematosus:
   a. is more common in females than males
   b. in most cases is characterised by circulating antinuclear antibodies, which mediate the tissue damage
   c. may be drug-induced
   d. causes renal abnormalities in almost all patients
   e. may be associated with a skin rash that is limited to the trunk

7. The following statements are correct:
   a. patients with dermatomyositis have an increased risk of developing visceral malignancies
   b. cANCA is often detected in the serum of patients with polyarteritis nodosa
   c. cranial (temporal) arteritis may lead to blindness if untreated
   d. systemic sclerosis is characterised by excess deposition of collagen
   e. skin involvement, which is characteristic of systemic sclerosis, is not seen in patients with CREST syndrome

8. The following statements are true:
   a. ankylosing spondylitis is the commonest joint disease
   b. seronegative spondyloarthropathies are associated with seronegativity for HLA-B27
   c. arthritis occurs in the majority of patients with psoriasis

   d. osteoarthritis never occurs in young people

   e. tophi are skin lesions characteristically seen in patients with rheumatoid arthritis

9. The following are features of rheumatoid arthritis:

   a. radial deviation at the wrist joint and ulnar deviation at the finger joint in patients with joint deformities

   b. widening of the joint space on X-ray

   c. lymphadenopathy

   d. vasculitis

   e. heart disease

Case history questions

Case history 1

A 60-year-old woman attends the accident and emergency department complaining of pain in her left hip following a trivial fall. A history reveals that she has been getting backache for some time. She is otherwise well but has been on steroids for Crohn's disease for some time. An X-ray demonstrates a fractured femoral neck.

1. What underlying diagnoses would you consider?
2. How would this patient be managed?

Case history 2

A 71-year-old man with a 20-year history of rheumatoid disease regularly attends an outpatient rheumatology clinic for investigation, physiotherapy and adjustment of his drug treatment. He is presently on non-steroidal anti-inflammatory drugs and cyclophosphamide. At his last clinic appointment he complained of increasing shortness of breath on exertion. Auscultation of the chest revealed late inspiratory crepitations. A chest X-ray shows a finely reticulated appearance. Serum haematology showed a normocytic normochromic anaemia.

1. What deformities might you expect to see in the hands of this patient?
2. What might be the cause of his increasing shortness of breath?
3. What are the possible causes of his anaemia?

Short note questions

Write short notes on:

1. The aetiology of osteomalacia.
2. The pathogenesis of osteomyelitis.
3. CREST syndrome.
4. Autoantibodies.

Viva questions

1. What functions does bone perform?
2. How are bone tumours classified?
3. What features do the seronegative spondyloarthropathies have in common as a group of disorders?

Self-assessment: answers

One best answer

1. d. Bone tumours can be bone-forming (such as osteoid osteoma) or cartilage-forming (such as enchondroma and chondrosarcoma). Ewing's sarcoma is a tumour arising in bones of children and adolescents; the tumour has 'small, round, blue cells' and is thought to be of neuroectodermal origin. Leiomyosarcoma is a malignant tumour of smooth muscle; it can arise in many sites, such as the gut, uterus and skin.

2. d. The ankle signs suggest an acute arthritis; the diuretic use and alcohol consumption are factors associated with hyperuricaemia and triggering of monosodium urate crystal deposition with joints. The ankle is a common site for gout. Tuberculous arthritis typically presents with gradual development of joint pain and limitation of movement in a patient with established infection elsewhere in the body. Osteomyelitis presents with localised bone pain and soft tissue swelling; in adults it most commonly involves the diaphysis rather than joints. Osteosarcoma also presents with bone pain and soft tissue swelling; symptoms are usually present for several months before diagnosis. Paget's disease may be asymptomatic, or present with symptoms including bone pain, heart failure, pathological fracture and nerve compression.

True-false answers

1. a. **False.**
   b. **False.** Osteoporosis occurs in both males and females.
   c. **False.**
   d. **False.** In osteomalacia the shape of the bone is not affected.
   e. **False.** Affected bones are more vulnerable to fracture because the enlarged bone is structurally unsound.

2. a. **True.**
   b. **True.**
   c. **True.**
   d. **False.** Metastases are the most common tumours of bone. Osteosarcomas are the most common primary bone cancers.
   e. **True.**

3. a. **False.**
   b. **False.**
   c. **False.** Pannus formation is seen in rheumatoid arthritis.
   d. **True.**
   e. **True.**

4. a. **True.**
   b. **False.**
   c. **True.**
   d. **True.**
   e. **False.**

5. a. **True.**
   b. **False.**
   c. **False.**
   d. **True.**
   e. **True.**

6. a. **True.**
   b. **True.**
   c. **True.**
   d. **True.**
   e. **False.** The skin rash is not limited to the trunk.

7. a. **True.**
   b. **False.** pANCA (not cANCA) is often detected in PAN.
   c. **True.**
   d. **True.**
   e. **False.**

8. a. **False.** Osteoarthritis is the most common joint disease.
   b. **False.** The term 'seronegative' in this context denotes seronegativity for rheumatoid factor.
   c. **False.** Psoriatic arthropathy occurs in a minority of patients, around 5%.
   d. **False.**
   e. **False.** Tophi are characteristically seen in gout. The skin lesions seen in rheumatoid arthritis are called rheumatoid nodules.

9. a. **True.**
   b. **False.** The joint space is typically narrowed.
   c. **True.**
   d. **True.**
   e. **True.** The heart may be involved by pericarditis, vasculitis, rheumatoid nodules or amyloidosis.

Case history answers

Case history 1

1. In this situation, a number of underlying pathologies should be considered. Most cases of fractured neck of femur are due to underlying osteoporosis. The recent history of backache and the fact that this woman is taking steroids would support this diagnosis. The other main diagnosis to consider is a pathological fracture secondary to bony metastases. The recent history of backache may be due to the presence of metastatic deposits in the spine. It is also important to realise that bones

affected by Paget's disease and osteomalacia are prone to fracture. The appearance of the bone adjacent to the fracture on X-ray may help establish the diagnosis.

2. The patient would need to have surgery to remove the head of the femur and replace it with a prosthesis. It is unlikely that the fracture would have healed by itself since fractures through the neck of the femur interrupt the blood supply to the head, which makes fracture healing difficult. Surgery is performed as soon as possible so that patients can be mobilised quickly. Patients immobilised after hip fractures are prone to developing pneumonia, which can be rapidly fatal.

Case history 2

1. This man has had rheumatoid arthritis for some time now and so many deformities may be present in the hands including swelling of the interphalangeal joints, flexion and hyperextension deformities of the fingers, radial deviation at the wrists and ulnar deviation at the metacarpophalangeal joints. In elderly individuals, you may also see changes related to osteoarthritis.

2. Increasing shortness of breath associated with coarse crackles on auscultation of the lung fields and a ground-glass appearance on chest X-ray would raise the suspicion of interstitial lung disease, which patients with rheumatoid arthritis are at increased risk of developing. Lung function tests could be performed to confirm this.

3. A normocytic normochromic anaemia is seen in anaemia of chronic disease, which is the most likely cause of the anaemia in this case. However, in the presence of anaemia in a patient on long-term non-steroidal anti-inflammatory drug treatment, the possibility of chronic blood loss owing to drug-induced peptic ulceration should be considered, but this would characteristically induce a microcytic anaemia.

Short note answers

1. Osteomalacia is caused by vitamin D deficiency. To give a full account of the aetiology, you must understand how vitamin D deficiency may arise. There are two main sources of vitamin D – diet and endogenous synthesis in the skin. Hence, poor diet, intestinal malabsorption and reduced exposure to sunlight may all lead to osteomalacia. Newly synthesised vitamin D is biologically inactive and conversion to its active form occurs in the liver and kidneys. Hence renal disease and liver disease may also lead to osteomalacia.

2. Remember that the term 'pathogenesis' refers to the process of production and development of a lesion, i.e. the mechanism through which the aetiology operates to produce the pathological and clinical

manifestation. Hence, a sequence of events linking the aetiological agent to the end lesion is what is wanted here. The aetiological agent in osteomyelitis is a microorganism, which may gain access to bone via several routes. When the infection has been localised in bone, the ensuing inflammation causes a sequence of events culminating in bone necrosis.

3. CREST syndrome is associated with systemic sclerosis. There are two main forms of systemic sclerosis: diffuse and localised. The diffuse form is characterised by widespread skin involvement and early visceral involvement. The localised form is characterised by usually localised skin involvement and late visceral involvement. Calcinosis, Raynaud phenomenon, oesophageal dysmotility, sclerodactyly and telangiectasia are features often seen in the localised form, and affected patients are then sometimes said to have CREST syndrome (CREST being an acronym of these five features).

4. *Comment*: Start by giving a definition of what an autoantibody is: an antibody directed against self-antigens (or autoantigens). Interactions between autoantibodies and autoantigens evoke an immune response against the individual's own tissues, a process known as autoimmunity. The immune reaction is self-perpetuating, causing chronic inflammatory disorders, which are known as autoimmune diseases. At this point, it would be a good idea to list the main autoimmune diseases, such as SLE and rheumatoid arthritis, remembering also to include some 'organ-specific' autoimmune diseases such as Graves' disease, Hashimoto's thyroiditis and myasthenia gravis.

Viva answers

1. Bone performs a number of functions other than just providing structural support. It is protective to certain organs, and it is involved in mineral homeostasis and haematopoiesis.

2. *Comment*: You should devise a system that enables you to classify all tumours. A simple one is to divide them into primary tumours and secondary tumours. Primary tumours are then subdivided into benign and malignant. Further classification is usually according to the cell of origin or histological appearance, and for bone tumours this means dividing them into those that are bone-forming, those that are cartilage-forming, and miscellaneous tumours such as Ewing's sarcoma and fibroblastic tumours.

3. The seronegative spondyloarthropathies are a group of disorders characterised by an inflammatory arthritis associated with disorders (usually infectious) in other systems. They include ankylosing spondylitis, Reiter's syndrome, enteropathic arthropathy and psoriatic arthritis. Patients are seronegative for rheumatoid factors, and many are HLA-B27 positive.

Skin

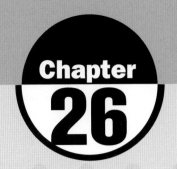

Chapter 26

Chapter overview

The skin is a multifunctional organ involved in structural support, protection from injury and infection and temperature regulation. When these functions are dramatically disturbed – in extensive burn injuries, for example – patients are at risk of fatal metabolic and fluid homeostasis disruption or overwhelming bacterial infection. Skin neoplasms are very common in white-skinned races, with malignant melanoma rising rapidly in incidence. There are many inflammatory diseases of the skin that cause significant morbidity and cosmetic problems.

26.1 Inflammation and infection

Learning objectives

You should:
- understand the terminology used to described skin lesions macroscopically
- know how inflammatory skin diseases can be classified according to the pattern of microscopic changes; this will help your understanding of clinical dermatology
- understand the classification and complications of burns.

One of the common difficulties students encounter when learning about skin diseases is the large number of specific terms used to describe both macroscopic and microscopic appearances. Common naked-eye and microscopic descriptive terms are shown in Box 31.

Eczema

Eczema is a common inflammatory skin disease presenting clinically with red papules or plaques containing small vesicles, which may itch, ooze and crust. There are several clinical subtypes. The characteristic histological feature is intercellular oedema in the epidermis (spongiosis), which separates the keratinocytes and can cause vesicle formation. Chronic inflammation with lymphocytic infiltration of the epidermis and dermis is often seen. Pathogenesis is variable and includes:

- direct toxic effects (irritant contact dermatitis)
- delayed hypersensitivity reaction (allergic contact dermatitis)
- combination of IgE-mediated and T cell-mediated reaction (atopic eczema).

Psoriasis

Psoriasis is a common chronic relapsing dermatitis that classically manifests as circumscribed red skin plaques often several centimetres in diameter, with silvery surface scale. Extensor surfaces of knees and elbows, the sacral region and the scalp are common sites. Nail changes are common and arthritis develops in a small percentage of patients. Onset is usually in early adult life. The pathogenesis is unclear but there is hyperproliferation of keratinocytes, with the epidermal turnover time reduced from the normal 13 days to 3–4 days. The histological features of classical psoriasis are:

- regular epidermal hyperplasia (thickening)
- parakeratosis (retained nuclei within the surface keratin layer)
- thinning of the granular layer
- neutrophil microabscesses
- increased mitotic activity (cell turnover).

Lichen planus

Lichen planus presents clinically as multiple small itchy violet papules, around the wrist and elbows. Oral and genital lesions also occur. Skin lesions often resolve after several months or years. Histological features include:

- irregular epidermal hyperplasia
- damage to the basal epidermis with vacuolation and apoptotic epidermal cells
- band-like ('lichenoid') chronic inflammatory infiltrate at the dermo-epidermal junction.

Erythema multiforme

Erythema multiforme (EM) is an uncommon but potentially serious hypersensitivity response to certain infections (herpes simplex and *Mycoplasma*) and drugs (including sulphonamides, penicillin and aspirin). Clinical lesions include red macules, papules and vesicles. The characteristic 'target' lesion has a pale, raised or eroded centre and erythematous (red) rim. Symmetrical involvement of the limbs is most commonly seen. Stevens–Johnson syndrome is severe erythema multiforme with oral mucosal lesions. Toxic epidermal necrosis is the most serious manifestation of EM, with a high risk of systemic

sepsis and fluid imbalance due to extensive loss of skin and mucosal epithelium; mortality is 35%. Histological examination shows a lichenoid inflammatory infiltrate with epidermal cell apoptosis.

Vesico-bullous diseases

Vesico-bullous diseases are classified according to the site of the vesicle formation, which may be within the epidermis or at the dermo-epidermal junction. The pathogenesis in many cases involves immune complex formation with autoantibodies. Examples are shown in Table 61. Many of these diseases are described further below.

Burns

Burns can be caused by hot liquids (scalds), gases or solids, as well as fire. Burn injuries are classified as:

- partial thickness (first and second degree burns)
- full thickness (third degree burns).

In first degree burns there is endothelial injury and leakage of intravascular fluid into the surrounding tissue. There is vascular congestion with pain and erythema, but no skin necrosis. Second degree burns show epidermal necrosis with blistering as the epidermis separates from the dermis. Regeneration of the skin surface cells can occur from adjacent viable epidermis or from surviving skin adnexal structures. More severe damage occurs in third degree burns, with necrosis of the epidermis and dermis. As the extent of severe burn injuries increases, so does the risk of serious or fatal complications, including:

- septic shock
- renal failure
- adult respiratory distress syndrome (ARDS)
- scarring and contractures.

Skin grafting is often required for healing of third degree burns.

> **Box 31** Descriptive terms
>
> Naked-eye:
>
> - **Macule** – flat area of altered colour
> - **Papule** – small raised lesion
> - **Plaque** – slightly raised, flat-topped lesion
> - **Erythema** – reddening of the skin
> - **Vesicle** – small fluid-filled lesion
> - **Bulla** – larger fluid-filled lesion
> - **Blister** – non-specific term that includes vesicle and bulla
>
> Microscopic:
>
> - **Hyperkeratosis** – increased thickness of the superficial keratin
> - **Parakeratosis** – presence of residual nuclear material within the superficial keratin (implies abnormal maturation)
> - **Spongiosis** – intercellular oedema in the epidermis, characteristically seen in eczematous lesions
> - **Acanthosis** – thickening of the epidermis
> - **Acantholysis** – discohesion, 'falling apart', of epidermal cells
>
> Inflammatory skin diseases can be classified according to the pattern of histological changes (Table 60).

Table 60 Major skin inflammatory disease patterns

Spongiotic	Spongiosis – intraepidermal oedema	Eczema
Psoriasiform	Regular epidermal hyperplasia (thickening)	Psoriasis
Lichenoid	Damage to basal epidermis, often with chronic inflammatory infiltrate along dermo-epidermal junction	Lichen planus
		Lupus erythematosus
		Erythema multiforme
		Graft-versus-host disease
Vesico-bullous	Vesicle or blister (bulla) formation	Pemphigoid
		Dermatitis herpetiformis
		Pemphigus
Granulomatous	Chronic inflammation with aggregates of enlarged (epithelioid) histiocytes	Sarcoidosis
		Infection (tuberculosis, fungal)
		Reaction to foreign material
Vasculitis	Inflammation of vessel walls	Primary cutaneous vasculitis
		Skin involvement by systemic vasculitis
Panniculitis	Inflammation of the subcutaneous fat	Erythema nodosum

Table 61 Vesico-bullous skin diseases

Site of blistering	Disease example	Pathogenesis
Within epidermis	Impetigo Staphylococcal scalded skin syndrome	Bacterial infection
	Pemphigus	Autoantibody formation
	Spongiotic dermatitis	Extreme intercellular oedema
At dermo-epidermal junction	Epidermolysis bullosa	Hereditary defect in proteins that anchor basal epidermis cells to basement membrane
	Porphyria	Enzyme deficiency causing skin fragility
	Dermatitis herpetiformis	IgA antibody deposition
	Pemphigoid	Autoantibody formation

Infectious disease

Skin infections are common, with a wide variety of potential pathogens, including:

- Bacteria
  - *impetigo (staphylococcal or streptococcal infection, particularly in children)*
  - *staphylococcal scalded skin syndrome (infants and children)*
  - *furuncles ('boils')*
  - *cellulitis*
  - *cutaneous tuberculosis.*
- Viruses
  - *varicella zoster (chicken pox and shingles)*
  - *verrucae (common warts – human papilloma virus infection)*
  - *molluscum contagiosum (poxvirus).*
- Fungi
  - Candida
  - *tinea (ringworm, athlete's foot).*
- Arthropods
  - *scabies*
  - *lice.*

26.2 Immunological disorders

Learning objective

You should:
- appreciate that certain skin diseases are immunologically mediated (specialist immunofluorescence tests may be needed for precise diagnosis in these lesions).

Lupus erythematosus

Lichenoid inflammatory pattern skin lesions may be part of systemic lupus erythematosus or more commonly isolated cutaneous disease, called discoid lupus erythematosus. Immunoglobulins and complement are deposited along the dermo-epidermal junction.

Graft-versus-host disease

Recipients of immunocompetent bone marrow transplants often develop lesions in the skin, gastrointestinal tract and liver, when grafted lymphocytes attack host tissue. Cutaneous graft-versus-host disease has a lichenoid pattern.

Bullous pemphigoid

Bullous pemphigoid is a blistering skin disease that occurs in the elderly. Up to 90% have IgG autoantibodies against the bullous pemphigoid major antigen located in the epidermal basement membrane. The vesicles and bullae usually contain eosinophils.

Pemphigus

Pemphigus is an intraepidermal blistering disease with autoantibodies to various structural proteins involved in intercellular adhesion.

Dermatitis herpetiformis

Dermatitis herpetiformis is a subepidermal blistering disease characterised by IgA antibody deposition, although the exact pathogenesis is unclear. There is a strong association with coeliac disease.

26.3 Genetic disorders

Learning objective

You should:
- understand that inherited skin disease can manifest as inflammatory disease or neoplastic disease.

Epidermolysis bullosa

Epidermolysis bullosa is a rare, blistering, skin disease with several subtypes that have dominant or recessive inheritance. Some variants are lethal in early life, others cause disfiguring scars with increased risk of developing squamous cell carcinoma. Blisters develop at sites of skin trauma or rubbing.

Xeroderma pigmentosum

Xeroderma pigmentosum is a rare, autosomal-recessive disease with defective DNA repair. There is extremely high incidence of epidermal and melanocytic malignancies.

Porphyria

Porphyria describes a group of rare diseases with deficiencies of enzymes involved in haem production. Porphyrins are pigments present in haemoglobin, myoglobin and cytochrome enzymes. In the skin, vesicle formation and scarring occurs, and symptoms may be precipitated by exposure to sunlight.

26.4 Neoplasia

Learning objectives

You should:
- know the pathology of the common skin cancers – basal cell carcinoma, squamous cell carcinoma and malignant melanoma
- understand the spectrum of benign and malignant melanocytic lesions in the skin and be able to recognise clinically suspicious 'moles'
- be able to interpret the prognostic information provided in a histopathology report of a malignant melanoma.

Neoplasms of the skin can arise from many of the component cells and tissues. The most common tumours arise from the epidermal cells and from melanocytes. The adnexal structures – eccrine sweat glands, sebaceous glands, hair follicles and apocrine glands – can give rise to a huge range of tumours, both benign and malignant (see Table 62).

Table 62 Skin tumours – a simple classification

	Benign	**Malignant**
Epidermal	Basal cell papilloma	Basal cell carcinoma
	Squamous cell papilloma	Squamous cell carcinoma
Melanocytic	Naevus (junctional, compound, intradermal, Spitz)	Malignant melanoma
Adnexal	Syringoma	Adnexal carcinomas (rare)
	Pilomatrixoma	
	Cylindroma	
Lymphoid		Cutaneous T cell lymphoma
		Cutaneous B cell lymphoma
Connective tissue	Dermatofibroma	Dermatofibrosarcoma protuberans
	Lipoma	Liposarcoma
	Haemangioma	Kaposi's sarcoma
		Angiosarcoma
	Neurofibroma	Malignant nerve sheath tumours
	Leiomyoma	Leiomyosarcoma

Basal cell papilloma

Basal cell papilloma is also known as seborrhoeic keratosis or seborrhoeic wart. It is a common benign warty tumour, arising in adults. It occurs almost anywhere on the body and is often pigmented. Microscopically the tumour consists of papillary projections of uniform cells resembling normal basal epidermal keratinocytes. There is hyperkeratosis and frequent formation of keratin nodules (horn cysts).

Basal cell carcinoma

Basal cell carcinoma is the commonest human malignant neoplasm. It typically arises in chronically sun-exposed skin of older adults; 80% develop on the head or neck. Metastasis is rare but, if untreated, basal cell carcinoma may cause extensive local tissue erosion, hence the historical name of 'rodent ulcer'. Basal cell carcinoma has several microscopic growth patterns:

- nodular – commonest (70%)
- superficial multifocal
- infiltrative (morphoeic) – highest risk of recurrence.

The tumour cells resemble those of the normal basal epidermis and are recognised histologically by their small hyperchromatic nuclei, mitotic figures and palisading (regular arrangement) of cells at the periphery of the tumour nests.

Squamous cell carcinoma

Squamous cell carcinoma is also a common tumour arising on sun-exposed skin of older adults. The tumour cells resemble those of the suprabasal epidermis in normal skin. Well-differentiated squamous cell carcinomas produce keratin and microscopically show thin cytoplasmic extensions or 'prickles', which represent desmosomal cell junctions, between the tumour cells. Squamous cell carcinomas have a low incidence of metastasis to local lymph nodes and distant sites (approximately 1%).

Squamous cell carcinoma often develops within a pre-existing dysplastic epidermal lesion, such as actinic keratosis or Bowen's disease (epidermal carcinoma in situ). Rarely, squamous cell carcinoma can arise in a chronic ulcer (Marjolin's ulcer), burn or scar. Immunosuppressed patients (e.g. following renal transplantation) have an increased incidence of squamous cell carcinoma.

Keratoacanthoma

Is a rapidly growing keratotic nodule that resembles well-differentiated squamous cell carcinoma, both clinically and microscopically, and the distinction between the two lesions can be very difficult. Keratoacanthomas tend to involute spontaneously, but can leave marked scarring.

Melanocytic lesions

Pigmented skin lesions can be due to:

- increased melanin pigmentation of the epidermis without melanocytic proliferation (pigmented basal cell papillomas, lentigo simplex)

- benign proliferation of melanocytes (naevi)
- malignant melanoma.

Clinical features that raise suspicion of melanoma in a pigmented lesion include:

- itching, crusting or bleeding
- change in size
- change in colour
- change in shape (irregularity of lesion border)
- size >7 mm – although malignant melanomas can be smaller than this.

Benign naevi (singular = naevus)

Benign naevi are extremely common and may be congenital or acquired. Most arise in childhood or adolescence. Naevi are classified according to the distribution of the melanocytic cells:

- junctional (naevus cells confined to epidermis)
- compound (naevus cells in epidermis and dermis)
- intradermal (naevus cells found only in dermis)
- blue naevi (intradermal, composed of spindle cells with marked melanin pigmentation).

Malignant change in acquired naevi is rare. However, large numbers of moles (>50 per individual) do appear to confer an increased risk of melanoma. Up to 10% of giant congenital naevi (>20 mm diameter) will develop melanoma within them.

Malignant melanoma

The incidence of melanoma in the UK is rising more rapidly than that of any other malignancy. The pathogenesis is clearly linked to UV-induced cell damage. Individuals with fair skin and hair, a history of sunburn and repeated high-intensity sun exposure are at particular risk. A strong family history is also significant.

Traditionally, classification of melanoma has been by architectural type:

- lentigo maligna melanoma
- superficial spreading melanoma (commonest, >50%)
- acral lentiginous melanoma (palm and soles – rare)
- nodular melanoma.

Lentigo maligna arises mainly on the chronically sun-exposed skin of the head and neck in the elderly. Atypical melanocytes replace the normal basal epidermis. The tumour may be present as an irregular pigmented macule

for several years before invasive dermal malignancy with metastatic potential develops.

Superficial spreading melanoma is characterised by atypical melanocytes scattered irregularly at all levels of the epidermis; this pattern is also known as 'pagetoid spread'. It can develop at any age, and is commonest on the back in males and lower leg in females.

More recently, melanomas have been classified according to their growth pattern into **radial growth phase** or **vertical growth phase**. It is proposed that only tumours showing evidence of proliferation in the dermis (vertical growth phase) have the capacity to metastasise (Table 63).

Classical melanoma cells are 'epithelioid' – large polygonal or cuboidal cells with copious cytoplasm and a large single eosinophilic nucleolus. Pigmentation is often found in a percentage of cells, but amelanotic lesions do occur and may be misdiagnosed clinically. Melanoma cells can also be spindle shaped. The histological diagnosis can be confirmed with immunocytochemistry with antibodies to S100 (a marker of neural crest origin) and HMB45 (see Box 32).

The most important prognostic factor in melanoma is the depth of invasion (Breslow thickness), measured from the top of the granular epidermal layer to the deepest dermal melanoma cell. The anatomical depth of invasion is also expressed as the Clark level (Figure 71). More recently, the prognostic importance of sentinel lymph node status in melanoma has been realised. The sentinel node is the specific node (or sometimes nodes) draining the area of a tumour. It can be identified by injecting coloured dye and radioactive tracer into the region of the primary tumour, and then locating the specific draining lymph nodes which take up the dye and radioactivity. The sentinel node status is a powerful prognostic indicator in melanoma and is included within the most recent staging system for the tumour. The sentinel node technique is also being utilised in the management of other tumours, particularly breast cancer, in order to reduce the morbidity associated with total axillary lymph node removal. Other adverse prognostic factors include:

- ulceration
- vascular invasion
- lack of a host inflammatory response
- male gender

Twenty six

Table 63 Melanoma growth phase classification

Radial growth phase melanoma	Vertical growth phase melanoma
Tumour grows within epidermis, with only single cells or small nests of melanocytes in the papillary dermis	Tumour usually involves the reticular dermis
Melanocyte cell groups in the epidermis larger than those in the dermis	Melanocyte cell groups in the dermis larger than those in the epidermis
No dermal mitoses are present	Dermal mitoses are often present

---

Box 32 Immunohistochemistry

What is it?

Immunohistochemistry is a histological technique in which labelled antibodies to specific proteins are applied to tissue sections. If the protein antigen is present in the cells they will bind the antibody, which can be detected on microscopy by the attached coloured label.

When is it used?

- To confirm the nature of a cell or tumour when the morphological appearances alone are not diagnostic.
- For prognosis and treatment, e.g. oestrogen receptor status in breast carcinoma.

Examples of commonly used immunohistochemical antibodies

Epithelial markers

- Cam 5.2 (low-molecular-weight cytokeratin)
- AE1/AE3 (a 'cocktail' of cytokeratins)

Lymphocyte markers

- LCA (leucocyte common antigen)
- CD3 (T cells)
- CD20 (B cells)

Melanocytic markers

- S100 (also stains neural tissue)
- HMB45 (a marker of melanosomes)

Muscle

- Desmin, myoglobin, anti-smooth muscle actin

Vascular endothelium

- Factor-8-related antigen

Nerve

- S100

Others

- Prostatic-specific antigen (PSA)
- α-Fetoprotein (hepatocellular carcinoma and certain germ cell tumours)
- Oestrogen receptor, *HER2* – breast cancer prognosis

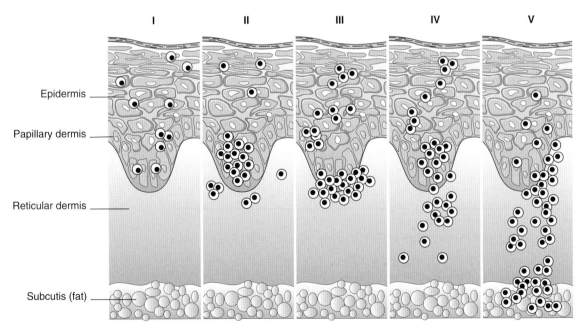

Figure 71 Clark levels (I–V) for staging of malignant melanomas: I, confined to epidermis; II, papillary dermal invasion; III, papillary-reticular dermis junction invasion; IV, reticular dermis invasion; V, subcutis invasion.

- anatomical site (lesions on the back have worse prognosis than those on the extremities)
- high mitotic rate
- the presence of satellite lesions (cutaneous metastases) in adjacent skin.

Survival in malignant melanoma is improving as a result of greater public and medical awareness with earlier clinical presentation. Radial growth phase lesions have virtually 100% 5-year survival. When the Breslow thickness exceeds 1.5 mm, 5-year survival drops to 34%.

Metastatic tumours

Deposits in the skin most frequently arise from:

- melanoma
- carcinoma (particularly breast, bronchus and large-intestine adenocarcinomas).

Cutaneous infiltration by lymphoma and leukaemia can also occur.

Twenty six

Self-assessment: questions

One best answer questions

1. Which immunohistochemical antibody stain is most helpful in confirming a tissue diagnosis of malignant melanoma?
   a. LCA (leucocyte common antigen)
   b. S100
   c. α-fetoprotein
   d. cytokeratin
   e. oestrogen receptor

2. A 29-year-old woman asks for advice about her risk of developing malignant melanoma, as one of her friends has just been diagnosed with this lesion. Which of the following are not of clinical relevance?
   a. number of benign naevi (moles)
   b. family history of skin cancer
   c. cigarette smoking
   d. fair hair colouring
   e. history of childhood sunburn

True-false questions

1. Granulomatous inflammation is typically seen in:
   a. tuberculosis
   b. ulcerative colitis
   c. erythema multiforme
   d. foreign body reaction
   e. sarcoidosis

2. In psoriasis:
   a. the flexor surfaces are mainly affected
   b. the epidermis shows regular thickening
   c. epidermal turnover time is increased
   d. nail changes are common
   e. skin lesions consist of red plaques with silvery scale

3. The following are correctly paired:
   a. Spongiosis – dermal oedema
   b. Erythema multiforme – lichenoid inflammation
   c. Xeroderma pigmentosum – squamous cell carcinoma
   d. Pemphigoid – bullae formation
   e. Dermatitis herpetiformis – granulomatous inflammation

4. In a pigmented lesion, the following clinical features are suggestive of malignant melanoma:
   a. irregular border
   b. uniform pigmentation
   c. itching
   d. changing size
   e. bleeding

5. The following are risk factors for squamous cell carcinoma:
   a. Bowen's disease
   b. chronic skin ulceration
   c. psoriasis
   d. actinic keratosis
   e. irradiation

6. Regarding basal cell carcinoma:
   a. 15% of tumours metastasise
   b. it is commonest on the lower limbs
   c. the microscopic growth pattern influences the risk of local recurrence
   d. if left untreated, it can erode into underlying bone
   e. it occurs exclusively in patients aged over 50

Case history questions

Case history 1

A 34-year-old man presents to his general practitioner (GP) with an enlarging lesion on his back which has recently bled. On examination there is a 7 mm papule with variable pigmentation and an irregular border. The GP decides to perform an incisional biopsy for diagnosis. Histopathology shows an ulcerated vertical growth phase superficial spreading malignant melanoma, Breslow thickness 2.1 mm, Clark level IV.

1. Is incisional biopsy appropriate for the initial diagnosis in this situation?
2. What do Breslow thickness and Clark level mean?
3. What does the histopathology report tell you about the likely behaviour of this tumour?

Case history 2

A 43-year-old woman presents to her GP with a linear vesicular rash around the left flank and back, which is painful. On examination, the GP also notes several warty growths on the hands, arms and neck. The patient underwent renal transplantation 2 years earlier and is taking immunosuppressive drugs to prevent rejection of the transplanted kidney.

1. What is the likely cause of the rash?
2. Give the differential diagnosis for the warty growths.

Viva questions

1. What advice would you give to a group of healthy school children about skin cancer prevention?
2. Discuss the classification and complications of burns.

Self-assessment: answers

One best answer

1. b. S100 antigen is commonly present on cells of neural crest origin – which includes peripheral nerves and melanocytes. Leucocyte common antigen is expressed by most white blood cells. α-Fetoprotein can be expressed by certain germ cell tumours and liver malignancies. Cytokeratins are a group of antigens expressed on epithelial cells. Oestrogen receptor immunostaining is most helpful in breast cancer, not just for diagnosis but also for prognosis and patient management.

2. c. Environmental risk factors for melanoma are clearly linked to UV exposure; pale-skinned individuals who burn easily in the sun are at highest risk. Although common benign naevi do not have an appreciable rate of transformation to malignant tumours, it does appear that individuals with large numbers of moles are at increased risk of melanoma, particularly if these moles are clinically or histologically atypical. A family history of melanoma also increases risk.

True-false answers

1. a. **True.** Often with central caseous necrosis.
   b. **False.** Granulomas are a feature of Crohn's disease.
   c. **False.**
   d. **True.** Common foreign bodies may be exogenous, such as surgical sutures, or endogenous (liberated keratin from inflamed hair follicles or sebaceous cysts).
   e. **True.**

2. a. **False.** Extensor surfaces are typically involved.
   b. **True.**
   c. **False.** Cell turnover time is decreased.
   d. **True.**
   e. **True.**

3. a. **False.** Spongiosis is intra-epidermal oedema.
   b. **True.**
   c. **True.** Xeroderma pigmentosum confers a greatly increased risk of all forms of skin cancer.
   d. **True.**
   e. **False.** Dermatitis herpetiformis is a vesico-bullous disease, which microscopically shows neutrophilic inflammation.

4. a. **True.**
   b. **False.** Uniform pigmentation can be seen in benign and malignant lesions.
   c. **True.**

d. **True.**
e. **True.**

5. a. **True.**
   b. **True.**
   c. **False.**
   d. **True.**
   e. **True.**

6. a. **False.** The rate of metastasis is less than 1 in 1000.
   b. **False.**
   c. **True.**
   d. **True.**
   e. **False.** Although commonest in the elderly, basal cell carcinoma does occasionally occur in young adults, particularly white adults with a history of high sun exposure. Rare inherited skin disease syndromes can give rise to basal cell carcinoma in childhood.

Case history answers

Case history 1

1. As the clinical features here are very suspicious of melanoma, the lesion should initially be excised complete with a narrow margin rather than biopsied, to allow accurate histological diagnosis. If this confirms melanoma, a further wider excision of the surrounding skin will be required.

2. *Comment*: These are described in the text and Figure 71.

3. The tumour is in the vertical growth phase, and therefore there is a risk of lymph node and distant metastasis. The Breslow thickness of over 2 mm is a poor prognostic factor as is ulceration. Statistically, male gender and lesion location on the back are also adverse features. This patient's chance of being alive 5 years from diagnosis is probably less than 50%.

Case history 2

1. This description of a painful, linear, vesicular rash arising in an immunosuppressed patient is virtually diagnostic of herpes zoster ('shingles'). The patient may recall a previous episode of chicken pox, representing initial infection with varicella-zoster virus. The virus persists as a latent infection in dorsal root ganglia and may become reactivated at any time, but particularly with increasing age and in periods of 'stress' or reduced immune-system functioning. The virus travels via sensory nerves to the skin, where it replicates, causing the characteristic lesions.

2. Many skin lesions can manifest as warty growths – including true viral warts and hyperkeratotic lesions. The latter include benign tumours (seborrhoeic warts/basal cell papillomas), dysplastic epithelial growths (actinic keratoses) and squamous cell carcinoma. Many of these lesions occur with increased frequency in immunosuppressed patients, reflecting the role of human papilloma virus infection in their pathogenesis.

Viva answers

1. *Comment*: Points to discuss include:
   - the danger of episodic high sun exposure throughout life but particularly in childhood and young adulthood
   - the rapidly increasing incidence of malignant melanoma, which is clearly linked to the increasing popularity of foreign holidays in hot places
   - the need to apply appropriate sun protection products to exposed skin, and to reapply these regularly, especially before and after swimming, even on hazy days
   - covering exposed skin with hats, sleeves, skirts, long trousers, etc.
   - avoiding sun beds and tanning salons; the long-term reward of a manufactured 'healthy' tan is skin damage and tumour formation.

   You could also discuss the features of a changing mole that should prompt the patient to seek medical help; these are discussed in the text.

2. *Comment*: Burns are discussed in the text in Section 26.1.

Nervous system

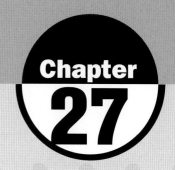

Chapter 27

Chapter overview

Diseases of the central nervous system (CNS) – particularly strokes, head injuries and dementia – are major causes of morbidity and mortality. Neurones do not divide in post-natal life (they are 'permanent' cells), and neuronal cell death is repaired by proliferation of supporting cells and 'gliosis' (the CNS equivalent of scarring). Children and young adults are not immune to serious CNS pathology – meningitis, congenital malformations, birth injuries, multiple sclerosis and certain neoplasms can particularly affect this population group.

The fixed available volume within the rigid skull means that an expanding mass lesion often results in raised intracranial pressure, which is frequently fatal without prompt medical intervention. Primary and secondary tumours are not uncommon in the CNS, and again the anatomical confines of the skull and vertebral column are important factors in prognosis, due to the effects of raised intracranial pressure and the physical limitation imposed on surgical resection.

27.1 Infection and inflammation

Learning objectives

You should:
- know the spectrum of organisms that can cause meningitis and encephalitis
- understand the pathology of acute bacterial meningitis and the information that can be obtained from investigation of cerebrospinal fluid in suspected meningitis
- be aware of how human immunodeficiency virus (HIV) infection can manifest in the CNS
- understand the basic pathology of spongiform encephalopathies.

Intracranial infection

Intracranial infection can affect the arachnoid and pial membranes (meningitis) or the underlying brain itself (encephalitis). Viral, bacterial, protozoal, fungal and protein (prion) agents all contribute. Routes of entry into the CNS include:

- blood-borne spread from distant site of infection
- direct inoculation of organisms (traumatic or iatrogenic)
- local extension of sepsis (e.g. dental or sinus infection)
- via the peripheral nervous system (viral agents including herpes simplex and rabies).

Meningitis can be:

- pyogenic (bacterial)
- aseptic (viral)
- chronic (bacterial or fungal).

The microorganisms likely to be responsible vary with age and immunocompetence. Clinical symptoms include headache, neck stiffness, photophobia, irritability and altered consciousness. A skin rash may only be present with certain strains of meningococcal bacteria causing systemic sepsis. Biochemical analysis and microscopic examination of cerebrospinal fluid (CSF) obtained at lumbar puncture is helpful in discriminating the causative agent (Table 64). Bacteria and protozoa may be directly identified by microscopy.

Acute bacterial meningitis

This can be fatal if not treated at an early stage. Complications include:

- extension of infection into brain tissue with abscess formation
- venous thrombosis with cerebral infarction
- meningeal fibrosis with hydrocephalus.

The infective organisms vary with the age of patients and immunisation status but include: *Escherichia coli*, group B streptococci and *Haemophilus influenzae* in infants; *Neisseria meningitidis* and *Streptococcus pneumoniae* in older children and young adults; and *Listeria monocytogenes* in the elderly.

Viral meningitis

Viral meningitis is clinically less important and usually self-limiting.

Table 64 CSF analysis in meningitis

Infectious agent	Predominant cell content	Protein	Glucose
Pyogenic bacteria	Neutrophil polymorphs	Increased	Marked decrease
Viral	Lymphocytes	Mild increase	Normal, occasionally decreased
Tuberculosis	Lymphocytes	Marked increase	Decreased or normal

Chronic meningitis

Tuberculous meningitis is rare, but is increasing in frequency among acquired immune deficiency syndrome (AIDS) patients. The onset is clinically more insidious with non-specific symptoms such as headache, confusion and vomiting. Chronic meningeal inflammation with granuloma formation and fibrosis can cause hydrocephalus and cranial nerve damage. Syphilis is a rare cause of neurological disease in the UK today, but a small percentage of those with tertiary syphilis develop chronic meningitis, sensory spinal cord damage (tabes dorsalis) or brain infection (dementia, Argyll Robertson pupils). The risk of developing neurosyphilis is increased in AIDS.

Viral encephalitis

Viral infections can cause encephalitis, with lymphocytic inflammation of the brain parenchyma and proliferation of glial cells. Intraneuronal inclusions may be seen in herpes simplex type 1 (HSV-1), cytomegalovirus (CMV) and rabies encephalopathy. Viral infections can be particularly damaging if acquired in fetal life (e.g. rubella, CMV-related congenital malformations) or during delivery (e.g. HSV-2-related neonatal sepsis).

Specific areas of the brain may be damaged, for example HSV-1 encephalitis particularly affects the temporal lobe.

Human immunodeficiency virus infection

HIV infects CNS macrophages and microglial cells. HIV infection and AIDS can cause numerous neurological lesions including:

- mild meningitis at seroconversion
- dementia-like illness
- spinal cord damage
- neuropathies
- congenital AIDS (microcephaly, motor delay and learning disabilities)
- opportunistic infections
  - *toxoplasmosis*
  - *CMV*
  - *cryptococcal meningitis*
  - *progressive multifocal leucoencephalopathy (PML) – a papovavirus infection, which affects oligodendrocytes, causing demyelination and multifocal white-matter damage.*

Rabies virus

The rabies virus gains entry to the brain by ascending along peripheral nerves. Symptoms arise weeks after initial infection and include abnormal CNS excitability (excessive pain on light touch, convulsions), paralysis, mania, stupor and coma. Local paraesthesia around the entry wound is a diagnostic pointer.

Poliomyelitis

Poliomyelitis is now very rare in industrialised countries. It initially occurs in the gut but in a small number of cases there is spread to lower motor neurones in the spinal cord, leading to muscle wasting and paralysis. Death can occur acutely due to a myocarditis or chronically due to respiratory muscle involvement.

Fungal infections of the CNS

Fungal infections of the CNS mainly occur in immunocompromised patients. The responsible organisms include *Candida*, *Mucor*, *Aspergillus* and *Cryptococcus*.

Spongiform encephalopathies

Spongiform encephalopathies are characterised by spongiform change (vacuolation) in the cerebral white matter. They are transmitted by prion protein, an abnormal form of a cellular protein that has undergone a conformational change and is able to induce a further conformational change in native protein when inoculated into previously normal cells. The prion protein gene is located on chromosome 20. It is highly conserved across species, and infectious particles in one species can corrupt the normal protein in other species. Spongiform encephalopathies include:

- scrapie in sheep
- bovine spongiform encephalopathy (BSE) in cattle
- transmissible encephalopathy in mink
- Creutzfeldt–Jakob disease (CJD), new variant CJD and kuru in humans.

Prions are neither destroyed by most normal disinfectants nor by formalin fixation.

Until the past decade, the incidence of CJD was approximately 1 per million, occurring sporadically in older adults. Iatrogenic transmission via corneal grafts, cadaveric growth hormone extracts or implanted electrodes has been documented. Recently there has been extensive debate about new variant (nv)CJD, which is thought to represent human infection by BSE transmitted by ingestion of contaminated meat products. Both CJD and new variant disease are characterised by rapidly progressive dementia with movement disorder (myoclonic jerks) and death usually occurs within 2 years of symptom onset. The eventual number of individuals likely to be affected by nvCJD remains unknown.

Brain abscesses

Brain abscesses can occur secondary to:

- acute bacterial meningitis
- direct extension of sepsis from outside brain
- penetrating injury
- blood-borne infection (infective endocarditis, cyanotic congenital heart disease, pulmonary sepsis).

The bacteria responsible are usually streptococcal or staphylococcal. Clinical symptoms include progressive focal neurological deficit and raised intracranial pressure.

27.2 CNS trauma and raised intracranial pressure

Learning objectives

You should:
- know the patterns of tissue damage and intracranial haemorrhage that can follow head injury
- understand the causes and consequences of raised intracranial pressure.

Mechanisms of traumatic brain injury

Contusion

Brain tissue is bruised on impact with the bony skull surface. A 'coup' injury occurs to the brain tissue underlying the point of external injury. A 'contre-coup' injury affects an area of brain directly opposite the impact. For example, a fall backwards onto the occiput causes contre-coup injury to inferior frontal lobes and inferior poles of temporal lobes (which is often more severe and clinically significant than the coup injury to the occipital lobe directly underlying the point of impact).

Laceration

Brain substance is torn, usually as a result of penetrating injury.

Diffuse axonal injury

Deceleration and rotational forces to the brain cause shearing injury to neurones and axonal processes. If extensive, this can cause coma and death. Diffuse axonal injury (DAI) is graded according to the extent of damage and the presence of grossly visible brain haemorrhage. Severe DAI can occur in the absence of any externally evident head trauma.

Tissue displacement following head injury damages blood vessels, causing haemorrhage and oedema with consequent mass effect (see below). Vascular injury and subsequent haemorrhage can be extradural, subdural, subarachnoid or intraparenchymal.

Intracranial haemorrhage

Extradural haemorrhage

Extradural haemorrhage is classically seen in association with a skull fracture involving the temporal bone with laceration of the middle meningeal artery. The typical clinical history includes a 'lucid interval' of several hours between the injury and neurological deterioration.

Subdural haemorrhage

Subdural haemorrhage usually originates from tearing of bridging veins that pass through the subdural space between the brain and the dural sinuses. The elderly are at increased risk, as brain atrophy increases stretching of the bridging veins and allows greater movement of the smaller brain within the skull following trauma. The precipitating head injury may be so trivial so as to have gone unnoticed. Subdural haemorrhage usually becomes clinically evident within hours, with non-specific signs (diminishing consciousness, headache) but may present chronically. Re-bleeding is common, and may occur from vascular granulation tissue within the organising haematoma.

Subarachnoid haemorrhage (SAH)

Subarachnoid haemorrhage occurring after trauma is usually secondary to brain tissue disruption. Non-traumatic SAH is more common and is discussed later in Section 27.3.

Raised intracranial pressure

The fixed skull volume allows very little room for the intracranial contents to expand in the presence of haemorrhage, tumour, abscess or oedema. Therefore a mild increase in intracranial mass can lead to increased intracranial pressure with serious consequences. Brain tissue becomes displaced (herniation). The site of herniation partly depends on whether mass increase is focal or diffuse (Figure 72):

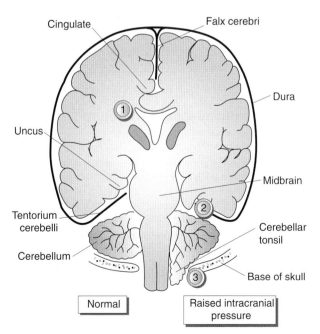

Figure 72 Sites of brain tissue herniation in presence of raised intracranial pressure.

- cingulate gyrus (inferior frontal lobe) can herniate across the midline under the dural fold of the falx cerebri, compressing the anterior cerebral artery
- uncal gyrus (inferior temporal lobe) can herniate under the tentorium cerebelli and compress the midbrain (leading to altered consciousness), oculomotor nerve, contralateral cerebral peduncle, aqueduct and posterior cerebral artery
- cerebellar tonsils can herniate through the foramen magnum, compressing the brainstem ('coning').

Compression of blood vessels supplying the midbrain causes venous stagnation with haemorrhage, necrosis and irreversible neuronal injury in this vital area.

Cerebral oedema

Cerebral oedema can be focal or diffuse. Oedema often makes a significant contribution to the mass effect of tumours and abscesses. The development of cerebral oedema indicates impaired function of blood–brain barrier, which normally tightly controls fluid movement within the brain. Mechanisms of cerebral oedema include:

- increased vascular permeability (vasogenic oedema)
- altered cell regulation of fluid (cytotoxic oedema)
- movement of fluid from the ventricular system into the brain.

Hydrocephalus

Hydrocephalus describes an increased volume of cerebrospinal fluid, usually due to a blockage in the CSF pathway. If occurring prior to the fusion of skull bone sutures in young children, hydrocephalus will result in head enlargement. The development of hydrocephalus may result from blood, post-inflammatory fibrosis or tumour blocking cerebrospinal fluid (CSF) flow. Apparent hydrocephalus in older adults due to atrophy of brain tissue and expansion of the ventricular system is sometimes called 'hydrocephalus ex vacuo'.

27.3 Cerebrovascular disease

Learning objectives

You should:
- understand the pathogenesis of thrombotic and embolic stroke, and be able to identify clinical risk factors
- know the causes and consequences of subarachnoid and intracerebral haemorrhage.

Cerebral infarction

Normal brain function ceases within a few seconds of loss of oxygen supply; irreversible neuronal damage occurs after 6–8 minutes of anoxia. Most cerebrovascular disease results from focal impairment of blood supply causing cerebral infarction. This manifests clinically as a 'stroke' – a neurological deficit of sudden onset but lasting more than 24 hours, caused by vascular insufficiency (neurological symptoms caused by lack of blood flow but resolving within 24 hours are known as transient ischaemic attacks or 'TIA'). Stroke can be due to thrombosis or embolus.

Thrombotic stroke usually complicates atherosclerosis in the basilar artery, proximal middle cerebral artery or at the carotid bifurcation. As thrombotic stroke arises on a background of atheroma, risk factors include hypercholesterolaemia, hypertension, diabetes mellitus and ischaemic heart disease.

When stroke occurs secondary to embolism, the source of the embolus is usually the heart. Cardiac mural thrombus can complicate myocardial infarction and atrial fibrillation. Thrombus may also embolise from abnormal heart valves, arterial walls (especially atherosclerotic carotid arteries) or from sites of cardiac surgery. Less commonly the embolus may consist of fat, air or tumour. Cerebral fat embolus should be suspected when neurological signs develop following non-head trauma with multiple bone fractures. Most embolic strokes affect the middle cerebral artery territory. Identification of the embolus at post mortem is often not possible, as a high percentage will have lysed.

Cerebral infarction can be haemorrhagic or non-haemorrhagic, as demonstrated by computed tomography (CT) or magnetic resonance imaging (MRI). The distinction is of therapeutic importance, as anticoagulation therapy is contraindicated in the presence of intracerebral bleeding. Thrombotic strokes are not usually complicated by bleeding. Haemorrhage can be secondary to reperfusion following an embolic stroke, but is more commonly seen in spontaneous intracerebral haemorrhage (ICH) associated with hypertension. ICH usually arises in:

- deep white matter of cerebral hemispheres/basal ganglia (>50%)
- pons (10%)
- cerebellum (10%).

Microscopically, the small arterial branches that rupture may show fibrinoid necrosis of the vessel wall and formation of microaneurysms known as Charcot–Bouchard aneurysms. Severe bleeding can cause rapid mass effect with an acute fatal rise in intracranial pressure. Haemorrhage may rupture internally into the ventricular system or externally into the subarachnoid space.

Hypertension can also result in small, often multiple lacunar infarctions (<15 mm in diameter) in the basal ganglia, deep white matter and pons. In accelerated or malignant hypertension, an encephalopathy may develop with headaches, vomiting, convulsions and altered conscious level.

The sequelae of stroke depend on the area of the brain involved and the extent of the infarction. Anterior circulation infarcts (internal carotid supply) affect cerebral hemispheres and can cause hemiparesis, sensory loss, dysphasia, incontinence and hemianopia. Posterior circulation infarcts (vertebrobasilar circulation) affect the brainstem and cerebellum. Neurological deficits may include ataxia and gaze abnormalities. Even small posterior circulation infarcts can cause coma and death due to involvement of vital regulatory centres in the brainstem.

Multiple small strokes can cause vascular (multi-infarct) dementia, with a stepwise deterioration in cognitive function. Cerebrovascular disease is the second commonest cause of dementia in the UK.

Rarer causes of intracerebral haemorrhage include:

- arteriovenous malformations
- tumours
- bleeding diatheses or anticoagulation therapy
- amyloid angiopathy.

Cerebral amyloid angiopathy occurs in the elderly and is associated with Alzheimer's disease (see Section 27.4). Haemorrhage is usually peripheral (lobar) in distribution.

Diffuse cerebral ischaemia can result following profound systemic hypertension. Clinically this may manifest as transient confusion with no permanent damage, or may result in widespread cerebral infarction with coma and death. The watershed areas of the brain – at the margins of perfusion by the major circle of Willis arterial branches – are particularly susceptible to such global ischaemia. Other brain regions particularly sensitive to hypoxia include:

- cerebellar Purkinje cells
- pyramidal neurones of hippocampus
- deeper neuronal layers of the cerebral cortex.

Subarachnoid haemorrhage

Subarachnoid haemorrhage is a relatively frequent natural cause of sudden unexpected death in young and middle-aged adults. The pathogenesis involves a congenital defect in the muscle wall of the cerebral arteries, which becomes manifest in later life as saccular dilatations known as 'berry aneurysms'. There is an association with adult polycystic renal disease (see Ch. 23) and hypertension. The aneurysms develop mainly in the anterior part of the circle of Willis (Figure 73), around the origin and proximal branches of the anterior and middle cerebral arteries. In 25% of cases there are multiple aneurysms. Rupture causes subarachnoid haemorrhage and clinically manifests with a sudden very severe headache. Bleeding may be precipitated by an acute rise in blood pressure (e.g. during sexual intercourse). Females are more frequently affected than males.

As with aneurysms elsewhere in the vascular system, the risk of rupture increases in proportion with the aneurysm size. Re-bleeding is common in those who survive the initial insult. As the haemorrhage resolves, fibrosis of the meninges at the base of the brain can lead to subsequent hydrocephalus.

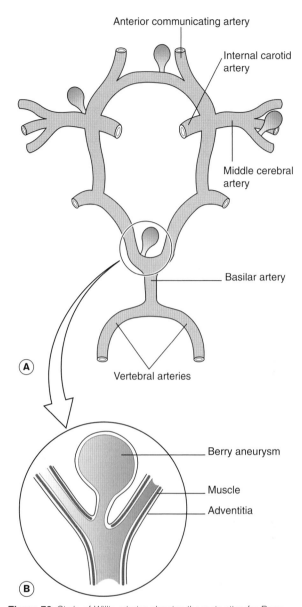

Figure 73 Circle of Willis arteries showing the main sites for Berry aneurysms.

27.4 Degenerative and demyelinating diseases

Learning objective

You should:
- understand the pathology of Alzheimer's disease, Huntington's disease and multiple sclerosis.

Dementia

Alzheimer's disease

Dementia is the progressive loss of cognitive function, manifest by memory loss and global intellectual impairment without diminished consciousness. The commonest cause of dementia in the UK is Alzheimer's disease (AD). AD is uncommon in people under 75 but thereafter its incidence increases dramatically. Up to 10% of cases are familial. Down's syndrome patients can develop AD changes at an earlier age, but seem to progress at a slower rate. CT head scan and brain examination at autopsy show cortical atrophy with widened sulci and compensatory dilatation of the ventricular system ('hydrocephalus ex vacuo'). Microscopically, three lesions are seen:

- neurofibrillary tangles
- senile plaques
- amyloid angiopathy.

Neurofibrillary tangles are bundles of intracytoplasmic filaments present within neurones. The tangles are often rounded or flame shaped. They can be seen on routine histological staining (haematoxylin and eosin (H&E)) but are better demonstrated with silver impregnation stains or by immunocytochemistry. Senile (neuritic) plaques are collections of neuronal processes surrounding an amyloid core. The main protein component of the core is β-amyloid protein, derived from amyloid precursor protein (APP). β-Amyloid protein is also present in the vascular amyloid deposits of amyloid angiopathy.

Plaques, tangles and amyloid angiopathy can all be seen to a certain extent in 'normal' brains and in individuals without clinical signs of AD. Amyloid angiopathy is a cause of peripheral intracerebral haemorrhage (see Section 27.3). It is the increased number and wide distribution of plaques and tangles that correlates with clinical dementia. In AD, cortical neurones, hippocampus and the amygdala are commonly involved sites.

Pick's disease

Pick's disease is a much less common form of dementia. There is severe atrophy of the frontal and temporal lobes, with basal ganglia involvement. Cytoplasmic Pick's bodies (filamentous structures similar to those seen in AD) are present within neurones.

Huntington's disease

This is a progressive inherited dementia associated with uncontrolled movements (chorea). Onset is in middle age. Atrophy occurs in the caudate, putamen and frontal lobes. The involuntary movements result from loss of GABA-utilising inhibitory neurones, which regulate motor output in the basal ganglia. Huntington's is an autosomal dominant condition with full penetrance, and new mutations are very rare. The gene responsible lies on chromosome 4 and contains repeats of the trinucleotide base sequence CAG. The normal allele contains 11–34 CAG copies, but in Huntington's there is amplification of this base sequence, with up to several hundred copies. The age of onset of disease decreases with each successive generation as the number of CAG copies increases (this phenomenon is known as 'anticipation'). A similar mechanism of disease is seen in X-linked spinal muscular atrophy, which is linked to trinucleotide repeats in the androgen receptor gene.

Parkinson's disease

Parkinson's disease is a movement disorder characterised by:

- abnormal gait and facial expression
- rigidity
- pill-rolling tremor
- difficulty in initiating movement
- dementia in a proportion of cases.

There is damage to dopamine-utilising neurones in the nigrostriatal tract. Loss of substantia nigra pigmentation can be identified at autopsy. Microscopically, Lewy bodies (cytoplasmic neuronal inclusions) can be seen in the brainstem nuclei, the cingulate gyrus and the hippocampus.

Motor neurone disease

This is clinically manifest by progressive muscular atrophy, fasciculation and symmetrical weakness. There is atrophy of anterior motor roots of the spinal cord (lower motor neurones) and of corticospinal tracts (upper motor neurones). Patients are usually middle-aged men. Death is often due to respiratory complications.

Toxic and metabolic disorders

Toxic and metabolic disorders of the nervous system include thiamine (vitamin B_1) deficiency and B_{12} deficiency. The latter affects long tracts with lower-limb weakness, ataxia and sensory loss (known as subacute combined degeneration of the cord). Other uncommon but important causes of neurological damage include hypoglycaemia, hepatic encephalopathy and ethanol.

Fetal alcohol syndrome

Fetal alcohol syndrome, which is caused by excess maternal ethanol intake during pregnancy, comprises:

- growth restriction
- cardiac septal defects
- facial abnormalities
- learning disabilities.

Demyelinating disorders

Demyelinating disorders affect oligodendrocytes in the CNS or the myelin sheath of peripheral nerves.

Multiple sclerosis

Multiple sclerosis (MS) is characterised by repeated episodes of demyelination within the central nervous system. Neurological deficit is variable. It may be relatively mild, with relapses and remissions, or severe and chronically progressive. Unilateral optic neuropathy causing sudden visual deterioration is the commonest presentation, but the diagnosis is based on finding CNS lesions disseminated in time and space. The aetiology of MS is unknown. No specific infectious agent has been implicated, although there are increased serum and CSF antibody titres to common viruses. The pathogenesis may involve an immune reaction against myelin, possibly triggered by viral infection.

Epidemiology

- Incidence of MS increases with increasing distance from the equator, particularly in the northern hemisphere
- Peak onset age 20–35
- More common in women
- Increased risk for first degree relatives but no pattern of inheritance.

CSF analysis shows normal or increased protein and there is often an oligoclonal increase in IgG. Lymphocytes are usually increased in number. The pathological lesions are plaques, a few millimetres in diameter, which can be seen on MRI scans and on examination of the brain and spinal cord at autopsy. Typical sites include:

- periventricular cerebral white matter
- optic nerves
- brainstem
- cervical cord.

Myelin is destroyed and oligodendrocytes lost but axons are preserved. There is a chronic inflammatory infiltrate. Older plaques become scarred ('gliotic').

27.5 Congenital malformations and genetic disease of the CNS

Learning objective

You should:
- know the common types of congenital malformation in the CNS.

Neural tube defects

Neural tube defects (NTDs) affect 2 per 1000 pregnancies in the UK, although their frequency in live births is much lower (many such pregnancies are terminated). Many NTDs can be detected antenatally by serum α-fetoprotein measurement and ultrasound. Defects include anencephaly, encephalocele and spinal fusion defects (Table 65). The rate of recurrence in subsequent pregnancies is approximately 5%. The incidence of NTDs varies in different ethnic groups. Folate deficiency is a recognised aetiological factor. Spinal defects are commonest and usually involve the lumbosacral region, predisposing to infection and cord damage. Table 66 details other more common CNS malformations.

Cerebral palsy

Is a non-progressive neurological defect arising in the perinatal period. The cause may not be apparent but intrauterine hypoxia, infection, birth trauma, kernicterus and hypoglycaemia may contribute. In premature babies, development of cerebral palsy is associated with cerebral haemorrhage and ischaemic damage to white matter (periventricular leucomalacia).

Inborn errors of metabolism in the CNS

Inborn errors of metabolism in the CNS include neuronal storage diseases and white matter diseases (leucodystrophies) involving damage to myelin or oligodendrocytes. Storage diseases usually have an autosomal recessive pattern of inheritance. Enzyme deficiencies cause accumulation of substrate (e.g. mucopolysaccharides, sphingolipids) within neuronal lysosomes and ultimately cell death.

Friedreich's ataxia

Friedreich's ataxia is an inherited spinocerebellar degeneration with axonal loss in long tracts. Onset is usually in late childhood, with boys more commonly affected than girls. Symptoms include ataxia, dysarthria, sensory loss and progressive paralysis. There may be associated cardiomyopathy.

27.6 Neoplasms

Learning objectives

You should:
- appreciate how the anatomy of the skull and spinal column influences the prognosis of both benign and malignant primary CNS tumours
- know the types of tumours that can arise within the central and peripheral nervous systems.

Table 65 Neural tube defects

Anencephaly	Absence of brain and skull
Encephalocele	Occipital bone defect with herniation of brain tissue
Meningomyelocele	Spinal column bony defect with exposed CNS tissue
Meningocele	Spinal column defect with herniation of meninges but no involvement of neural tissue
Spina bifida	Vertebral body bony defects but no involvement of spinal cord tissue

Table 66 CNS malformations

Microcephaly (small brain)	Fetal alcohol syndrome HIV Cytomegalovirus
Holoprosencephaly (incomplete separation of cerebral hemispheres)	Trisomy 13
Arnold–Chiari malformation	Multiple abnormalities involving cerebellum, medulla, aqueduct (stenosis) and lumbosacral spinal column (myelomeningocele)
Dandy–Walker malformation	Absent central cerebellum replaced by midline cyst

Primary nervous system tumours arise from:

- glial cells – astrocytes, oligodendrocytes and ependymal cells (60%)
- meningeal cells (20%)
- choroid plexus epithelium
- lymphoid cells
- nerve sheath (Schwann cells).

Central nervous system tumours

Intracranial tumours are 10 times more frequent than spinal neoplasms. About 20% of childhood cancers arise in the CNS. Primary tumours of the CNS cannot be labelled as 'benign' or 'malignant' using the same criteria as for tumours arising elsewhere in the body. Cytologically benign tumours can show locally extensive growth patterns preventing surgical excision. Slow-growing lesions can prove fatal due to their location or mass effect (e.g. benign tumour of the brainstem). Even microscopically high-grade tumours rarely metastasise outside the CNS, although dissemination can occur via the subarachnoid space and CSF pathways. Up to half of all CNS neoplasms are primary. The rest are metastases arising largely from carcinoma of the lung, breast, kidney, gastrointestinal tract and from malignant melanoma.

Astrocytomas

Astrocytomas are the most common adult primary brain tumours (Table 67). High-grade tumours (glioblastoma multiforme) have a very poor prognosis. Low-grade astro-

Table 67 Cancer checklist: astrocytoma

Incidence	Commonest in middle-aged and elderly adults (cerebral hemispheres); cerebellar astrocytomas in children
Risk factors	Not established
Protective factors	Not established
Associated lesions	Occasional gliomas are part of neurofibromatosis or inherited cancer syndromes (e.g. Turcot syndrome)
Common clinical presentation	Seizures, focal neurological signs Headache and vomiting if raised intracranial pressure
Location	Cerebral hemispheres most common, but can arise in brainstem, cerebellum and spinal cord
Macroscopic appearance	Poorly defined mass infiltrating adjacent brain
Histological features	Vary from low to high grade according to mitotic activity, nuclear pleomorphism and necrosis
Pattern of spread	Local brain infiltration
Prognosis (per cent 5-year survival)	Approximately 5–10 years' survival for low-grade astrocytoma; 8–10 months' average survival in glioblastoma multiforme (high-grade tumour)

cytomas often dedifferentiate to high-grade tumours over the course of several years.

Oligodendrocytomas

Oligodendrocytomas account for up to 15% of gliomas, and occur in middle-aged adults. Tumours arise in the cerebral hemispheres. Survival averages 5–10 years post-diagnosis.

Ependymomas

Ependymomas most commonly occur in the fourth ventricle in children, causing hydrocephalus. Their prognosis is poor as surgery is difficult and there is a tendency to dissemination via the cerebrospinal fluid.

Choroid plexus papillomas

Choroid plexus papillomas mainly occur in the lateral ventricle during childhood. They cause hydrocephalus due to obstruction of CSF flow and increased CSF production.

Medulloblastoma

Medulloblastoma is a primitive neural tumour which accounts for 20% of childhood brain tumours. It is a rapidly growing lesion in the central cerebellum, which can cause hydrocephalus. Medulloblastoma spreads along CSF pathways, but is highly sensitive to radiotherapy.

Primary brain lymphoma

Primary brain lymphoma is increasing in incidence. The pathogenesis is linked to Epstein–Barr virus infection and immunosuppression, but the frequency of lymphoma is also rising in immunocompetent individuals. Tumour deposits are often multiple. Histologically, these are high-grade, B lymphocyte, non-Hodgkin's lymphomas.

Meningiomas

Meningiomas are usually benign tumours of adulthood, arising from meningothelial cells of the arachnoid. Meningiomas are commoner in women and occur in young and middle-aged adults. Meningiomas can compress and invaginate into the brain substance but remain separate from it, which may permit surgical excision. Overlying bone can be eroded or infiltrated. There are many histological subtypes.

Metastatic tumours

Metastatic tumours frequently found in the CNS include lung and breast carcinomas and malignant melanomas.

Paraneoplastic symptoms

Paraneoplastic symptoms are defined as clinical phenomena associated with malignancy but not directly attributable to tumour infiltration. Paraneoplastic symptoms involving the CNS most commonly occur with small cell lung carcinoma. The pathogenesis is uncertain but may be immunologically mediated by antibodies against tumour expressed antigens cross-reacting against nervous system cells. CNS paraneoplastic syndromes include:

- cerebellar degeneration (antibody-mediated damage to Purkinje cells)
- spinal cord damage
- limbic encephalitis (a form of subacute dementia).

Peripheral nerve sheath tumours

Schwannoma

Schwannoma is a benign tumour of cells that produce myelin in the peripheral nervous system. Schwannomas can involve cranial nerves, especially the VIIIth nerve, which gives rise to the name 'acoustic neuroma'. Schwannomas are encapsulated tumours attached to the nerve. Malignant change is very rare.

Neurofibroma

Neurofibroma is a common tumour composed of Schwann cells, fibroblasts and perineural cells. Neurofibromas are unencapsulated, and cannot be separated from nerve in which they arise. Neurofibromas occur sporadically or in patients with neurofibromatosis (Box 33).

Malignant peripheral nerve sheath tumours

Malignant peripheral nerve sheath tumours arise de novo or from transformation of neurofibromas in neurofibromatosis.

Box 33 Neurofibromatosis

Type I

- Mutation in tumour suppressor gene on chromosome 17.
- Autosomal dominantly inherited or spontaneous mutation.

Characterised by:

- multiple neurofibromas (cutaneous and visceral)
- pigmented skin macules (café-au-lait patches)
- pigmented nodules on the iris (Lisch nodules).

There is an increased incidence of other tumours including acoustic neuromas, gliomas, meningiomas, phaeochromocytomas. Learning disabilities and skeletal abnormalities are common.

Type II

- Bilateral acoustic schwannomas, with or without cutaneous neurofibromas.
- No iris nodules.
- Tumour suppressor gene involved is on chromosome 22.

Twenty seven

Self-assessment: questions

One best answer questions

1. A 23-year-old woman presents with rapid onset of severe headache, photophobia and altered consciousness. Lumbar puncture is performed and subsequent cerebrospinal fluid analysis shows increased protein and decreased glucose, with neutrophil polymorphs present on microscopy. The likely diagnosis is:
   a. acute bacterial meningitis
   b. intracerebral tumour
   c. cerebral abscess
   d. viral meningitis
   e. subarachnoid haemorrhage

True-false questions

1. Prion protein:
   a. Is degraded by formalin
   b. is present in plaques of Alzheimer's disease
   c. is highly conserved across species
   d. causes cell damage by inducing a conformational change in normal protein
   e. can be transmitted by corneal grafts

2. Berry aneurysms:
   a. are usually multiple
   b. classically cause subdural haemorrhage
   c. are associated with polycystic kidney disease
   d. are present at birth
   e. have a high risk of re-bleeding following rupture

3. In multiple sclerosis:
   a. there is loss of both myelin and axons
   b. unilateral optic nerve involvement is a common presentation
   c. the incidence is highest in equatorial countries
   d. the cerebrospinal fluid often contains an oligoclonal increase in IgM antibodies
   e. plaques are characteristically found in the periventricular white matter of the cerebral hemispheres

4. Subdural haemorrhage:
   a. is commonest in the elderly
   b. may not become clinically evident until several weeks after the event
   c. is always preceded by a significant head injury
   d. usually originates from the subdural sinuses
   e. is rarely complicated by re-bleeding

5. The following are correctly paired:
   a. Huntington's disease – trinucleotide repeats
   b. Parkinson's disease – neurofibrillary tangles
   c. Pick's disease – frontal lobe atrophy
   d. Alzheimer's disease – amyloid angiopathy
   e. fetal alcohol syndrome – cardiac septal defects

6. The following are causes of non-traumatic intracranial haemorrhage:
   a. hypertension
   b. thrombocytopenia
   c. cerebral embolism
   d. arteriovenous malformations
   e. glioblastoma multiforme

7. Concerning meningitis:
   a. cerebrospinal fluid neutrophils are always increased
   b. cerebral infarction is a complication
   c. *Neisseria meningitidis* is the commonest causative organism in infants
   d. cryptococcal meningitis is increasing in incidence
   e. viral meningitis is associated with markedly low CSF glucose

8. Neural tube defects:
   a. affect 2 per 1000 live births in the UK
   b. can be detected by measurement of serum carcinoembryonic antigen
   c. of the spine are commonest in the cervical region
   d. recur in 10% of subsequent pregnancies with the same parents
   e. are associated with folate deficiency

9. Concerning CNS tumours:
   a. the commonest primary glial tumours are astrocytomas
   b. 20% of childhood malignancy occurs in the CNS
   c. glioblastoma multiforme metastasises widely outside the CNS
   d. medulloblastoma is usually radiosensitive
   e. primary brain lymphoma is associated with herpes simplex virus

10. The following are risk factors for cerebral infarction:
    a. Myocardial infarction
    b. infective endocarditis
    c. fat embolism
    d. diabetes insipidus
    e. septic shock

Case history questions

Case history 1

A 56-year-old man presents with a 9-month history of worsening concentration and forgetfulness. He is anxious because his wife has noticed his behaviour has changed and he is worried that he has a brain tumour.

1. What clinical diagnosis do these symptoms suggest?
2. What further information would you seek from the history and clinical examination to help determine the underlying cause?

Case history 2

You are a consultant histopathologist, and have been asked by the coroner to carry out a post-mortem examination on a 19-year-old man who died unexpectedly. The deceased had been out with friends the night before his death and had consumed several pints of lager. He had been involved in a fight and had briefly been knocked unconscious but appeared to recover within a few minutes and did not seek medical help. He had later felt tired and had been taken home to bed by his friends, where he was found dead the morning after.

1. What causes of death would you consider likely in this scenario?
2. On exposing the skull, you identify a fracture of the right temporal bone. What other abnormalities do you now expect to find inside the cranial cavity?

Case history 3

A 32-year-old woman presents with a 2-week history of headaches and recent onset of left-arm weakness. A CT head scan (with contrast) shows an intracerebral mass with rim enhancement and a low-density centre.

1. What is the differential diagnosis?
2. What further information would you seek from the history and clinical examination to help determine the underlying cause?

Viva question

1. How can tumour involvement of the CNS present clinically?

Self-assessment: answers

One best answer

1. a. The cerebrospinal fluid (CSF) findings are typical of pyogenic bacterial infection. In viral meningitis, lymphocytes predominate in the CSF. Cerebral abscess typically presents with symptoms of focal neurology and raised intracranial pressure; meningeal irritation is not present unless the abscess has ruptured. Brain tumours also present with localising or mass effects, often developing over weeks or months. In neoplastic infiltration of the meninges, lymphocytes are the predominant white blood cell in the CSF. In subarachnoid haemorrhage, the CSF may be macroscopically blood stained or appear yellow after centrifugation (xanthochromia) due to red blood cell lysis; large numbers of erythrocytes would be seen on microscopy.

True-false answers

1. a. **False.**
   b. **False.**
   c. **True.**
   d. **True.**
   e. **True.**

2. a. **False.** Twenty-five per cent are multiple.
   b. **False.** Subarachnoid.
   c. **True.** In a proportion of cases.
   d. **False.** The weakness of the arterial wall is present at birth but the aneurysms develop in later life.
   e. **True.**

3. a. **False.** Axons are not damaged.
   b. **True.**
   c. **False.**
   d. **False.** There may be oligoclonal IgG antibody increase.
   e. **True.**

4. a. **True.** Alcoholics are another high-risk group.
   b. **True.**
   c. **False.** The injury may be trivial and may have gone unnoticed or not be remembered.
   d. **False.** From bridging veins.
   e. **False.** Re-bleeding from vascular granulation tissue in the organising thrombus is common.

5. a. **True.**
   b. **False.**
   c. **True.**
   d. **True.**
   e. **True.**

6. a. **True.**
   b. **True.**
   c. **True.**
   d. **True.**
   e. **True.**

7. a. **False.** Neutrophil polymorphs are inconsistently present in tuberculous meningitis and are absent in viral meningitis.
   b. **True.**
   c. **False.** *Haemophilus influenzae* in young children and *Escherichia coli* in babies.
   d. **True.** Through its association with HIV infection.
   e. **False.** CSF glucose is usually normal in viral meningitis.

8. a. **False.** Many are detected antenatally and may be aborted spontaneously or by medical intervention.
   b. **False.** Maternal serum α-fetoprotein may be raised.
   c. **False.** They are most common in the lumbosacral region.
   d. **False.** Recurrence rate is less than 5%.
   e. **True.**

9. a. **True.**
   b. **True.**
   c. **False.**
   d. **True.**
   e. **False.** It is associated with Epstein–Barr virus infection in HIV-positive patients.

10. a. **True.** Cardiac mural thrombi are a source of cerebral emboli.
    b. **True.** Embolisation of valve vegetations.
    c. **True.**
    d. **False.**
    e. **True.** Profound hypotension can cause global cerebral ischaemia.

Case history answers

Case history 1

1. The symptoms are those of a chronic decline in cognitive function, suggesting dementia. The commonest causes in the UK are Alzheimer's disease and multiple cerebral infarctions. The age of onset in this patient is unusually young for Alzheimer's but this certainly does not exclude the diagnosis. A family history of dementia, especially with decreasing age of onset in successive generations, should raise the suspicion of Huntington's disease; a history of movement disorders should also be sought. CJD and nvCJD are very rare conditions (at least currently) and the typical history is of a more rapidly progressive dementia often with psychiatric

symptoms and muscle disease (myoclonia or wasting).

2. The history and clinical examination must also include assessment of cerebrovascular and cardiovascular disease (previous strokes, hypertension, atrial fibrillation, etc.). Bear in mind other conditions in which dementia can arise, such as HIV infection.

Case history 2

1. The history raises the suspicion of traumatic injuries, either to the head or the viscera. Catastrophic haemorrhage could have occurred from a ruptured spleen. Acute alcohol intoxication certainly needs to be excluded (post-mortem blood samples for alcohol and drugs would be taken).

2. The history of brief loss of consciousness followed by a 'lucid interval' and the finding of a temporal bone fracture are highly suggestive of extradural haemorrhage. The bleeding is arterial in nature, with origin from a torn middle meningeal artery. At post mortem you would expect to see the extradural haematoma, and if this is the cause of death, there will almost certainly be signs of raised intracranial pressure.

Case history 3

1. The radiological appearances here suggest either an abscess or a tumour (primary or secondary).

2. You should specifically ask about and look for sepsis – either a local infection (middle ear or sinuses) or a distant source of septic embolism (infective endocarditis from congenital heart disease, intravenous drug use, etc.). You must establish whether the patient is immunosuppressed (diabetes, HIV, steroid therapy, organ transplant), which would increase the risk of brain abscess following infection with virulent and opportunistic organisms. Although metastatic tumour is rare in this age group, remember that breast cancer and melanoma in particular can affect young adults and are common tumours to metastasise to the CNS. Primary glial malignancies are most frequently seen in older adults but can present at any age.

Viva answer

Comment: Think logically:

- Localising neurological signs of gradual onset – focal weakness or sensory deficit, hearing loss (acoustic neuroma), spinal cord level of dysfunction for intravertebral tumours. Sudden severe neurological deficit may be caused by haemorrhage from the tumour.

- Focal or generalised epilepsy.

- Local mass of tumour with or without oedema causing raised intracranial pressure with headaches and vomiting.

- Remember that primary brain malignancies very rarely metastasise outside the CNS, but some will disseminate along the CSF pathway.

- Remember that some paraneoplastic syndromes occur in the CNS.

Glossary

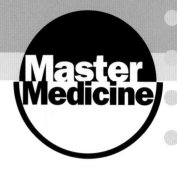

Adenocarcinoma A carcinoma of glandular epithelium, e.g. adenocarcinoma of colon.

Adenoma A benign tumour of glandular epithelium.

Aetiology The cause of a disease.

Allergen An agent that causes IgE-mediated hypersensitivity reactions, e.g. pollen, house dust mite.

Allergy Common term for a type I hypersensitivity reaction.

Alternative pathway The complement cascade pathway which starts with C3. It is triggered by a variety of factors such as tissue damage, but does not require antibodies.

Anaemia A reduction in the oxygen-carrying capacity of the blood, almost always the result of abnormalities of red cells, e.g. iron deficiency, premature destruction (haemolysis) and abnormal haemoglobins.

Anaphylaxis The antigen-specific immune reaction mediated by IgE which results in systemic vasodilatation and constriction of smooth muscle (including those of the bronchus), leading to shock and sometimes death.

Anoxia Complete loss of oxygen supply.

Antibody Also known as immunoglobulin, an antibody is a molecule produced by B cells or their mature progeny (plasma cells) in response to antigen with which it can specifically bind.

Antibody-dependent cell-mediated cytotoxicity A cytotoxic reaction where Fc receptor-bearing cells recognise and kill target cells via specific antibodies. Natural killer (NK) cells are principally responsible, but other cells with Fc receptors can participate.

Antigen A molecule which reacts with the B cell or T cell receptor to induce a specific adaptive immune response.

Antigen-presenting cell This cell can process and present antigen to lymphocytes. Examples are the dendritic reticulum cells in follicle centres, and the Langerhans' cells of the skin and B cells.

Apoptosis A form of programmed individual cell death which occurs normally during embryological development. It also occurs in pathological processes such as atrophy, ischaemic injury and neoplasms. It is an energy-dependent process which is not associated with an inflammatory reaction.

Atrophy The reduction in size of an organ or tissue because of either natural ageing (e.g. gonads) or a pathological process (such as ischaemia).

ATP ATP (adenosine triphosphate) is manufactured by cells to act as the source of energy for most biochemical reactions.

Atypia Changes in the histological appearances of cells, usually suggesting neoplastic transformation. Thus, dysplastic and malignant cells are atypical.

Autolysis The changes that occur in an organ or tissue after removal from the body, and in the whole body after death. No vital (inflammatory) reaction seen.

Basophil Basophilic polymorphonuclear leucocytes. A white blood cell with a multi-lobated nucleus and coarse cytoplasmic granules. Comprises 1% of the total white cell count in peripheral blood. Have the same properties as mast cells.

BCG (Bacille-Calmette-Guérin) An attenuated strain of *Mycobacterium tuberculosis* used as a vaccine.

Biopsy A sample of tissue removed from the body for histological examination by a pathologist.

Blood group, blood group antigen The result of the expression of an antigen at the red cell membrane. There are many different 'groups' but the most important in clinical practice are the ABO and the rhesus systems.

Cachexia The term used to describe the clinical appearance of a patient with advanced cancer. There is often marked weight loss and the patient is emaciated and wasted. Probably cytokine induced.

Cancer Any form of malignant tumour.

Carcinogenesis The process/processes by which neoplasms develop. Often qualified by the causative agents, e.g. viral carcinogenesis, chemical carcinogenesis.

Carcinoma A malignant tumour showing epithelial differentiation.

Carcinoma in situ An epithelial neoplasm with all the histological characteristics of malignancy but which has not (yet) invaded through the basement membrane. An example is high-grade cervical intra-epithelial neoplasia (CIN).

Carcinomatosis Carcinoma in many different organs following extensive metastases from a primary tumour.

CD markers Cluster differentiation markers are molecules on leucocytes and other cells that can be recognised with monoclonal antibodies and may be used to differentiate different cell populations.

cDNA Complementary DNA. When a single strand of DNA acts as a template, the new strand synthesised from it is complementary. If complementary strands are brought together they will bind to each other by adenine-thymine and guanine-cytosine bonds.

Cell cycle The process of cell division which comprises four phases G1, S, G2 and M. DNA replicates in the S phase and the cell divides in the M (mitotic) phase. Another phase, G0, contains cells that are no longer dividing but can return to the cell cycle if suitably stimulated.

Cell injury The consequence of a wide variety of different insults, e.g. bacteria, viruses or physical agents. Can be lethal (causing cell death) or non-lethal (producing degenerative changes).

Cell-mediated immunity Immune reactions which are mediated by cells (lymphocytes) rather than antibody.

Chemotaxis The purposeful movement of cells towards a chemical stimulus.

Ciclosporin A A T cell suppressive drug which is useful in the suppression of graft rejection.

Classical pathway The pathway by which antigen–antibody complexes can activate the complement system, involving complement proteins C1, C2 and C4.

Clone A family of cells which is genetically identical. The progeny of a single stem cell form a clone.

Clot A solid mass involving fibrin produced by the coagulation cascade. A clot that forms in a blood vessel during life is a thrombus.

Complement C1–C9 are the serum protein components of the complement cascade which are responsible for mediating inflammatory reactions, opsonisation of particles and cell lysis. The cascade can be activated by the immune system (classical pathway) or by tissue damage and micro-organisms (alternative and MBL pathways (see separate entries)).

Congenital Present at birth. Includes inherited abnormalities and diseases acquired during pregnancy or delivery.

Cytokines A family of messenger proteins which stimulates the maturation or activation of a variety of cells including lymphocytes and macrophages. Originally known as lymphokines, when it was thought that they were only secreted by lymphocytes, cytokines have a wide variety of different physiological and pathological effects, including the maturation of haemopoietic stem cells.

Degeneration The changes which may follow non-lethal cell injury.

Desmoplasia The reaction of the body to invading malignant cells characterised by active fibroblasts and inflammatory cells.

Dysplasia Changes in the histological appearance of cells which suggest that they have become neoplastic. Usually applied to epithelia.

EBV (Epstein–Barr virus) Causal agent of Burkitt's lymphoma (a malignant proliferation of immortalised B cells) and infectious mononucleosis (glandular fever).

Embolus Material which circulates in the blood and lodges in a blood vessel and occludes it. Examples of emboli are air, thrombus, fat and amniotic fluid.

Emigration The process by which inflammatory cells leave blood vessels and enter the tissue.

End artery An artery that is solely responsible for the blood supply of a particular zone of tissue.

Endocytosis The physiological mechanism by which fluid is taken in small discrete amounts into the cell cytoplasm from the interstitial tissues.

Endophytic Growing inwards, producing a mass beneath a surface.

Endoplasmic reticulum This organelle is a labyrinth of tubules and vesicles in the cytoplasm. It has a wide variety of functions which mostly involve the processing of proteins.

Eosinophil Eosinophilic polymorphonuclear leucocyte. A white blood cell, often with a bilobed nucleus and eosinophilic cytoplasmic granules. They have many functions, including breakdown of histamine and killing of parasites. Comprise 2–3% of total white cell count in peripheral blood.

Epithelioid cell A macrophage commonly found in tuberculous and other granulomatous lesions. In histological preparations, these cells have eosinophilic cytoplasm and superficially resemble epithelial cells – hence their name.

Exophytic Growing outwards from a surface, producing a polyp or fungating mass.

Exudate An abnormal collection of fluid within tissues, or in a body cavity. The protein concentration of an exudate is usually high and there is almost always associated inflammation.

Fatty change (fatty degeneration) A potentially reversible form of cell injury, most often seen in the liver. The result of impaired cytoplasmic metabolism of fat.

Fibrosis Synonymous with scarring. Repair by replacement with collagen-rich tissue.

Fistula An abnormal connection between two epithelial-lined surfaces. For example, a colovesical fistula connects the colon to the bladder, while a cholecysto-cutaneous fistula connects the gall bladder to the skin. A fistula has an opening at both ends, unlike a sinus, which has only one opening.

Fungating An exophytic tumour with extensive necrosis and ulceration.

Gamete Reproductive cell that is haploid (contains half the genetic material of a diploid cell). One derived from the female and one from the male fuse to produce a diploid zygote which develops into the embryo. In humans, the gametes are the ova and spermatozoa.

Gangrene A characteristic 'blackening' of necrotic tissue. Produced by infection with bacteria and tends to occur in tissues which have a resident bacterial flora, e.g. skin and large bowel. In limbs, the term wet gangrene refers to this process, whereas dry gangrene refers to 'mummification' with little or no infection.

Genotype The set of genes possessed by an organism.

Giant cell A large cell with many nuclei. In chronic inflammation, giant cells are formed by the fusion of macrophages. These must be distinguished from tumour giant cells – cancerous cells with multiple nuclei and a bizarre histological appearance.

Granulation tissue The richly vascular tissue containing inflammatory cells, endothelial cells and myofibroblasts which is laid down in the first stages of repair. Granulation tissue matures into scar tissue.

Granuloma A localised aggregate of macrophages. There are many examples of 'granulomatous diseases' including tuberculosis, leprosy, schistosomiasis and Crohn's disease.

Growth factors Polypeptides which stimulate protein synthesis within individual cells. They attach to specific receptors on the cell surface and are involved in cell proliferation. Good examples include the cytokines PDGF (platelet-derived growth factor) and epidermal growth factor.

H&E Haematoxylin and eosin, the common stain used routinely by most histopathology laboratories for tissue sections. Haematoxylin is a blue dye and stains acidic molecules such as nucleic acids, whereas eosin is a red-pink dye and stains basic molecules such as proteins.

Hapten A molecule too small to be recognised by the receptors on B cells and T cells unless bound to a larger immunogenic molecule.

Healing by first intention The normal process by which surgical wounds heal. The close apposition of the edges of the wound is essential. Only small amounts of granulation tissue are laid down and there is minimal scarring.

Healing by second intention The process by which large wounds whose edges cannot be apposed heal. There is abundant granulation tissue formation and consequent scarring.

Histiocyte Another name for macrophage.

Hyperplasia The increase in the size of an organ or tissue as a result of an increase in the number of constituent cells. Can only occur in labile or stable tissues, i.e. tissues which can undergo mitotic division.

Hypertrophy The enlargement of a tissue or organ resulting from an increase in the size of the constituent cells, not an increase in number.

Hypoxia A shortage of oxygen, but not an absolute lack (anoxia).

Immune complex The product of an antibody–antigen reaction, which may also contain components of complement.

Immunoglobulin *See* antibody.

Infarct An area of necrosis produced by a localised reduction in blood supply. Common examples result from obstruction of end-arteries (e.g. myocardial infarction), venous outflow obstruction (e.g. torsion of the testis) and watershed infarcts at the boundaries between the territories of two circulations (e.g. in the brain after hypotension).

Inflammation A mechanism by which the living body reacts to many different forms of injury. It has both vascular and cellular components. Acute inflammation usually lasts for days or a few weeks. In chronic inflammation the process can last for months or years.

Interferons/interleukins Types of cytokine involved in signalling between cells of the immune system.

Ischaemia Shortage of blood flow, often a result of an obstruction to the circulation. Causes hypoxia.

Kupffer cells Phagocytic macrophages found in the liver sinusoids.

Ligand Any molecule which binds to a receptor.

Lymphoma Malignant tumour of lymphocytes or macrophages. Chiefly involves lymph nodes, spleen and bone marrow, but can affect many other organs.

Lysosomes Cytoplasmic organelles completely enclosed by membranes and containing a wide variety of enzymes. The release of these enzymes after cell death in living tissue produces some of the changes of necrosis.

Macrophage A cell derived from blood monocytes with phagocytic properties. Prominent in the chronic inflammatory response.

Margination The process by which inflammatory cells come to lie at the margins of blood vessels, just before emigrating to the adjacent tissue. Mediated by adhesion molecules.

MBL pathway The mannose (mannan) binding lectin (MBL) pathway activates complement. When MBL recognises and binds to a bacterial carbohydrate, it interacts with a serine protease that cleaves C4.

Mediator A chemical substance which instigates, or controls, a physiological or pathological response, such as those which modulate the inflammatory reaction (e.g. histamine).

Mesenchymal Mesenchyme is the undifferentiated embryonic connective tissue derived from the mesoderm. It is found in the embryo and fetus, and develops into various adult tissues, including muscle, fat, blood vessels, lymphatics, fibroblasts, bone and cartilage. Sometimes, the term 'mesenchymal' is used as shorthand for this group of adult tissues.

Metaplasia The adaptive transformation of one adult cell type into another.

Metastasis Transfer of tumour from one site (the primary) to another (the secondary), usually via the blood or lymphatic systems. Defines a malignant tumour.

MHC (major histocompatibility complex) A genetic region encoding molecules involved in presenting peptides to cells of the immune system. The term 'histocompatibility' derives from the fact that these molecules can act as foreign antigens in transplants and are responsible for the rapid rejection of grafts between individuals. In the human the MHC is also known as the human leucocyte antigen (HLA).

Mitochondria Organelles that are the principal site of ATP synthesis. They also have a role in initiating apoptosis. Mitochondria have their own DNA, which encodes some (but not all) of their components.

Monocyte A mononuclear white blood cell, derived from precursors in the marrow. After migration into the tissues they are known as macrophages or histiocytes.

Myofibroblast A specialised cell characteristically seen in granulation tissue. The cytoplasm of these cells contain contractile filaments and they are largely responsible for closing up the gap between the edges of wounds.

Necrosis The morphological changes which occur in organs or tissues after cell death in a living body. Sometimes used to imply passive cell death (oncosis) as opposed to apoptosis.

Neoplasm A tumour, either benign or malignant.

Neutrophils Neutrophil polymorphonuclear leucocytes. The commonest form of white cell in the blood (about 50–60% of the total), actively phagocytic, important in the acute inflammatory response.

NK (natural killer) cells These lymphocytes can kill other cells through a number of mechanisms, including antibody-dependent cell-mediated cytotoxicity, membrane-bound complement component C3b, and receptors for various proteins expressed by stressed cells. Reduction of major histocompatibility complex (MHC) class I receptors on the target cell (seen in some infections and neoplasms) also act as a kill signal. NK cells are particularly important in defence against viruses, intracellular bacteria and spontaneously arising neoplastic cells.

Oedema The accumulation of abnormal amounts of fluid in tissue. Occurs when the normal balance between the hydrostatic pressure of the circulation and the oncotic pressure of the plasma proteins is upset.

Oncogene, proto-oncogene, viral oncogene An oncogene is a gene which codes for a protein that contributes to the tumorous characteristics ('phenotype') of a neoplastic cell. They are derived from proto-oncogenes, which have important roles in normal cellular physiology, especially in the control of cell growth. Viral oncogenes are fragments of genetic material carried by viruses into normal cells, which then influence the expression of the tumorous phenotype. In both humans and animals, genes are given short code names and written in italics. Human genes are generally written in upper case: *RAS*, *MYC*, *ABL*.

Oncogenesis The production of neoplasia. It refers to the stepwise development of the neoplastic phenotype. Literally, it means 'production of a swelling'.

Oncoproteins The proteins encoded by oncogenes. For example, some can mimic the action of growth factors.

Oncosis Passive cell death characterised by the destruction of membranes.

Oncotic pressure The osmotic pressure exerted across a semi-permeable membrane by dissolved colloids. In medicine, it usually refers to the force tending to drive water into the vascular space due to the presence of plasma proteins. Oncotic literally means 'swelling'.

Opsonisation A process whereby phagocytosis is helped by the coating of a micro-organism with any of a number of substances, including antibody, complement components (principally C3b), and substances such as the lectins and pentraxin proteins (e.g. C-reactive protein and serum amyloid P) which bind to various bacterial components.

Organisation The conversion of inert material to scar tissue via granulation tissue. Macrophages in the granulation tissue digest the inert material (blood clot, necrotic tissue, etc.) while the blood vessels and fibroblasts migrate into it. The granulation tissue then matures into a scar.

Oxidative phosphorylation The series of reactions that occur on the inner mitochondrial membrane in which oxygen is used to produce ATP. Can only occur if oxygen is available.

Papilloma A protuberance composed of fibrovascular cores covered by endothelium. Usually have a polypoid pattern of growth with finger-like excrescences, but occasional types of papilloma show an endophytic (inverted) pattern.

Pathogen An organism which causes disease.

Pathogenesis The mechanism(s) by which a disease is produced.

Phagocytosis The process by which material is ingested by cells.

Phagosome The 'bag' of inverted cell membrane enclosing the phagocytosed material or particle.

Phenotype The sum of the structural and functional characteristics manifested by a cell or by an organism.

Polyp Any structure that rises above the normal level of an epithelial surface. If it has a stalk, it is pedunculated. If it has no stalk but lies flat on the surface, it is sessile.

Prognosis The expected course of a disease; the likely outcome for the patient.

Putrefaction The process of decomposition of animal or vegetable matter by bacteria and fungi. Often has an associated foul odour.

Pyknosis The dark, condensed appearance of a nucleus, typically seen in cells undergoing apoptosis.

Pyogenic bacteria Bacteria that are commonly associated with a vigorous acute inflammatory reaction. The term pyogenic literally means 'pus-producing'. Examples include *Staphylococcus aureus*, species of *Streptococcus* and *Neisseria*, and some Gram-negative rods.

Resolution The restoration of normal anatomy in damaged tissue.

Repair The healing process that occurs when resolution is not possible. In most areas of the body, the result is fibrosis. However, in the brain and spinal cord, glial tissue is laid down (gliosis).

Sarcoma A malignant tumour showing mesenchymal differentiation (e.g. fibrosarcoma, osteosarcoma, liposarcoma, angiosarcoma).

Scar *See* fibrosis.

Serology The detection of antibodies by laboratory methods. For example, antibodies to blood group antigens, self antigens and micro-organisms can be identified.

Shock A systemic failure of circulation due to inadequate blood pressure, caused by either a fall in cardiac output or a reduction in the effective circulating blood volume.

Sinus A blind-ending track leading from an epithelial-lined surface. For example, an abscess cavity may drain from deeper tissues onto the skin surface via a sinus.

Stasis Stagnation of a fluid; the failure of the normal flow of a fluid. Can predispose to infection and stone formation.

Stem cell A dividing cell capable of producing a variety of different mature forms.

Stricture A narrowing of a tube due to a thickening of its wall.

Telomere A length of repetitive DNA at the ends of each linear chromosome.

Teratoma Tumour with elements derived from all three germ layers – often arise in ovary (usually benign) or testis (usually malignant).

Thrombus An aggregate of platelets and fibrin with enmeshed leucocytes formed in living vessels. Sometimes has a banded light and dark appearance (lines of Zahn), suggesting formation in flowing blood. Thrombi may fragment and embolise (thromboembolism).

Translocation The transfer of a gene from its normal position to one on another chromosome. Occurs regularly in some tumours (e.g. chronic myeloid leukaemia and Burkitt's lymphoma), involving sites of chromosomes occupied by proto-oncogenes. The rearrangement of these segments is, therefore, a key step in the development of neoplastic characteristics.

Transudate An accumulation of fluid with a low protein content in the tissues or the body cavity. In contrast to an exudate, there is usually no associated inflammation – the fluid usually accumulates because of circulatory factors.

Trauma Damage to tissues by mechanical forces. Sometimes the concept is expanded to include other physical injuries like burns.

Tuberculosis A chronic inflammatory disorder produced by infection with *Mycobacterium tuberculosis*. The classical disease involves the lungs and can spread to many other organs.

Ulcer A localised area of loss of epithelium. Many different causes including inflammation (inflammatory ulcer) and tumour (neoplastic or malignant ulcer).

Ultrastructure The internal structure of a cell. In particular, cell structure that requires the electron microscope for visualisation.

Index

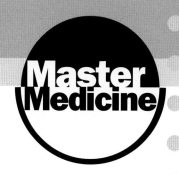

Note: Question and Answer Sections are referenced in the form '14Q/16A'. Entries such as '7Q/8A:9A' indicate that there are 2 separate parts in the answers section about a topic implying that there is more than one question on page 7 about that topic. Occasionally a topic is mentioned in the answer though not in the associated question. In such cases references appear in the form '9A'. References in italics are to the glossary (definitions).